# UNDERSTANDING CHRONIC FATIGUE SYNDROME

# UNDERSTANDING CHRONIC FATIGUE SYNDROME

## An Introduction for Patients and Caregivers

**Naheed Ali**

ROWMAN & LITTLEFIELD
Lanham • Boulder • New York • London

Published by Rowman & Littlefield
A wholly owned subsidiary of
The Rowman & Littlefield Publishing Group, Inc.
4501 Forbes Boulevard, Suite 200, Lanham, Maryland 20706
www.rowman.com

Unit A, Whitacre Mews, 26-34 Stannary Street, London SE11 4AB

British Library Cataloguing in Publication Information Available

**Library of Congress Cataloging-in-Publication Data**

The hardback edition of this book was previously cataloged by the Library of Congress as follows:

Ali, Naheed, 1981-
Understanding chronic fatigue syndrome : an introduction for patients and caregivers / Naheed Ali.
pages cm
Includes bibliographical references and index.
ISBN 978-1-4422-2657-9 (cloth : alk. paper) — ISBN 978-1-4422-2658-6 (electronic) — ISBN 978-0-8108-9595-9 (paper : alk. paper)
1. Chronic fatigue syndrome—Popular works. 2. Caregivers—Popular works. I. Title.
RB150.F37A45 2015
616'.0478—dc23
2015011442

Printed in the United States of America

*Understanding Chronic Fatigue Syndrome* is dedicated to my readers, to chronic fatigue syndrome sufferers, and to all who provided encouragement and support for my research.

Also by Naheed Ali

*Understanding Lung Cancer:*
*An Introduction for Patients and Caregivers*

*Understanding Celiac Disease:*
*An Introduction for Patients and Caregivers*

*Understanding Parkinson's Disease:*
*An Introduction for Patients and Caregivers*

*Understanding Alzheimer's:*
*An Introduction for Patients and Caregivers*

*The Obesity Reality:*
*A Comprehensive Approach to a Growing Problem*

*Arthritis and You:*
*A Comprehensive Digest for Patients and Caregivers*

*Diabetes and You:*
*A Comprehensive, Holistic Approach*

## Disclaimer

This book represents reference material only. It is not intended as a medical manual, and the data presented here are meant to assist the reader in making informed choices regarding wellness. This book is not a replacement for treatment(s) that the reader's personal physician may have suggested. If the reader believes he or she is experiencing a medical issue, professional medical help is recommended. Mention of particular products, companies, or authorities in this book does not entail endorsement by the publisher or author.

# Author's Note

*Understanding Chronic Fatigue Syndrome* isn't meant entirely for medical professionals, yet the nonmedical reader may encounter advanced medical terminology. This is necessary to keep the book in line with the intended comprehensive review of chronic fatigue syndrome, and because certain medical concepts necessitate clarification well beyond a modest introduction. A glossary at the back of the book defines the complex lexicon to those who aren't familiar with the language of medicine.

# CONTENTS

## 14 Conclusion                                              155

# PREFACE

Chronic fatigue syndrome, otherwise known as CFS or myalgic encephalomyelitis (ME), is a complicated disorder that's primarily designated by a feeling of severe exhaustion that doesn't get better with sleep
or rest and that persists for at least six months.[1] Chronic fatigue syndrome has also been called post-viral fatigue syndrome, chronic fatigue
and immune dysfunction, as well as the "yuppie flu."[2] Severe exhaustion follows stressors such as physical activity and intense mental exertion.[3]

The syndrome can affect anyone—at any age and of either sex—but
it's usually diagnosed in more women than men.[4] Likewise, it's seen in
people who are obese or partake in a sedentary lifestyle.[5] Chronic fatigue syndrome affects about two out of every 1,000 individuals in the
United States and about four of every 1,000 in the United Kingdom.[6]
People who are diagnosed with chronic fatigue syndrome are said to
have significantly lower activity levels when compared to the time before they became unwell.[7]

Chronic fatigue syndrome can be described as mild, moderate, or
severe.[8] Mild CFS involves difficulty or trouble doing simple tasks, but
the individual is capable of moving as well as tending to necessities of
life. Moderate CFS involves a termination of things that require labor
or exertion, difficulty in sleeping, and moving around alone. Severe
CFS embroils (a) the inability to do anything alone, (b) serious struggles
regarding mental concentration, learning, and understanding, (c) the

inability to move at all, and (d) sensitivity or irritability to noise and brightness.[9]

As of this writing, researchers have yet to identify a direct, significant cause of CFS or even a single test to diagnose CFS.[10] However, specialists theorize that chronic fatigue syndrome may be prompted by a combination of factors such as underlying medical conditions, infections, immune system problems, nutritional deficiencies, and stresses of psychological origin.[11] A series of tests may be needed to suitably diagnose chronic fatigue syndrome, as a number of other health conditions present matching symptoms that include sleep apnea, anemia, diabetes, insomnia, bipolar disorder, hypothyroidism, depression, and schizophrenia.[12] These tests take in full medical history and examination, mental status examination, full blood count (FBC), gluten sensitivity, erythrocyte sedimentation rate (ESR), creatinine kinase, and urine evaluation.[13]

Shared symptoms expressed by patients suffering from chronic fatigue syndrome include distended lymph nodes in the armpit or neck, persistent sore throat, muscle pain of unknown origin, unexplainable headache, severe feeling of exhaustion that continues for at least twenty-four hours following mental or physical stress, difficulty with memorization, joint pain, non-revitalizing rest or sleep, and, most importantly, fatigue.[14]

Before reading any further, the reader should understand that an individual is said to be suffering from chronic fatigue syndrome when he consistently experiences at least four of these symptoms for at least six months concurrently with, and not before, the fatigue itself.[15] Also, the fatigue shouldn't have been brought about or caused by in-progress physical or mental effort and the fatigue must impede simple everyday tasks. Other associated symptoms include chills and night sweats, allergies, irritable bowel, dizziness, fainting, balance problems or difficulty in standing up and maintaining proper posture, abdominal pain, panic attacks, chest pain, and shortness of breath.[16]

In general, the treatment for CFS is focused on relieving the symptoms, which can be accomplished by either medication or therapy.[17] Medications include antidepressant drugs that can partially alleviate or completely ease associated pain and sleeping pills that can help enhance sleep. Therapies include gradual physical exercise and psychological counseling.[18] In other cultures, especially Asian, one resorts to acupuncture, massage, yoga, or tai chi for symptom relief.[19] These methods are used to manage the symptoms but not to completely assuage the condition, so the most that they can do is to improve the quality of life of the individuals who have CFS. Unfortunately some clients don't fully recover.[20]

By now the reader might also wonder why CFS is a syndrome and not officially a disease. In reality, a condition, a term by which CFS is often correctly identified, is also classified as a syndrome when it's characterized by a set of symptoms occurring together, concurrently, and/or changing over time and when its cause is unknown.[21] On the other hand, a disease is present when the symptoms impair normal bodily function resulting in a sense of pain that has a proven source.[22] Since chronic fatigue syndrome is really a conglomerate of symptoms with no known cause, it's categorized as a syndrome and not a disease.

Moreover, a comprehensive approach to chronic fatigue syndrome, such as this book, is important, since individuals with chronic fatigue syndrome react to or handle the signs and symptoms differently; pain that's tolerable for one person could be debilitating for another, and depression brought about by the syndrome might be too much to take for an individual who doesn't know that he has CFS.

Needless to say, when this disorder is left ignored and unmanaged, it can be debilitating or incapacitating to the individuals who have it; it may significantly affect their livelihood as difficulty in moving, loss of concentration, social isolation, and depression become typical in un-compromising cases.[23] A comprehensive approach is also important since patients need to be aware of the real dangers of CFS—especially those who don't even realize that they suffer from it—so that it can be managed effectively, thus avoiding further possible complications.

# Part I


# Groundwork

# I

# ENERGY AND THE HUMAN BODY

Energy is defined as the exertion of power or the aptitude to do work.[1] Other definitions include the capacity to cause change and the ability to rearrange a collection of matter. In its different forms, energy can be kinetic energy or potential energy. Thermal energy, which implies movement of atoms or molecules, is kinetic in nature. However, chemical energy that's released in a chemical reaction is a form of potential energy.

## BENEFITS OF HAVING ENERGY

Many unfortunate events are reported in the news every day, and for that reason, it's important to know that car accidents from drowsiness happen more frequently than those due to alcohol intoxication. In a recent survey, 27 percent of the participants admitted to dozing off at some point while they were driving.[2] That's because they lack energy to do their jobs properly and end up falling asleep at the wheel on their way home. There are also many reported suicide incidents caused by depression. That's in part because some people lack the energy to live when they face difficult challenges in their life. They become so hopeless that they resort to suicide as their way out.

The realities are alarming and these things happen mostly because of a lack of energy. Simple unfortunate events can also befall chronic fatigue syndrome (CFS) patients' daily lives. Some students taking im-

portant tests in school don't pass because they lack the energy to rumi-
nate answers correctly. They feel tired and reckon their minds aren't
functioning properly. Again, this happens because of lack of energy.[3]

The benefits of CFS patients having energy are virtually endless
because everything that they do requires energy. Without it, the examples mentioned earlier are just a few of the terrible scenarios that could
result at any time. These are some of the reasons why it's beneficial for
people to have bursts of energy. The good news for everyone is that
most accidents, failures, and calamities can be prevented with just a
simple rule: every person should have the energy to live gainfully, especially if these tasks are easy to do. Energy can be obtained by getting
ample sleep and consuming nutritious foods. There are simple benefits
of having energy. These advantages can be divided into three catego-
ries: physiological, occupational, and social and personal benefits.[4]

## ENERGY AND METABOLISM

### Energy in Relation to the CFS Patient's Body

Energy is necessary for learning and carrying out psychomotor skills
involving psychological processes associated with muscular movements
and the production of voluntary movements.[5] Examples of these skills
are running, swimming, jogging, bicycling, tennis, walking, golfing, driving a car, standing or sitting, and sleeping.[6] Energy buildup occurs by
increasing the intake of foods that are high in energy, by having adequate rest and sleep, and by treating pain.[7] Even when the CFS sufferer sits still, his heart continues to pump blood throughout his body.
Great amounts of food and energy aren't needed to keep it pumping,
but even so, more work requires more energy.[8]

Anyhow, the body uses some nutrients for energy. With it, a person
can move his muscles and be active. It helps him in repairing injuries to
his body. Whatever he does, nutrients serve up energy. Lastly, nutrients
are like the building provisions for a human body. They become a part
of the muscles, skin, bones, and other parts. Basically, they're essential
for growth.[9]

To conserve normal body functions (body temperature regulation,
muscular movement), the average person requires 2,000 to 3,000 calo-

ries per day. Calories in excess of what the CFS patient's body uses are stockpiled as fat, which then contributes to weight gain, whereas using more calories than are ingested fuels weight loss. As a general rule, 3,500 calories are equivalent to approximately a pound of body weight. Certain activities burn body weight to yield energy such as running, which has an energy output of 0.110 calories per minute, per pound of body weight.[10]

## ENERGY AND THE NERVOUS AND ENDOCRINE SYSTEMS

Since neurologists often see chronic fatigue syndrome patients, it's prudent for the reader to understand how energy plays a role in the nervous and endocrine systems.

### The Nervous System's Role in Energy Production

Cerebrospinal fluid formed in the brain by filtration of blood circulates slowly through the central canal and ventricles of the brain and then drains into the veins, assisting in the delivery of nutrients and hormones to unique regions of the brain and in the removal of waste. This is one way in which the CFS patient garners energy.[11]

Sensory neurons send information about the internal and external environment to the brain while the motor neurons control the muscles and glands. Brain cells connect the motor and sensory pathways, monitor body processes, take action on the internal and external stimuli, maintain *homeostasis*, and orchestrate psychological, biological, and physical activities.[12]

### The Endocrine System's Role in Energy Production

The endocrine system is the interconnected network of glands. Due to its links to the nervous system and the immune system, the endocrine system has far-reaching energy-producing effects in the chronic fatigue syndrome patient. The hormones emitted by this system are affected greatly by organs such as the hypothalamus. Other structures in the brain, some of which are endocrine system glands, also manipulate the function of other endocrine glands. The energy-providing hormones secreted by the endocrine system affect the nervous system, but at times, the latter system also intervenes. For example, norepinephrine and epinephrine, which are secreted by the adrenal medulla, act as neurotransmitters.

## ENERGY AND THE RESPIRATORY AND CIRCULATORY SYSTEMS

The upper and lower respiratory tracts constitute the respiratory system. Together, the two tracts are responsible for ventilation, the movement of air in and out of the airways. The upper respiratory tract, also known as the upper airway, warms and filters air so that the lower respiratory tract, the lungs, can accomplish gas exchange. The process of gas exchange involves delivering oxygen to the tissues through the bloodstream and expelling waste gases such as carbon dioxide during expiration. The respiratory system works together with the circulatory system. The former is accountable for ventilation and diffusion while the circulatory system is responsible for *perfusion*.[13]

### Breathing Control and Energy

Humans can voluntarily hold their breath, but most of the time, automatic nervous mechanisms oversee breathing. Without inhalation, individuals with CFS wouldn't have any energy at all. This ensures that the work of the respiratory system is coordinated with that of the heart and with metabolic demands for oxygen. The main breathing control centers are located in two regions of the brain, the medulla oblongata and the pons.[14]

Breathing control is effective only if it's coordinated with control of the cardiovascular system so that there's a good match between lung ventilation and the amount of blood flowing through the alveolar capillaries. For instance, during exercise, increased cardiac output is matched to the increased breathing rate that enhances oxygen uptake and carbon dioxide removal as blood traverses through the lungs. By extension, this is how the CFS patient's body regulates its own energy.[15]

## ENERGY AND THE MUSCULOSKELETAL AND DIGESTIVE SYSTEMS

The musculoskeletal system includes the bones, joints, muscles, tendons, ligaments, and *bursae*. These components function in an integrated manner. The health and proper functioning of this system is interdependent with that of the other body systems. The system, which is fundamental for the use and buildup of energy, also (a) provides protection for vital organs, including the brain, heart, and lungs, and (b) offers a resilient framework to support body structures. It makes moving possible.[16]

## ANALYSIS

All of the cells of the body require nutrients, and energy production is the denouement. Without energy, CFS patients can't carry out daily functions properly. Food that contains proteins, fats, carbohydrates, vitamins, minerals, and cellulose fibers and other vegetable matter is the birthplace of these nutrients and therefore serves as the foundation of energy for the CFS sufferer.

There's no dependable formula for simultaneously attaining happiness and satisfaction, enjoying a long life, getting a job promotion, or becoming famous. Nonetheless, if a CFS patient has adequate energy for everything he does, he'll get more or less all of the benefit there is to receive in the physiological, occupational, personal, and social aspects of his life.

# 2

# HISTORY OF CHRONIC FATIGUE SYNDROME

In recent years, chronic fatigue syndrome (CFS) has been popularized as an illness of the twentieth century. However, the disorder isn't entirely novel. In fact, there are a number of reports of diseases similar to chronic fatigue syndrome dating back as early as two hundred years ago.[1]

## EVOLUTION OF THE TERM "CHRONIC FATIGUE SYNDROME"

The long history of CFS has been surrounded by rightful controversy in both defining and naming it. Naming a disease such as CFS imposes a great challenge because the selected name can influence how the patients are perceived and treated by society, including by those involved in their treatment and their families, friends, and coworkers. Since its discovery, the syndrome has undergone many name changes before a trove of scientists coined the name "chronic fatigue syndrome" in 1988. Even in recent years, its name is controversial.[2]

### Febricula and Neurasthenia

In 1750, Sir Richard Manningham reported a syndrome that was known as *febricula*, otherwise called little fever, a disease characterized by a copious number of symptoms that were difficult to diagnose objective-ly.[3] In the nineteenth century, an American psychiatrist and neurologist, George Miller Beard, popularized the concept of *neurasthenia*. This disease was thought to be nervous system mayhem characterized by enfeeblement of nerve forces.[4] Fatigue, anxiety, headache, and impotence, as well as neuralgia and depression, were among neurasthenia's reported symptoms.[5] It seemed that young women were more susceptible to the disease and its onset was most often triggered by an infection.[6] Lasting tiredness was seen as the primary symptom with the cardinal sign being an inordinate sense of physical or mental fatigue.[7]

One of the most famous historical figures who might have been victimized by CFS was Florence Nightingale, known as the mother of modern nursing.[8] In fact, Nightingale's birthday (May 12) is International ME/CFS and Fibromyalgia Day. It was reported that her illness started after returning from the Crimean War, when she spent years lying on a bed too exhausted to talk to more than one visitor at a time.[9]

She suffered from obdurate pain and fatigue for a large part of her life. Fascinatingly, shortly after her death, medical opinion favored the idea that she'd been suffering from neurasthenia. The concept of neurasthenia was actually commercialized by Beard in the 1880s, who described the illness prevalent among young women with a great resemblance to the disease that's now embedded in medicine as fibromyalgia.[10]

The censures of neurasthenia involved widespread pain, fatigue, dizziness, palpitations, and psychological problems. Neurasthenia, in fact, literally means "nervous exhaustion." The wide gamut of symptoms experienced by Florence Nightingale led to speculation that she suffered from CFS, fibromyalgia, or even post-traumatic stress disorder. Others refuted this view and claimed that Florence Nightingale was suffering from brucellosis, a chronic bacterial infection with nonspecific symptoms.[11]

Although it's difficult to ascertain an accurate diagnosis for Nightingale's condition, research suggests that bacterial or viral infections are risk factors for the development of chronic fatigue syndrome. Furthermore, recent findings assert that chronic bacterial infection may in fact be a cause of CFS.[12]

In current times, neurasthenia is perceived as a behavioral rather than a physical condition. However, it isn't considered a medical diagnosis.[13] As of this time, the World Health Organization's ICD-10 system categorizes neurasthenia under category F48 ("other neurotic disorders"), which specifically excludes chronic fatigue syndrome. As neurasthenia began to lose popularity, two episodes of CFS, which involved doctors and nursing staff, occurred in successive decades and grabbed hold of the public's attention. These outbreaks also gave rise to various names for CFS.[14]

## Poliomyelitis

The first-ever recorded outbreak of CFS known widely occurred at the Los Angeles County General Hospital in 1934. Symptoms included muscle pain of long duration, tenderness, weakness, and sensory symptoms, lapses in memory, difficulty in concentration, sleep disturbance, instability of emotions, and inability to walk short distances without suffering fatigue. Around two hundred members of the hospital staff acquired the disorder, due to which more than half of them were still unable to work six months later.[15] Initially, it was thought the unknown illness might be related to polio. However, the patients' muscles didn't waste away as they did with polio. This all subsequently provided a scrupulous explanation of what unfolds in a CFS patient's organs.

Similar outbreaks of the disease initially thought of as poliomyelitis also underwrote the long history of the syndrome before it finally came to be known as chronic fatigue syndrome. At a Wisconsin convent, apprentices and administration candidates were detected with a disease that they called encephalitis in 1936. In 1937, two towns in Switzerland had outbreaks of "abortive poliomyelitis." Two years later, more than seventy Swiss soldiers were diagnosed with the same.[16] In 1938, Alexander Gilliam reviewed medical records and interviewed patients affected by the outbreak in Los Angeles Country General Hospital. Gilliam referred to the disorder that infected staff as "atypical poliomyelitis."[17]

## Iceland Disease

More than a decade since the Los Angeles epidemic, an outbreak of a disorder very similar to poliomyelitis occurred in Akureyri in northern Iceland.[18] That explains why CFS is also called Akureyri disease or Iceland disease. The first case of the outbreak was reported in Iceland on September 25, 1948. The spate of disease there affected more than 1,000 people. Interestingly, a successive polio epidemic on the island in 1955 didn't affect the town. Speculators then argued that the virus, which may have caused the CFS outbreak, resulted in providing a level of immunity to polio.[19]

The main clinical offshoots were tiredness and exhaustion and the disorder was still diagnosed as poliomyelitis. Between the third and fourth weeks of November, the outbreak was differentiated from epidemics of poliomyelitis. It lasted for more than three months and yielded hundreds of reported cases.[20]

## Royal Free Disease

Miniature outbreaks occurred in the United Kingdom: Middlesex in 1952, Newscastle in 1959, and London from 1970 to 1971. The number of cases recorded reached 150. As a result, the United Kingdom, together with the United States, is now arguably at the crest of CFS research.[21] In late spring of 1955, an outbreak occurred at the Royal Free Hospital, probably the most well-known incidence of chronic fatigue syndrome on a large scale in the United Kingdom. The incident, which commenced when the hospital admitted a number of people with bizarre symptoms, lasted more than four and a half months. Events drastically unfolded when in July of the same year, around 300 staff members fell ill, of whom 255 needed to be quarantined on hospital grounds. To this end, the hospital was forced to go bust in the early part of October.[22]

Interestingly, only 12 percent of the nearly 300 people affected were in-hospital subjects at the time of the epidemic. Symptoms developed initially from a flu-like malaise that later became more prominent after a short remission, with a new group of symptoms arising. The most noticeable clinical sign of the disorder was extreme muscle fatigue after minimal exertion. Other symptoms were related to brain function, specifically with short-term memory and concentration. Headaches, blurred vision, and unusual skin sensations were also reported as indications. The medical examination conducted afterward concluded that roughly 70 percent of the patients had their central nervous systems bungled by CFS.[23]

The disorder now known as chronic fatigue syndrome was later coined by Melvin Ramsay, who was the medical consultant in charge at the time. Based on this outbreak, "myalgic encephalomyelitis" was defined by Donald Acheson in an editorial entitled *A New Clinical Entity?* that was published in *The Lancet* in 1956. Acheson named the disorder "benign myalgic encephalomyelitis," with *benign* denoting a zero mortality rate.[24]

The article covered selected epidemic outbreaks that happened in the years prior, according to the description of Ramsay and others. In 1981, Ramsay finally published his designation of the disease, naming it myalgic encephalomyelitis. The definition included four central tenets: (1) fatigue after minimal exertion and delay of recovery of muscle power after exertion ends, (2) one or more symptoms indicating circulatory impairment, (3) one or more symptoms indicating involvement of the central nervous system, and (4) wavering symptoms.[25]

## Tapanui Flu

In Australia, one of the earliest occurrences of CFS happened in Adelaide in 1949. Hundreds of unwitting patients were confined to the hospital due to a CFS-like infirmity. Australia had also been piloting research on CFS, especially in regard to immunology, infection, and management. In 1998, they created a working group that provided instructions to best diagnose and manage people with CFS.[26]

Chronic fatigue syndrome disembarked on the South Island region of Otago, New Zealand, in 1984. Due to the location of the outbreak, CFS was dubbed the Tapanui flu. The patients initially developed a flu-like malaise and suffered from fatigue that incapacitated them for several weeks. A ten-year study was conducted following the outbreak on twenty-one of the patients who were affected. The journal *Archives of Internal Medicine* reported that sixteen of twenty-one victims who had the illness achieved a nearly perfect degree of functioning by the culmination of the ten-year period.[27]

## Epstein-Barr and the Yuppie Flu

In 1984, another similar outbreak unraveled in the Lake Tahoe locale of Nevada, which caught significant attention from the U.S. public and media. In the latter part of 1984 a number of healthy adults suddenly displayed symptoms of an unusual flulike affliction followed by symptoms related to myalgic encephalomyelitis or chronic fatigue syndrome, namely, muscular fatigue and cognitive degeneration. Doctors examining the patients affected were skeptical about whether the latter were physically ill since blood tests failed to bring anything unusual to light.[28]

Around that time, researchers started to ponder whether the disorder was related to the Epstein-Barr virus (the virus linked with gland-based fever) or infectious mononucleosis. However, clinical research findings demonstrated that even though three-quarters of the patients had high levels of Epstein-Barr virus antibodies, the rest had no virus or no E-B virus antibodies at all. Their theory also appeared questionable because E-B virus antibody tests were difficult to deduce. The various test results were highly similar to the anticipated results from normal, healthy adults coming from similar backgrounds. In addition, by age thirty, most people had been exposed to the E-B virus with only a selected few developing glandular fever.[29]

Despite the incongruence, CFS grew in popularity as the U.S. media publicized it unsparingly. *Newsweek* labeled it the malaise of the '80s. Others called it "yuppie flu" because most of the affected population were young and active professionals. Although its relationship with glandular fever virus was also uncertain, it seemed that the public's curiosity about the disorder was satiated with the new aliases they had given it: chronic Epstein-Barr virus (CEBV) or chronic mononucleosis. These two terms became widely accepted.[30]

Another trendy U.S. magazine, *Hippocrates*, publicized the epidemic at Lake Tahoe when it published an issue with a cover story about the epidemic. However, despite its established title—CEBV—the magazine used another name—Raggedy Ann syndrome—to reflect the fatigue and loss of muscle power experienced by the patients.[31]

The National Institute of Allergy and Infectious Diseases held a consensus conference in 1985 when chronic Epstein-Barr virus or CEBV was used to describe the CFS-like symptoms. CEBV became the well-known term for the disorder at that time, and academic journals considered it a legitimate medical disorder. In 1987, two years after chronic Epstein-Barr virus gained popularity as the name of choice for the disorder, the CEBV Association was established by Mark Iverson and Alan Goldberg.[32]

The group's name was later on changed to the CFIDS Association of America. This was the suggestion of Seymour Grufferman, an immunologist who recommended the name "chronic fatigue immune dysfunction syndrome" in order to reflect more on the immune anomalies of the condition rather than fatigue as the prominent symptom.[33]

## Issues with Nomenclature

In 1988, researchers primarily from the Centers for Disease Prevention, or CDC, coined the term *chronic fatigue syndrome* to describe the most prominent symptom of the illness. A new case definition was also developed using the Holmes criteria.[34] Other "medical-sounding" terms were also suggested but dismissed due to the lack of definitive evidence of a causative agent. Even though the syndrome was finally called by a name that's most appropriate for it, the naming of CFS still didn't come easy, as issues continue to surface from time to time.

In 1996, Kenneth Calman, then the United Kingdom's chief medical officer (CMO), requested a commentary from the Royal Colleges of Physicians, Psychiatrists, and General Practitioners. This soon led to the release of a report supporting that "chronic fatigue syndrome" was found to be the most fitting term. This was further supported by a follow-up report in 2002 by Liam Donaldson, the new CMO.[35]

However, CFS terminology still remains highly divisive.[36] There are a remarkably high percentage of patients affected by this illness who have received disrespect and poor treatment by the medical world. The name of an illness, therefore, is very important in how it's perceived by the general populace. It's essential to know and review the issues concerning the terminology of CFS to understand the public's cynicism and stigma toward the patients.

Although the term *chronic fatigue syndrome* was chosen because fatigue was considered the apex symptom of the illness in question, the new phrase received only negative feedback from the patients.[37] They believe that naming the disorder CFS belittled its seriousness. This is due to the fact that the illness is typified by many severe symptoms aside from fatigue. Fatigue is also a common symptom in the general population, even for healthy individuals.[38]

In 2001 and 2002, two consecutive studies were announced to determine whether the alternative names of CFS—chronic fatigue syndrome and myalgic encephalopathy—affected the academic efforts of college undergraduates and medical trainees concerning the syndrome.[39] Participants were randomly divided into two groups, each with different diagnostic labels used in a case description of a patient with symptoms of chronic fatigue syndrome. The studies concluded that the characteristics that participants attributed to CFS depended on the different diagnostic labels used to characterize it. The results showed that the diagnostic name myalgic encephalopathy (ME) paralleled the worse prognosis.[40]

Myalgic encephalopathy was also more likely to be linked with a physiological rather than psychosocial origin, thus requiring nonpsychiatric treatment when compared with those with the title "CFS."[41] A high number of patients believed that changing the name from myalgic encephalomyelitis to chronic fatigue syndrome was a major contributing factor to the stigma this disorder received.

Due to these issues surrounding CFS, there have been continual studies regarding its name. During the summer of 2000, the CFS Coordinating Committee (CFSCC) of the Department of Health and Human Services appointed a name change workgroup (NCW). The group aimed to change the name from "chronic fatigue syndrome" to one that perfectly reflected the severity of the syndrome and the organ systems affected.[42]

One alternative that NCW considered was NEID, or neuro-endocrine immune disorder, due to the growing scientific evidence of neurological, neuroendocrine, and immune system dysfunctions in patients shaken by this syndrome. Myalgic encephalomyelitis or myalgic encephalopathy was also suggested as an official label for the syndrome, considering that myalgic encephalomyelitis had been used prior to the term CFS. According to a study in 2001, most of the roughly 430 respondents (85 percent) indicated that they wanted a name change. However, both the patients and the physicians were split between adopting a name such as myalgic encephalopathy (ME) or one such as neuro-endocrine immune disorder (NEID). The survey also indicated that the acronym NEID had certain pejorative characteristics. Thus the NCW members were compelled to think of a better name for the syndrome.[43]

Since the results of the studies showed that the previous labels for the syndrome weren't the preferred choices, the NCW negotiated the umbrella term "chronic neuroendocrine immune syndrome," or CNDS, under which patients could be classified into subgroups according to their symptoms and pathophysiology.[44]

One of these subgroups would be myalgic encepahalomyelitis or myalgic encephalopathy. This recommendation was based on (a) the frequency of the reported symptoms of patients with the syndrome, (b) chronicity of the illness, (c) the lack of an understanding of its causes, and (d) insufficient published evidence supporting an abnormality in the neurologic, endocrine, and immune systems. In 2002, researchers facilitated two surveys that found that between 57 and 66 percent of patients and health care providers endorsed the term CNDS.[45]

Still, there are CFS experts who argue that the current name still factors in the invalidation and stigmatization of the disease. Due to the controversy revolving around the name and diagnosis of CFS, patients affected with the syndrome face skeptical attitudes, and many of them suffer great losses in their support system.[46]

## CHRONIC FATIGUE SYNDROME AND FAME

Celebrities are no exception to the far-reaching outcomes of CFS. Here is a synopsis of celebrities who have been known to battle this syndrome.

### Michelle Akers

Born February 1, 1966, in Santa Clara, California, Michelle A. Akers is a former American soccer star despite her long-term battle against chronic fatigue syndrome. She was born to Robert and Anne Akers and grew up in a suburb in Seattle, Washington, where she attended and played soccer for Shorecrest High School. She was dubbed an All-American three times during her high school career. After her retirement, she continued to promote the game of soccer. One of her books chronicled her battle with chronic fatigue syndrome, the disorder that hampered her training during the last eight years of her career.[47]

## Susan Blackmore

A renowned figure in England, Susan Blackmore is the author and contributor of more than sixty academic articles and forty books.[48] She's also famous for her book *The Meme Machine*. Aside from being a writer, Susan is a lecturer, skeptic, and broadcaster on psychology and the paranormal. She's a contributor to *The Guardian* newspaper, and she earned degrees in psychology and physiology from Oxford University and a PhD degree in parapsychology from the University of Surrey. She spent decades proving to her colleagues at Oxford that the paranormal does exist. Afterward, she changed her beliefs, which was considered a devastating blow to her, ultimately turning her identity upside down.[49]

In 1995, she developed CFS after spending many long hours on different projects. She couldn't manage to walk and couldn't bring herself to a relaxing sleep. Reading and concentrating were also difficult for her, except for short periods. The syndrome, however, became a positive aspect of her life as it led to her discovery of a new branch of science: cultural evolution, or memes, in which humans store ideas, art, stories, technologies, and science and pass them to the next generation, just like that seen in genetics. Thankfully, CFS gave her a whole new perspective on life.[50]

## Cher

Cher is an American singer and actress and one of the world's most celebrated stars. Born May 20, 1946, as Cherilyn Sarkisian in El Centro, California, Cher was nicknamed the "goddess of pop." Cher has proven herself to be a consummate entertainer with platinum-selling albums, sold-out concerts, award-winning movies, and famed television shows. Cher started her career as half of a singing act with her then-husband Sonny Bono in the 1960s.[51]

In the 1990s, Cher suffered from chronic fatigue syndrome for three years. She developed bronchitis and pneumonia because of CFS. During this period, she had to drag herself to her performances and occasionally cancel her shows. In an interview in 1999, she told Larry King that no one believed her for a long time. Traditional doctors didn't have a clue as to what she was suffering from. It was only when a homeopathic physician believed her complaints and sympathized with her that she finally made her way to recovery.[52]

## Blake Edwards

Born as William Blake Crump in July 26, 1922, Edwards was an American film director, screenwriter and producer. Edwards started off as an actor in the 1940s, but his interest in acting soon waned, and he turned to screenplays and radio scripts and then to producing and directing film and TV shows. His most famous films are *Breakfast at Tiffany's*, *Days of Wine and Roses*, and the hit *Pink Panther*.[53]

He was famous for directing comedies, but he also directed other film genres, such as drama and mystery. Although he suffered from CFS for years, he was able to find ways to continue his career. Edwards died in December 15, 2010, at eighty-eight due to pneumonia.[54]

## Amy Peterson

Amy Peterson is an American short-track speed skater who competed in five consecutive Olympic Games, from the time that short-track speed skating was an exhibition sport in 1988 until 2002.[55] Peterson was only in her teens when she qualified for her first Olympics in 1988 in Calgary.[56] She had an ongoing battle against CFS, which eventually ended her participation in the Olympics. She returned to qualify for the Winter Olympics in Japan in 1998 after overcoming the syndrome. Peterson's career suffered at that time with her Olympic rankings tumbling.[57]

## Stevie Nicks

Stephanie "Stevie" Nicks, a well-known American singer and songwriter, produced more than forty top-fifty hits and unloaded more than 140 million in album sales. She was considered the "reigning queen of rock and roll" as well as one of the 100 greatest singers of all time.[58] In 1998, she was inducted into the Rock and Roll Hall of Fame. She also has won a total of eight Grammy Award nominations as a solo artist.[59]

Around 1986, Nicks developed an addiction to cocaine, which her doctor warned could lead to severe health problems. Although her cocaine consumption didn't directly lead to her CFS, in 1987, one of Nicks's tours was suspended due to her symptoms of chronic fatigue syndrome and slowly developing addiction to clonazepam. Nicks was still able to pull through with great career in the entertainment business in the following year.[60]

## ANALYSIS

The reason that chronic fatigue syndrome has gained the image of a new disorder can be traced to its long history of having various titles, leading it to be labeled as the disease of a thousand names.[61] A thousand may be an exaggeration, but there's indeed a long list of names that were used for this disorder in different parts of the world and during different eras.

# Part II

# Clinical Picture

# 3

# CAUSES AND RISK FACTORS

**A**lthough chronic fatigue syndrome (CFS) isn't a new medical discovery, its causes remain unknown today. Scientists and researchers have yet to determine a precise explanation for what triggers CFS due to the heterogeneous and inconsistent symptoms present in patients diagnosed with the disorder.

## SUSPECTED CAUSES

Patients with CFS have reported that they had experienced moderate to severe physical pain (possibly caused by viral infections) or emotional instability involving depression before developing CFS. These symptoms, whether alone or combined, have led medical experts to believe that the nervous system and a gene abnormality could possibly trigger CFS. However, medical experts haven't discovered a specific brain or nervous system hindrance that's consistent in every patient.[1]

Continuing studies are still in progress. As of late, only logged medical theories can provide information about the supposed sources of CFS. The symptoms listed in these medical theories have been observed to be the most common similarities among patients diagnosed with chronic fatigue syndrome. Medical speculations that attempt to resolve the causes of CFS state the following probable reasons: viral infection, genes, brain defects, an overreactive immune system, psychiatric or emotional conditions, and stress-related hormonal abnormalities. These are some of the more prevalent theories involving the grounds of CFS.[2]

## Viral Infections

Researchers believe that a viral infection may cause CFS because its symptoms are similar to that of an infection. Sadly, this claim is idiosyncratic since not all patients with CFS have had a serious infection. This led researchers to consider that there may be two causes of CFS: viral and nonviral causes. Medical studies haven't discovered a single viral infection that may have a direct relation with CFS even though these infections share the same symptoms with CFS. Some of the viruses that have been scrutinized include the following:[3]

- Epstein-Barr virus infection, otherwise known as mononucleosis;
- Human herpesvirus 6 infections, which is problematic for those with impaired immune systems;
- Enterovirus infection, a type of virus found in the gastrointestinal tract that isn't severe or deadly. This form of infection shows mild flu-like symptoms;
- Rubella, more commonly known as German measles;
- *Candida albicans*, a type of fungus that can cause yeast infections;
- Borna viruses, known to cause the infectious Borna disease;
- Mycoplasma, which causes atypical pneumonia;
- Ross River virus, a virus that begets Ross River fever, a mosquito-borne tropical illness;
- *Coxiellaburnetti*, the infectious agent that caused Q fever; and
- Human retrovirus infection, such as HIV or xenotropic murine leukemia virus-related virus (XMRV), a gamma retrovirus.

A study states that patients who have had stark viral septicity are more likely to be diagnosed with CFS than other patients, which leads medical pundits to believe there may be more than one way to contract CFS.

## Genetics

According to various clinical investigations, genetics may be a possible culprit lurking in the shadows of CFS.[4] These studies show that there are certain genetic characteristics that may put some patients at more risk than others. Researchers affirm that genes that are linked to infections and blood disease may cause CFS. Furthermore, genes overseeing the body's response to stressful and traumatic injuries may also be a contributing factor of CFS.[5]

Genetic components involved in the functions of the immune system, communication between cells, and the transfer of energy to cells are also listed as a possible cause. Many medical findings have indicated that a patient's immune system may lead to CFS. Unfortunately, despite studies claiming that viral infections may be a direct cause, a patient's immune system isn't the sole basis of CFS. Since the syndrome is held to have been brought about by viral infections, medical experts theorized that genetic predisposition could only exacerbate the development of CFS in a human being.[6]

When a patient encounters a viral infection, his body generates cytokines. Cytokines are a group of proteins relinquished by certain cells in the immune system.[7] Chronic fatigue syndrome patients have exhibited, possibly genetically, a significantly elevated level of circulating cytokines.[8] Antibodies in the immune system are proved to be positive among CFS patients, but again, there hasn't been a direct genetic link that would lead researchers to believe that such circumstances lead to the disorder.

No typical tissue disconcertion related to autoimmune disease has been indicated in CFS patients. Additionally, the human herpesvirus 6 (HHV-6), a microbe which also causes CFS, can be integrated via *chromosomes*.[9] This virus can be active or inactive in a person's body.[10] This means that there's a possibility that the virus is inherited by a CFS patient but doesn't cause any harm to the health system. Thus, a patient should try to figure out whether he inherited CFS. Identifying the genetic potential of CFS enlightens experts as to why the patient has CFS in the first place.

## Preexisting Immune Abnormalities

Chronic fatigue syndrome has a number of other medical names because of its oodles of unjustifiable causes. That being said, CFS is also known as chronic fatigue immune dysfunction syndrome because medical personnel also believe that the immune system could be a pivotal player in the explanation of the disorder. Some medical studies have discovered some preexisting (but not necessarily genetic) irregularities in the immune systems of patients diagnosed with CFS.[11]

Patients' immune systems respond inconsistently, sometimes over-reacting and other times underreacting. However, just like the other medical theories, this claim doesn't have any significant pattern that could justify the immune system idiosyncrasies as the actual roots of CFS. Medical research has also discovered that the majority of CFS patients have allergies to pollen, certain kinds of food, metals, and other types of substances. Just as is the case with the viral infection theory, allergies are a weak stand to explain the causes of CFS. Not all CFS patients are allergic, and neither do they all completely detest a distinct substance to which they're continually allergic.[12]

## Psychiatric Causes

Other medical investigations affirm that chronic fatigue syndrome isn't a viral infection at all. It is said to be a psychiatric condition instead.[13] Extreme tiredness and inactivity are unexceptional symptoms found in CFS patients as well as in people suffering from some mental disability. At least half of CFS patients experience depression. This has led researchers to tie CFS to mental disorder.

Since some theories state that CFS is caused by genes that manage the body's response to traumatic events and injuries, medical researchers have also pondered that genes are unrelated to the conundrums of chronic fatigue. Instead, CFS could be just a condition of the patient's mind. This theory has been controversial for academic dons involved in CFS research. Many are displeased about labeling CFS as a "mental" illness, primarily because declaring CFS as a mental disorder dismisses the reality of CFS as a "real" disease for some. Still, the syndrome hasn't been proven to be a purely psychological sickness.[14]

## Central Nervous System and Hormone Abnormalities

Research also indicates that the hypothalamus-pituitary-adrenal (HPA) axis could be a major factor causing CFS.[15] Hypothalamus-pituitary-adrenal disorder occurs when several chemicals in the brain system are at abnormal levels. This is significant for the study of CFS because the

HPA axis is responsible for several physical and emotional functions such as sleep, depression, and response to stress. All of these functions are related to the symptoms shown in chronic fatigue syndrome. A few of the more notable observations regarding this study are as follows:

- Significant changes in important neurotransmitters: CFS patients have been observed to have abnormally high levels of serotonin, a deficiency of dopamine, and an imbalance between the neuro-transmitters norepinephrine and dopamine.
- Interrupted circadian rhythm: Almost all CFS patients have trouble with sleep, particularly in sleeping and waking. The circadian clock regulates the sleep-wake cycle and an exposure to viral infections can cause stress and trauma, disrupting this cycle. This leads to difficulty in getting much-needed rest.
- Deficiency of stress hormones: CFS patients have a low level of cortisol; this may explain why patients have a low tolerance to both physical and psychological stresses, such as a viral infection or even exercise.

Some CFS patients tend to look for a quick fix to resolve their hormonal tribulations. This means turning to over-the-counter (OTC) drugs and other quick remedies instead of making the change holistically, a change to all aspects of life, from social activities, diet, daily regimen, and finally, the cessation of bad habits. Weight gain and increased cortisol have been found to have a deeper connection with the level of stress that the CFS patient experiences. Cortisol has a significant role in the different bodily and metabolic processes affecting internal organs.[16]

Stress hormones, a category that includes adrenaline, provide one with instant energy along with other hormones such as cortisol and CRH. Otherwise known as corticotrophin releasing hormone, CRH is secreted from glands whenever a person faces a certain stressor or stressful event. This is in connection with the "fight or flight" mechanism that the CFS patient has when facing high levels of stress. An advanced level of adrenaline and CRH would then decrease the person's appetite; however, this would be only ephemeral. Cortisol would then help to replenish the lost minerals from the CFS sufferer's body after the stressful incident.[17]

Generally speaking, cortisol is the body's fight-or-flight hormone that's released every time one is stressed or faced with a certain stressor. Its main purpose is to replenish the lost energy after exertion during the fight-or-flight stage. It's the hormone responsible for letting the body revert back into its normal functioning after a stressful event. Ancestors of the human race, who could be traced to primitive man, needed this hormone to fight off wild beasts and to compete for food, shelter, and other basic necessities. At present, humans (whether CFS patients or not) still respond to stress by either facing it (the "fight" mechanism), or running away from the perceived threat. [18]

Stressors for the modern man are more complicated than those for the primitive bloke, and sometimes continual strain has a detrimental effect on the person's health. When cortisol is forfeited by glands, the body's viscera and tissues are relieved of stress, but continuous discharge of cortisol in this manner can be harmful. This is because cortisol is continually being discharged within the body in high amounts, which then predisposes the patient to develop other illnesses or conditions such as high blood pressure and diabetes mellitus, thereby compromising the body's verve to fight off infection. [19]

## Low Blood Pressure

Another medical theory about the cause of CFS is the irregular blood pressure levels of patients. People who've been diagnosed with CFS also illustrate symptoms of neutrally mediated hypotension (NMH) that causes a dramatic drop in the patient's blood pressure level even during unpretentious motions such as standing up or moseying. This causes the patient to experience nausea, light-headedness, and proneness to fainting. [20]

## RISK FACTORS

Similar to the medical theories explaining the causes of CFS, the risk factors are also quite vague. Listed risk factors encompass a very broad and general audience, making it seemingly possible for everyone to have CFS. Of course, not all individuals with the same symptoms may be diagnosed with the syndrome. As long as medical investigations regarding CFS are still active, there's no single risk factor that could guarantee the syndrome in an individual. The CDC says that more than one million people in the United States are diagnosed with chronic fatigue syndrome. This number is quite alarming considering that the complete lineup of risk factors is still unknown.[21]

## Age, Gender, and Ethnicity

Chronic fatigue syndrome occurs in both sexes from all racial and ethnic groups. However, it's been observed that most of these CFS patients are between forty and fifty years old.[22] Studies also show that there are more women who suffer from CFS than men, even though the severity of pain doesn't differ from that of the men. Children and young adults may also have CFS but it isn't common. There are more girls diagnosed with the syndrome than boys.[23]

## Psychological Risk Factors

Many chronic fatigue syndrome patients are ill with depression. It's one of the most common symptoms pooled among CFS sufferers. Social factors such as the individual's personality and mental health are said to influence the onset of CFS. Those who aren't able to tolerate stress and have experiences with depression have a higher chance of developing the syndrome.[24]

Although the medical disorders flanked by physical factors and emotional factors are still quite complex, scientific researchers have discovered that personality disorders are consistent among patients. This is momentous information. Compared to other indicators, depression seems to be the highest similarity among chronic fatigue patients. This could be a key lead for those investigating the risk factors of chronic fatigue syndrome.[25]

## Stress

Psychological disabilities are promulgations for developing CFS, and researchers have also discovered relevant information regarding the patients' tolerance to stress. One of the possible causes of CFS includes a gene that handles the body's response to psychological tension. Studies have shown that patients who've experienced severe trauma and stress—especially those who've gone through a lot of abuse—are regrettably more prone to CFS.[26]

## ANALYSIS

The complex nature of CFS makes the medical investigation of its causes and risk factors a challenging study requiring further examination. These factors not only differ on a case-to-case basis for every patient, but they're also quite common and may not even be related to CFS in the long haul. Nonetheless, the CFS patient must understand that not all hope is lost.

# 4

# PATHOLOGY OF CHRONIC FATIGUE SYNDROME

Although pathology, by definition, pertains to diagnostics from a medical standpoint, diagnosis can present a discrete problem when it comes to chronic fatigue syndrome (CFS), because symptoms of the syndrome are similar to other medical complaints. There aren't any direct examination results that can verify the diagnosis, so confirmation of CFS involves a process of elimination.

## GENERAL PATHOLOGY OF CFS

Chronic fatigue syndrome, as the name suggests, is characterized by persistent fatigue or exhaustion. Fatigue is the main indicator for this disorder, but not the type of fatigue a person faces after a gruesomely tiring or stressful day. It's not the type of tiredness that persists for only days, weeks, or couple of months.[1]

It's an intense, lingering, debilitating fatigue that can't be treated by a surefire set of medications, and it doesn't resolve through rest. It often becomes worse when a person does any kind of physical or mental activity. Pathologically, CFS totally affects a person's stamina and activity level. It results in a considerable lessening of an individual's work, school, personal, and social activities.[2]

**Specific Set of Symptoms**

An individual is said to be afflicted with CFS if he presents with three main symptoms. First, he has severe, extended fatigue for six or more successive months. Second, the fatigue notably affects the patient's daily physical work and routine. Third, the individual suffers four or more symptoms from a general list of symptoms of CFS.[3]

The first criterion is an extreme and continued fatigue that occurs for six months or longer and for 50 percent of the time.[4] There are also other guidelines released by the National Institute for Health and Care Excellence (NICE) stating that physicians should consider a diagnosis of CFS if a patient's fatigue level: (a) is relatively new to the patient or has a definite starting point, (b) is constant and or frequent, (c) cannot be explained by other conditions, (d) greatly affects the activities of a patient by diminishing strength to carry on daily activities both physical and mental, and (e) worsens after intense physical activity.[5]

The second criterion is where the individual experiences severe exhaustion while engaging in a typical activity. The individual may experience what's known as post-exertional malaise, or a period of extreme lethargy, and other CFS symptoms that persists for more than twenty-four hours. There's been ongoing research into this. Upon post-exertional malaise, there's a marked change in the blood and genetic manifestation.[6] This can be considered a basis for identifying CFS. The third criterion is that the individual experiences at least four of the identified general symptoms of CFS. These universal symptoms of CFS are:

- Neurocognitive issues, which may include short-term memory loss, clumsiness, difficulty in concentration and thinking, trouble in finding words or speech impairment, struggling with planning or organizing thoughts, and problems in processing information;
- Non-refreshing sleep or difficulty in sleeping, such as disrupted sleep, an unstable sleep-wake pattern, insomnia or hypersomnia;
- Muscle or joint pains without swelling or inflammation;
- Headaches differing in intensity, severity, or pattern;
- Painful or tender axillary or cervical lymph nodes; and
- Frequent sore throat.

Although the draining symptom of CFS is indeed fatigue, individuals often state that the mental deficiencies—including difficulty in concentration and memory loss—are the most upsetting. Some physicians posit that idled mental performance is due to depression, which is common in individuals with CFS. Aside from these symptoms, other general symptoms of CFS include the following:[7]

- Mental fogginess or a state of a clouded consciousness, wherein an abnormality is observed in the control of the level of consciousness that's milder than delirium;
- Sudden plunging blood pressure resulting in dizziness or nausea, paleness, fainting, difficulty in maintaining an upright position, and balance problems;
- Aggravating allergies including sensitivity to foods, noise, odor, light, medications, or chemicals;
- Irritable bowel syndrome including abdominal pain, stomachaches, bloating, diarrhea, or constipation;
- Incessant night sweats and chills;
- Visual disturbances including eye pain, blurring or worsening vision, light sensitivity, and dry eyes;
- Mental snags that may include mood swings, irritability, depression, panic attacks, and anxiety;
- Palpitations or escalated heart rate or shortness of breath (dyspnea);
- Chronic or a long-lasting cough;
- Recurring flulike illnesses that may or may not implicate chest pain; and
- Undetermined reasons for weight change (usually rapid weight loss).

## Other Signs of Chronic Fatigue Syndrome

Apart from the symptoms of CFS listed above, there are specific biological signals found in most individuals with CFS. Notable changes affect the individual's central nervous system, hormones, and immune system. Many studies have connected chronic fatigue syndrome to the central nervous system. The nervous system is responsible for some important bodily functions such as slumber, response to stress, and depression. People with CFS have unusual levels of chemicals in the hypothalamus-pituitary-adrenal (HPA) axis, as elaborated in the preceding chapter.[8]

The hypothalamus decreases the production of corticotrophin discharging hormone, or cortisol, which is a steroid hormone released in reaction to stress, resulting in a reduction in the release of the pituitary gland, which then leads to *hypocortisolism*, or adrenal insufficiency. Mild hypocortisolism is one symptom consistently found in individuals with CFS, which may also explain the symptoms of slackened or weaker reaction to physical or psychological stresses, for instance, isometrics or infections.[9]

Neurotransmitters are chemical envoys of the brain. Other CFS signs noted are the changes in the major neurotransmitters, whereby patients have (a) remarkably high levels of serotonin, a compound supplying the sense of happiness and well-being, (b) deficits of dopamine, a neurotransmitter contributing to the sense of reward, or (c) inconsistencies between norepinephrine, a neurotransmitter responsible for attentive concentration, and dopamine. Studies also show that some individuals with CFS frequently exhibit disturbances in their sleep-wake cycles. The sleep-wake cycle is disciplined by the body's circadian clock, which is really a cluster of nerves found in the HPA axis. Stressful physical or mental events, such as illnesses or viral disease, can upset one's natural circadian rhythm. The inability to retune the circadian rhythm results in continual sleep instabilities.[10]

Some studies indicate that SPECT scans of individuals with CFS have diminished cerebral blood flow; PET scans have shown abridged metabolism of the brain; MRI scans have revealed the occurrence of small lesions.[11] These irregularities have been seen in clinical statuses of otherwise healthy folks. Anomalies in individuals with CFS most resemble those observed in AIDS encephalopathy.[12]

In addition, CFS is usually followed by substantial economic, social, and physical disability and dysfunction. Patients with CFS normally function at crucially lower levels, resulting in significant economic and personal stress. The high unemployment rates among the patients and the costs related to uninformed care are economic burdens faced by the patients that can result in depression. Chronic fatigue syndrome has been declared a form of infrequent depressive illness due to symptomatic overlaps.[13]

## Signs of CFS in the Immune System

Scientific inquiries have shown that the immune system shows many abnormalities in individuals with chronic fatigue syndrome.[14] Some elements appear to be under-reactive, whereas others tend to be overreactive. Studies continue to spitball the theory that the majority of individuals with CFS have allergies to pollen, food, metal, chemicals, and other substances. One hypothesis posits that allergens, similar to viral diseases, may activate a series of immune system irregularities that are linked to CFS. However, not all people with allergies suffer from CFS. The risk outline for CFS is identical to the risk outline for some autoimmune diseases. These findings are mutable in that autoantibodies (antibodies that infect the body's own tissues) are present in those with CFS. Scientists found that the range of immunological deficiencies imply that CFS is a form of acquired immunodeficiency.[15]

Inconspicuous symptoms of chronic fatigue syndrome that may be logged from laboratory reports may include immunoglobulin G, immune complexes, alkaline phosphatase, low-level antinuclear antibody titer, cholesterol, lactate dehydrogenase, and atypical lymphocyte (a genus of white blood cell) levels.[16] There may also be a special type of fat manifest in CFS patients. These chronic phase lipids (CPLs) may be akin to "acute phase proteins" such as C-reactive protein, which escalates in settings of trauma and inflammation.[17]

## Level of Symptoms

There are three levels of severity of chronic fatigue syndrome. First is a trifling presentation of symptoms, wherein an individual can take care of himself and perform light household tasks but with some difficulty. The patient might still report to work or go to school, but may often be absent periodically. It's likely that he's halted most social and leisurely outings, too. Days off from work or school and weekends are often spent reclining to recover from fatigue.[18]

Second is the moderate presentation of symptoms, wherein the individual experiences lessened agility and has limited ability in performing daily, routine tasks. The individual has difficulty sleeping at night and may experience other symptoms recurrently. Third is the severe presentation of symptoms, wherein the person can perform only nominal tasks daily. Any activity easily weathers the individual, and the symptoms experienced are heightened. He contends with mental processes such as concentrating. The CFS patient may require a wheelchair and won't be able to leave home most of the time. He might suffer from severe post-exertional malaise and may also be bedridden for long periods of time. He also becomes sensitive to noise, bright lights, odor, sounds, or what they call "overload phenomenon." The flexible cognitive, sensory, motor, or emotional overstrain may trigger a "crash," wherein the individual suffers an intense, debilitating mental and physical fatigue or weakness.[19]

## Symptoms of Chronic Fatigue Syndrome in Men

In earlier epochs dating back to the 1800s, neurasthenia (currently referred to as CFS) consistently plagued men in upper class society. This was attributed to their hard work and society's overwhelming pressure combined with minimal time for sleep and rest. During this period, chronic fatigue syndrome was considered a male disorder.[20] However, over the course of time, more women were diagnosed with CFS than men.[21]

The common symptoms experienced by men are similar to those suffered by women, but skeptics believe men are hesitant to admit to symptoms such as muscle and joint pains, headache, malaise, and others. The reason for this is that men have more difficulty verbalizing their symptoms, probably due to gender stereotypes, their cultural and social upbringing, or their belief that the symptoms will just go away by themselves. Physicians are encouraging men to be more open in expressing their symptoms for prompter intervention.[22]

## Symptoms of Chronic Fatigue Syndrome in Women

Symptomatically, there isn't much difference between chronic fatigue syndrome in women and men. Most women in their forties or fifties commonly mistake symptoms of menopause for CFS.[23] Some women with CFS report symptoms analogous to premenstrual syndrome. These include *dysmenorrhea*, pain felt in the lower abdomen, tension, irritability, headache, mood swings (emotional labiality), *dysphoria*, anxiety, stress, insomnia, tenderness in the breasts, bloating, constipation, and joint and muscle pain. It is possible that there are more women diagnosed with CFS than men because women are more likely to report symptoms of CFS early.[24]

## Symptoms of Chronic Fatigue Syndrome in Children and Adolescents

A small percentage of children or adolescents are afflicted with chronic fatigue syndrome, since the age bracket during which CFS commonly occurs is usually between twenty and fifty years of age. Diagnosis of CFS in childhood happens rarely because children and adolescents seldom experience stress and anxiety, but it does happen, especially if the parents have a history of CFS themselves.[25]

CFS in children is usually detected between the ages of twelve and seventeen. Kids, like men, have a hard time voicing their symptoms due to difficulty in describing the nature or level of their fatigue or pain. Confirming a CFS diagnosis in children is different from that of adults, in that children must experience consistent occurrences of fatigue and the symptoms should last about three months (unlike adults, who must experience it for six consecutive months), and a pediatrician should be consulted at once.[26]

It is also more difficult to determine CFS in adolescents and children because they don't necessarily look ill, so it's sagacious to note the symptoms that they complain about. For most children and adolescents, the typical symptoms are headache, sleep troubles, and neurocognitive impairment. The headaches or migraine they experience are generally draining and accompanied by vomiting, shaking, diarrhea, abrupt declivity of body temperature, and severe debility.[27]

The neurocognitive deficiencies usually include difficulty in reading and focusing; some even have dyslexia that materializes only when the child is exhausted; and cognitive deficiencies worsen with any physical or mental activity. The variation and severity of symptoms tend to vary more swiftly and dramatically in children or adolescents than in adults. Many youngsters also show signs of juvenile fibromyalgia, or pain and sore points in nerve fibers and muscles. There are also some findings that show children or teenagers with CFS tend to have hyper-flexible joints.[28]

Other signs of note in a child with CFS are anxiety or refusal to go to school. It may also be difficult to differentiate CFS from other conditions in children such as infectious mononucleosis, psychiatric disorders, Lyme disease, and so forth. Chronic fatigue syndrome is often mistakenly branded as "school avoidance behavior" in children or as Munchausen's syndrome by substitution (a condition wherein a parent invents their child's sickness).[29]

## RARE PATHOLOGY OF CHRONIC FATIGUE SYNDROME

There's a predetermined set of symptoms included in the evaluation for chronic fatigue syndrome and associated clinical perplexities. However, there are some individuals who demonstrate unusual pathology of the disease. Although these symptoms may be recognized, they're usually not omnipresent in CFS.

### Brain Fog

Although brain fog or mental fog is a common symptom in individuals with CFS, its levels and severity vary. Other patients may feel the following:[30]

- Difficulty in word recall and use, which includes forgetting known words;
- Delayed recollection of names;
- Directional disorientation or inability to recognize familiar surroundings;
- Failure to recall where things are, as well as getting lost easily;
- Multitasking problems, which include failure to pay attention to more than one thing;
- Failure to remember the task at hand when sidetracked;
- Number problems, where the CFS patients experience difficulty in doing simple math, recalling sequences, and transposing digits.

## Heart Abnormalities

Chronic fatigue syndrome, apart from being connected to nervous system, immune system, and hormonal dysfunctions, is conjoined with heart abnormalities as well. The following heart dysfunctions signal an onset of CFS: small left ventricle, low nocturnal heart rate inconsistency, quick QT interval, postural tachycardia, low blood volume, waning cardiac function, and irregular cardiac wall contraction. There are four chambers of the heart: the left ventricle, the right ventricle, the left atrium, and the right atrium. One study links an undersized left ventricle in a subgroup of CFS patients with a symptom known as orthostatic intolerance (OI).[31] According to this study, the individuals with OI have an undersized left ventricle that doesn't pump blood as steadily as it should, and this peculiarity is very distinguishable. Individuals who have OI usually feel dizzy while standing upright.

Blood pressure surges momentarily to oppose gravity and sustain the blood streaming to the brain when a person gets up from a lying or sitting position, but people with OI experience a drop in blood pressure when standing. This causes them to feel lightheaded, which at times can lead to semi-unconsciousness. Research has shown that an undersized small ventricle may increase the occurrence of OI and CFS symptoms due to the low blood flow to both body and brain. OI also was shown to be a precise subgroup of CFS.[32]

The sleep-wake configuration of people with CFS and their heart rates were observed overnight.[33] It was noted that low heart rate variability (HRV) was present in the individuals with CFS compared to a healthy group. When study members breathed in and out slowly, it was noted that the heart rate dithered, accelerating when breathing in and decelerating when breathing out.[34]

This is known as heart rate variability. Low HRV can denote (a) problems with the brain and nerve signals traveling to and from the heart, or (b) nuisances with the segment of the cardiac conduction system known as the sinus node. It was theorized that low HRV in CFS is related to the brain, since the autonomic nervous system controls the body's automatic functions. Deregulation of the autonomic nervous system is known as *dysautonomia* and is widely accepted among academics to be a characteristic of CFS.[35]

A common test concerning the heart's health is the EKG (electrocardiogram), wherein a machine plots the heart's electrical cycle on a graph. To be able to measure its specific characteristics, the points of the lines are marked. These intervals, or variances in points, provide useful information for doctors. The interval between points marked as Q and T is one of them. It was implied that a short QT interval rate, while uncommon in the general masses, is nearly ubiquitous in CFS patients because of its relevance to dysautonomia.[36] Another experiment also showed that QT intervals could differentiate cases of CFS from a similar disorder called fibromyalgia, with an 85 percent probability rate.[37]

Postural tachycardia is comparable to orthostatic intolerance, but it affects pulse rate rather than blood pressure. It's also linked to dysautonomia. Tachycardia is an unusually fast heart rate. Postural tachycardia therefore indicates that the heart rate increases irregularly upon standing. It is often observed as POTS, or postural orthostatic tachycardia syndrome, identified in individuals with CFS.[38] As a result of a research trial concerning the study of adolescents, CFS was deemed to be associated with symptomatic low vitamin D levels.[39] There are other speculative studies linking CFS to vitamin D deficiency.[40]

Investigators have noted that individuals with severe CFS have the lowest blood volume.[41] Further tests have shown that impaired heart function was a likely upshot of low blood volume and not due to structural deficiencies. Think tanks confer that low blood volume influences the many symptoms of CFS by removing oxygen from the cells, which they require to spawn energy, though this hasn't been confirmed by research.[42]

Furthermore, scientists have studied the correlation between irregular cardiac motion of the walls of the heart and CFS and examined the way the walls of the heart move to measure the success of treatment. However, the experts concentrated only on self-reported CFS subgroups. In the study, irregular motions (contract/relax) of the cardiac walls exist in some cases of CFS found with *cytomegalovirus* and Epstein-Barr virus infection.[43]

## Other Rare Symptoms of Chronic Fatigue Syndrome

Other uncommon symptoms of CFS include the following:[44]

- Morning stiffness;
- Numbness;
- Earache;
- Prickly sensations in the hands or feet (paresthesia);
- *Temporomandibular joint (TMJ) disorder*;
- Sensitivity to the cold or heat that worsens the other symptoms;
- Recurring respiratory illnesses;
- Low fever or low temperature of the body;
- Too much sweating, dry mouth or eyes (sicca syndrome);
- Difficulty in moving the tongue;
- Disordered feelings of the tongue;
- Mouth ulceration;
- Painful or repeated urination;
- Rashes on the body;
- Tinnitus or humming, ringing, hissing, or popping noises heard inside both ears;
- Muscle spasms;
- Seizure;
- Canker sores;
- Persistent infections;
- Herpes or shingles.

Chronic fatigue syndrome can be a perplexing disorder and its patholo-gy can be very difficult to ascertain. There are several tests to take, multiple benchmarks to meet, and several other sicknesses to rule out before anyone can be fully confirmed to be suffering from chronic fatigue. Symptoms should be carefully evaluated because CFS tends to coexist with other underlying illnesses. Although the main symptomatic feature of CFS is austere and incapacitating fatigue lasting for at least six months, the presence of other clues should be monitored as well to avoid mistaking CFS with other afflictions.[45]

It's important for patients and caregivers to note that additional re-search indicates that (a) orthostatic intolerance, which in some cases involves a virally-induced dysfunction of a patient's autonomic nervous system, (b) low red blood cell count and low plasma volume, (c) signs of left ventricular failure upon stress, and (d) left chamber damage when the patient is in an upright position, are among the prominent features and distinguishing patterns of CFS. Muscle weakness or delayed recovery of the muscles following exercise, orthostatic fainting, and decreased cardiac output are just the tip of the iceberg when it comes to symptoms of chronic fatigue syndrome.[46]

## ANALYSIS

In studying the pathology of CFS, it's vital to note the signs and symptoms rather than to concentrate on the diagnosis. There's no standard laboratory test or *biomarker* for identifying CFS, thus the signs and symptoms present in an individual become the benchmarks for the diagnostic formulas delineated in the next chapter.

# 5

# DIAGNOSING CHRONIC FATIGUE SYNDROME

Even though the fatigue isn't acute anymore, the chronic fatigue syndrome (CFS) patient is driven to change his lifestyle due to possible risk of relapse. Its incidence has taken its roots from both gene-to-gene relationships and environmental experiences. Various methods were used to decipher the spot-on root cause of CFS long ago, but these attempts were likely a failure. Most study designs are watered down with many possibilities, thus giving unreliable measures. With all the above in view, different attempts have been made to remove the obstacles and offer sound inferences and unified criteria for CFS diagnosis.[1]

Oxford University's criteria for chronic fatigue syndrome is similar to the diagnostic rules of the Centers for Disease Control and Prevention, except Oxford contends that the following should be excluded from diagnosis of CFS: patients with recognized medical situations with similar symptoms as those seen in CFS and in patients suffering from manic-depressive conditions, schizophrenia, eating disorders, longtime substance abuse, or other proven brain diseases.[2]

## DIAGNOSIS AT A GLANCE

There aren't any specific diagnostic run-throughs for determining whether an individual has CFS, but there's an extensive process to be followed. First, the physician needs to acquire a detailed medical history of the patient through a string of questions. The CFS patient has to undergo a complete physical exam. Next, the patient has to pass a mental status examination through an interview.[3]

There are tests that assess the effects of fatigue on cognitive skills, such as mental organization, memory, and concentration. These evaluations can also be beneficial in differential diagnostic processes or for verifying specific areas where therapy would be gainful. Afterward, the patient is subjected to a standard series of laboratory tests, including blood and urine tests. Additional scans and tests might be required to dismiss other possible medical conditions. These may include the following:[4]

- Full blood count;
- Blood urea nitrogen (BUN);
- Blood biochemistry (calcium, sodium, potassium, urea);
- Creatine kinase (to exclude muscle disease);
- Blood glucose;
- Urinalysis;
- Alanine aminotransferase (ALT);
- Electrolytes;
- Globulin;
- Phosphorus;
- Total protein;
- Albumin;
- Alkaline phosphatase (ALP);
- Erythrocyte sedimentation rate (ESR);
- Thyroid stimulating hormone (TSH); and
- Transferrin saturation and other liver function tests.

Second-line tests may also be required, depending on the discretion of the physician, in case other illnesses are present as well. These include antibody diagnostic tests for certain disorders such as the following:[5]

- Hepatitis B or C;
- Lyme disease or Lyme borreliosis and parvovirus;
- Screening for celiac disease for inexplicable anemia;
- Gastrointestinal indications or evidence of malabsorption;
- MRI scan if additional neurological illnesses such as multiple sclerosis are noted on the basis of symptoms and signs;

- Autoimmune and rheumatology screens if joint and muscular pains are pronounced; and
- Pituitary and adrenal function tests if there are indications that imply a specific endocrine disorder.

Oftentimes, CFS diagnosis is a thorny mission for a number of reasons:

- The beginning may be gradual, after an individual has experienced an illness or stressful episode, or all of a sudden;
- The scope of the exposing symptoms is wide, and fatigue and pain may not always be notable;
- The individual may have been checked thoroughly but with negative findings for varying physical symptoms; and
- Complaints vary in category and intensity over a period of time (either weeks or months), which might confuse both the caregiver and the client.

Therefore, much of the diagnosis of CFS relies on the signs and symptoms presented by a patient.

## Importance of Early Detection

Diagnosis of CFS is complicated because there aren't any sole lab tests, obvious indications, or inimitable biomarkers. Doctors must first rule out any other possible causes before diagnosing the patient with chronic fatigue syndrome. However, it's still important to detect CFS speedily if possible because it may lead to more severe psychological and physiological struggles.

## Onset of CFS and Diagnosis

Careful scrutiny of the symptoms and the pattern of illness can establish a diagnosis of CFS. Simply put, CFS isn't something straightforward from a diagnostic standpoint like depression. It's a syndrome wherein fatigue is the foremost earmark affecting the mind and body. For a period of six months, the patient must be observed and for at least 50 percent of the time, he must be experiencing fatigue. Persons with clinical history of concurrent diseases are excluded from this diagnostic definition.[6]

Seventy-five percent of people suffering from CFS report acute viral infections such as bronchitis, gastroenteritis, tonsillitis, and meningitis.[7] Chronic fatigue syndrome may also arise from chicken pox, glandular fever, and rubella. It could also just be a derivative of vaccinations or toxin exposure. In the end, it isn't fair that patients are often left hanging by medical practice due to diagnostic uncertainty.[8]

If a patient experiences a viral infection, persistent fatigue that'll last for almost six weeks should be observed and considered for further diagnosis. If the symptoms persist four months, the patient should be diagnosed with CFS provisionally and an initial treatment approach can be made. After six months, the provisional diagnosis can be confirmed, and clinical procedures should be driven forward. Through this method, the onset of the illness can be monitored and an early working diagnosis can be established. With some cases, the onset of CFS can fail to kick off a warning. The disorder slowly eats the patient's well-being in an insidious manner, different from one that starts from an infection. The prescriber might not be able to initiate a test and the CFS patient himself may not be aware of deviations from his normal mental and physical state.[9]

## A Patient's Experience

Treatment delays nurture frustration and severity of medical disorders. An unfit patient who registers a virus and hasn't received the right medical instruction will face a more classic range of symptoms and the physician may not be able to provide satisfactory explanation of the case. The absence of clear diagnostic supposition hinders the person from (a) the appropriate sickness benefits, (b) vital care, (c) precautionary measures, and (d) access and mobility of their needs. Around 25 percent of people with CFS are wheelchair bound, housebound, or even bedridden.[10]

A case study supporting the scrutiny of CFS as a "diagnosis of exclusion" occurred to a thirty-three-year-old man who for two years had been travailing with fatigue.[11] After two years of utilizing various modalities of clinical management, his suffering increased; later on, he was diagnosed with Lyme disease, which arose from a late infection associated with his CFS. He was unable to function well and became bed-bound. He didn't have a medical history of any disease and his health records were unremarkable. Late diagnosis of the disorder caused him to suffer drastic changes in his physical activities. The gentleman was a former police officer who practiced martial arts, yet his physical functionality deteriorated due to late detection.[12]

## Reasons for Delayed Diagnosis

There are many reasons for late detection of CFS in a clinical setting. Most patients would think that their fatigue was bred by overwork, so they tend to rest for a period of time and then return to their former routine. In due course, they discover that they're ill, and their disorders might have grown severe as they neglected their well-being. The following notes elucidate delayed detection:[13]

- People might believe that CFS is a nonexistent disorder that isn't taught in medical school.
- Clinical specialists tend to dismiss the possibility of the disease and therefore don't recommend such a diagnosis.
- Clinical criteria for diagnosis aren't completely established. Published papers pertaining to CFS methods and treatment vary, and research designs are rigid for clinical practice.
- Lab tests aren't possible since there's no abnormality that can be spotted through any clinical procedure. The symptoms of CFS are neither unique nor specific.
- One major hindrance for early detection is that the symptoms should be observed for a minimum of six months until the physician can conclude the CFS patient's diagnosis.

## THE PATIENT'S CLINICAL HISTORY

Assessment of the life events of the patient prior to the onset of CFS should be considered. The medical history of the CFS sufferer gives evidences for a more accurate medical diagnosis. In one experiment, nearly three hundred CFS patients said that they'd been sick for an average of sixty-three months before they were diagnosed with CFS.[14]

These people had been suffering with extreme stress that could have possibly contributed to their condition. Another study involved patients with infectious mononucleosis or upper respiratory tract infection initially, and, due to these adversities, development of chronic fatigue was made possible.[15] Additional health mishaps came from disorders of muscle function: *phonasthenia*, neurasthenia, and others concerning voice difficulties.[16] These studies occured during war, and the onset of the disease might have been triggered by trauma and psychological struggle.

## Medical History of the CFS Sufferer

A patient's medical history may provide clues that lead to the development of chronic fatigue syndrome. The history also gives a clear picture of the nature and characteristics of the patient's symptoms. Moreover, the importance of the clinical history is related to subsequent steps advised by the doctor. The patient's history would also help to determine whether he's really experiencing CFS or if there's already a lingering condition exacerbated by CFS.[17]

For example, early stages of hepatitis might lead to CFS-like illness. Every ounce of blood taken out of the body and other tests performed are relevant key indicators for diagnosis. Lyme disease, which is often part of a CFS diagnosis, is induced by tick bites. Such a medical past can add to the complication of the diagnosis of CFS. Due to numerous factors (*psychosomatic*, etc.) and previous activities and uncertainty in the disease definition, CFS really needed a lot more studies before it finally became established in the medical community.[18]

## Medical Overlaps in the Diagnostic Process

Chronic fatigue syndrome often occurs alongside fibromyalgia, a syndrome characterized by tender points throughout the body. Although the diagnostic characteristics of CFS and fibromyalgia are different, studies show that 20 to 70 percent of people with fibromyalgia have CFS.[19] Thus, researchers have considered that symptoms, patient characteristics, and treatments of functional somatic syndromes are manifestations of biomedical and psychosocial processes. The diagnostic overlays among these conditions can be explained by *pathophysiology*.

Therefore, the occurrence of one symptom might be able to expound the origins of another.[20]

## Age and Early Life Factors in Diagnosis

Chronic fatigue syndrome doesn't choose the age of its victim. The syndrome can occur in adults and children alike. Pediatric settings may cause delay in diagnosing CFS among youngsters. Chronic fatigue syndrome at a young age is suggestive of early life causative factors, and the instigators of the disease might be difficult to identify, but their presence is definite from the beginning. These are considered environmental inducers.[21]

Early life inducers increase the potential of developing CFS during adulthood. Prenatal and neonatal exposure to the environment may induce some factors leading to development of CFS, as well. There are also studies fastening childhood autism with prenatal inflammatory attacks. Prenatal (before birth) exposure to disruptive chemicals associated with the *endocrine system* can induce aberrant responses of the immune system, thereby muddying the diagnostic steps of CFS even further.[22]

## Role of the Immune System in Diagnosis

CFS detection and diagnosis needs a definite time frame in order to determine the "cause and effect" of the disorder. The likely causative factor of the onset of the disease might have occurred before the diagnosis of CFS. This leads to the fact that infectious agents, toxicants, viruses, or bacteria might already be present. This may mislead the medical findings and diagnostic results given to the patient. That in turn also evokes the assessment of blood levels of environmental chemicals and drugs and therefore pairs it with the postpartum biomarkers of CFS. Analyses suggest a strong correlation between the prenatal progress of the child and the critical window of the occurrence of CFS in later life.[23]

Heavy metals, lead, and polychlorinated biphenyls (PCB) are often found in the body during diagnosis. Clinical investigations concur that the toxicity induced by the chemicals causes an obtunded IQ. Lead is also demonstrable in blood. This lead-induced immune toxicity impedes some necessary body functions and can eventually lead to fatigue and other known CFS by-products. This is an important aspect to take into consideration diagnostically, since prenatal stages affect every dimension of childhood development.[24]

Immune dysfunction to date report facilitated abnormality across the *physiological* systems that have been appended by inflammatory cell damage during early life stages. It's also a result of stress, which is a postnatal stimuli of infections to which the CFS sufferer could have been exposed before.[25] Overall, immune dysfunction has an inordinate connection to CFS. Physiological systems can be interrupted by early life disruption of the *homeoregulatory* role of immunity cells in the neurons and endocrines.[26]

## INTRODUCTION TO EXAMS, DIAGNOSTIC TESTS, AND SCREENING PROCEDURES

Prior to any diagnosis, examinations and diagnostic tests should always be performed. These tests are influenced by the medical history and other therapeutic procedures prescribed for the patient in the past.

### Clinical Presentation

It's well founded that CFS is connected to recurring fatigue, but certain forms of fatigue (a) take shape after pre-illness conditions and (b) abruptly transpire a loss of energy to perform daily routines. Grown-ups with chronic fatigue syndrome have often experienced chronic headaches, difficulty in concentrating and other cognitive problems, attention deficit hyperactivity disorder (ADHD), interstitial cystitis, irritable bowel syndrome, sleep problems, and *temporomandibular joint (TMJ) disorder*.[27] Examinations or clinical procedures given to children are more likely based on the physiological attributes in growth such as any disruption in height, weight problems, disproportional size of the head, glandular or *tonsiliar enlargement*, evidence of chronic sinusitis, and *postural orthostatic tachycardia syndrome (POTS)*.[28]

## Clinical Evaluation

Although there isn't a single test that will provide a definitive CFS diagnosis, there are a lot of clinical evaluations recommended to eliminate other potential conditions, thereby marking CFS as the prime possibility. These methods are discussed later in this chapter, since these laboratory techniques often render unremarkable results.[29]

## Diagnostic Tests and Screening Procedures

The following diagnostic tests are performed before a full CFS diagnosis is afforded by the physician.[30]

- Full blood count and differential;
- ESR or acute phase protein changes;
- Blood biochemistry;
- Creatinine kinase;
- Thyroid function tests;
- Liver function tests; and
- Urine tests for renal disease and diabetes.

Anything significant found in these tests will impact the patient's diagnosis and his syndrome will be reassessed. The second clutch of diagnostic tests must be performed. These procedures include:

- Antibody screening tests for infection such as hepatitis B and C, Lyme disease, and the presence of parvovirus should be checked. Positive results for any of these possibilities require immediate treatment.
- If gastrointestinal symptoms are prevalent, the patient must be screened for celiac disease. This may also be present if the patient is suffering from malabsorption and arcane *anemia*.
- Prominent joint pains might be present for patients who are elderly or older than forty. They can be screened using accurate rheumatology procedures.
- Neurological illness needs to be tested using an MRI scan to screen for signs of multiple sclerosis.
- Endocrine-related disorder should be verified through pituitary and adrenal function tests.

## GENETIC TESTS

An important way to determine the cause, development, and progress of a medical condition is to know the genetic connection and environmental influences. Sundry studies have been made to demonstrate the connection between DNA and familiality with CFS. One study was based on the prevalence of the disease among family members.[31] Those with relatives suffering from CFS would likely have a higher risk of acquiring the same disorder. The subjects included twins ages fifty and older hailing from the Australian Twin Registry. Researchers found that fatigue can be hereditary when it occurs for a minimum duration of four weeks.[32]

In another study of twins with evidence of CFS, their data was used to examine nexuses of genetic involvement and DNA to chronic fatigue. Sustained fatigue and CFS-like illnesses should be probed based on the genetic and familial affinity factors. However, this situation might not be applicable for broader populations. There are several elements that need to be considered, including the due-process measures of fatigue, classification of CFS on the basis of environmental, social, emotional, and cultural setting, family interviews, and sampling within the family of each patient. Susceptible individuals are more likely to be those with genetic relation to those affected by the disorder.[33]

## CENTRAL NERVOUS SYSTEM DIAGNOSTICS OF CFS

The central nervous system might be a system of defect as suggested by numerous CFS-related symptoms such as fatigue, impaired concentration, impaired attention, and short-term memory loss, along with headaches. Several diagnostic procedures can assess the functionality of the central nervous system, like neuroimaging, cognitive testing, neuropeptide assays, and autonomic assessment.[34]

### Neuroimaging

Magnetic resonance imaging (MRI) is a method of seeing the brain's activities. This is done together with single photon-emission computed tomography (SPECT). Individuals facing trauma have fewer subcortical abnormalities compared to subjects with CFS. However, there are also dossiers that show the same MRI results among healthy and depressed people and CFS patients.[35] Using SPECT, researchers have found that people suffering from CFS have lower levels of local cerebral blood flow in the brain, unlike the healthy subjects.[36] *Hypoperfusion* is more evident in CFS patients compared to depressed subjects. However, another survey confirmed that cerebral blood flow for twins with chronic fatigue syndrome corresponds to the same blood flow of twins who are healthy.[37] Scientists believe that CFS has obvious abnormalities in the central nervous system. Conversely, this claim lacks functional significance and therefore remains inexplicit in the frontiers of medical science. Findings and more results are still awaiting further clarification and investigation.

## Neuroendocrine Tests

CFS patients were found to have evidence of hypothalamic-pituitary-adrenal (HPA) axis. There is also some occurrence of serotonin pathways, which make stress. Hypocortisolism also exists in some patients. Genetic mutation has also been found in a family with thirty-two members suffering from CFS. The mutation impacts the body's production of globulin, a protein that's detectable during diagnosis, which helps in the transport of cortisol in the blood.[38]

Serum prolactin levels produced in CFS patients are greater than in those who are depressed but healthy. Unlike other acknowledged symptoms of CFS, HPA abnormalities, hormonal stress responses, and serotonin neurotransmission offer more evidence and certainty, though the findings aren't yet conclusive.[39]

## Neuropsychiatric Tests

Some experts might believe that CFS is a psychiatric disorder. That's why doctors are sometimes reluctant to diagnose CFS. Chronic fatigue syndrome is actually related to various psychological disorders like somatization disorder, hypochondriasis, major depression, and atypical depression.[40] Obvious conditions for CFS patients are mood swings, which can last for a lifetime. Clinical studies note that chronically ill

CFS patients have current and lifetime major depression.[41] There are also high rates of anxiety disorders preceding the onset of CFS.[42]

Management of the patients with respect to diagnostic tests is imperative even when it comes to CFS sufferers without psychiatric issues. This helps physicians rule out other symptoms and may also be a way to assess any issues of maladaptive coping styles, psychopathological situations, and psychiatric disorders. Soon, this could be an integral part of the clinical evaluation for every patient.

Furthermore, cognitive problems involving attention, concentration, and memory malfunction are some of the disruptive and unsettling traits of CFS. Patients suffer with discrepancies in processing information, poor learning, and memory loss. Thus, the patients would have a gritty time with cognitive information processing, leading to poor performance on the job or elsewhere. This leads to suspicions that CFS can be associated to psychological impairment or psychiatric disorder. Despite all this, there are also countless cases where CFS patients show highly intellectual abilities and normal cognitive performance during the diagnostic process.[43]

One way of checking the patients who are affected by CFS is by use of exercise programs and cognitive therapy. This is based on the possibility that behavior and cognition play a major part in CFS diagnosis. These are all based on ruminant association of the symptoms to the disease. Thus, cognitive therapies are also readied to test the patients. Chronic fatigue syndrome sufferers undergoing advanced behavior therapy have shown applicable results of stagnated pain in the lower back as well as in the chest, and they can perform better coping exercises.[44]

## Sleep Tests

Sleeping pattern is a highly overlooked periphery of CFS diagnosis. Sleep is the unrivaled form of rest. People with fatigue are short of rest, and sleep can be one of the symptoms or drawbacks of being ill with the syndrome. Chronic fatigue syndrome patients have difficulty in their sleeping patterns, various sleeping disruptions, and inconsistent napping routines compared to healthy people. This is a highly observable piece of the diagnostic puzzle. Experts have found that CFS patients have *alpha-intrusion* that occurs during *non-REM sleep*. However, some studies didn't yield similar results. There are also cases where patients with CFS-like illness have been found to have a sleeping disorder called apnea, a condition that can be treated immediately, excluding any possibility of CFS.[45]

## IMMUNOLOGICAL TESTS OF CFS

Compared to a healthy person, CFS sufferers have been observed as having superfluous quantities of *autoantibodies*. This results in a sapped immune system and low levels of protection against foreign "invaders." The magnitude of the physical degradation, cognitive deficiencies, and physiological impairment is due to the body's inability to fight these conditions. Thus, there's a great need to check the antibody count and to provide the CFS patient with the necessary antibodies that can fight his specific symptoms. Immunological tests to date aren't yet fully established in the clinical arena.[46]

### Infectious Agent Screening

Although the Epstein-Barr virus has been indirectly connected to CFS, medical researchers have been trying to solidify a viral connection. However, there's still no tangible evidence to support the idea.[47] It's improbable for a CFS patient to have only one source of infection, so this arena must be scrutinized and scientists must delve more closely into it for immunological hints regarding the disorder.

## ANALYSIS

Cast-iron certainty of diagnostic results still lies afar. Researchers and the medical world continue to investigate how to clarify and support the diagnosis of CFS. In fact, difficulty in the diagnosis of CFS could arise from inadequate and poorly described sampling procedures, and sometimes the choice of comparison groups simply isn't diverse enough to draw conclusions. In summary, the diagnosis for this illness is established on the foundation of subjective clinical interpretation, exclusion, and the CFS client's rapport with the caregiver.

# 6

# ROLES OF THE FAMILY PHYSICIAN, INTERNIST, AND NEUROLOGIST IN CHRONIC FATIGUE SYNDROME

**A** physician is necessary to ensure the wellness of a patient with chronic fatigue syndrome (CFS). However, a doctor's role in regard to treating this syndrome must be clearly defined before seeking medical attention. This chapter is about the importance of finding the right physician and identifying the appropriate questions to ask. The research presented here discusses the usual functions of the three physicians who normally handle CFS cases—the family physician, the internist, and the neurologist—and also enumerates the questions a CFS patient should ask his healthcare professionals. Likewise, the following paragraphs also include possible questions a physician might ask a person who has CFS.[1]

## COMMON FUNCTIONS

The basic task of any physician depends on the education he's completed. People with CFS should learn about the roles played by their various physicians prior to their consultations in order to prevent misunderstandings and incorrect assumptions. This section defines the roles of a family physician, an internist, and a neurologist.[2]

## Family Medicine and CFS

A family physician is known to be a practitioner in general medicine. This doctor has wide medical training that can be of use to a diverse set of patients (including CFS sufferers) to provide primary care.[3] This means that a family physician has the ability to provide initial medical attention to anyone. Considered the backbone of the community health system, a family physician attends to any health concern that the CFS sufferer may have, whether it's a physical, mental, or emotional topic.[4]

Since a family doctor has knowledge about wide spectrum of medical areas, he's well-rounded in handling various maladies. Moreover, when it comes to CFS, one of the basic roles of a family physician is to prevent further illness of the patient.[5] An awareness about general medicine enables a family physician to guide patients to a proper and healthy lifestyle. As the family physician establishes a CFS patient's healthy immune system, he lessens the chances that the patient will suffer from other clinical disorders.

A family physician also acts as a role model who promotes professional attire, appropriate behavior, correct posture, proper speech, and auspicious habits in terms of health.[6] This helps the members of the community in attaining a healthy physical condition and well-being. Aside from assuring the patient's wellness, a family physician continually provides a personal patient-physician connection.[7] The profound relationship between a physician and a patient develops over the course of time, as a physician may treat his patient from birth to adulthood. This role enables the doctor to track and record the medical history of the CFS patient wholeheartedly.

Another function of a family physician is to refer and advocate specialists for his patients when necessary.[8] Depending on the complexity of the health concern of a patient, the family physician may seek the help of an appropriate specialist with across-the-board knowledge of a specific area of medicine. The family physician serves as a channel between two parties: the client and the specialist. Since a family doctor usually handles the primary record of the CFS client, this physician can provide important information that may help the specialist. At the same time, the family physician can help a patient to comprehend the specialist's findings by explaining them in simple terms.[9]

## Internists and CFS

Contrary to a family physician's wide range of patients, an internist focuses only on adults. Thus, an internist is often referred to as a doctor for grown-ups.[10] The core of an internist's medical training is an expansive field called adult medicine.

An internist practices almost all the basic functions of a family physician because an internist is also knowledgeable in general medicine. The family physician's role, such as maintaining and improving the quality of a patient's health, are also performed by an internist.[11] Enhancing the well-being of a person encompasses the prevention, immediate discovery, and treatment of a health problem such as chronic fatigue syndrome in a mature adult patient. Nonetheless, an internist implements a more scientific and logical approach when diagnosing a specific health concern.[12]

Aside from his knowledge of general medicine, an internist also has subspecialties of his choice.[13] Possible subspecialties include neurology, immunology, cardiology, ophthalmology, gastroenterology, dermatology, and many others.[14] An internist's métier provides deeper knowledge into a specific medical field, which in turn enables him to handle the more complex health concerns of CFS patients.

Most of the time, an internist acts as a consultant to other doctors such as surgeons, the family physician, and other specialists. These doctors refer their patients to an internist who can analyze serious medical issues. Due to a vast and more in-depth background in medicine, the internist can expertly evaluate the clinical indicators reported by his adult CFS patient. In addition to handling referrals, internists also assess whether a patient qualifies for surgery.[15]

Internists may attend to patients who are planning to undergo a surgery at the request of a surgeon or a family physician.[16] This role requires explanation of the potential risk of the surgery, preparing the CFS patient prior to the operation, and assisting the client after the surgical process.[17] Based on a study, an internist usually tries to reduce the patient's surgical danger when there's about 65 percent or more risk of CFS perceived.[18] This corroborates that an adult patient should consult with an internist to diminish the possible threat of surgery.

## Neurologists and CFS

Disorders involving the nervous system are commonly treated by a neurologist.[19] This physician has a medical expertise that focuses on diagnosing and managing the CFS patient's nerves, whether the problem involves the central or peripheral nervous system. In addition, a neurologist can have a diverse set of patients since this physician treats the neurological concerns of adults as well as children.[20]

Similar to a family physician and an internist, a neurologist is also conversant in general medicine.[21] This enables the neurologist to assess the health concerns of a CFS patient. However, a neurologist can provide a more thorough evaluation of the medical issues related to neurology. When a patient has a neurological issue such as Alzheimer's disease, peripheral nerve disorder, brain tumors, Parkinson's disease, or sleep disorders, a neurologist serves as the primary care provider for the patient.[22] As a primary care specialist, a neurologist has the overall control in managing the patient's health.

The neurologist also examines the cognitive ability of a patient.[23] This role involves testing the CFS sufferer's mathematical logic, memory, and language capacity to determine the condition of his motor system, cranial nerves, and sensory system.[24] Identifying the cognitive ability of a patient helps the neurologist to understand the patient's situation. In terms of diagnostic examinations, a neurologist also serves as a patient's guide.[25] This physician may request blood tests, electroencephalography, biopsy, spinal fluid analysis, and imaging tests.[26] The findings of the diagnostic examinations clarify the condition of the patient. With these diagnostic results, a neurologist gives a more comprehensive analysis of the patient's health situation. When a neurologist finally identifies the extent of the CFS patient's nerve-related disorder, he forms a plan on how to pursue treatment.[27] This protocol enables the patient to recover from his neurological issue. Depending on the patient's condition, the neurologist may include a recommendation for surgery.[28] This means that another role of a neurologist is to refer the CFS patient to a neurosurgeon as necessary.

## QUESTIONS FOR THE DOCTOR

When a doctor diagnoses a patient with chronic fatigue syndrome, the patient should ask some questions to completely understand his health condition. Aside from knowing the definition of this syndrome, individuals with CFS must also learn about its causes and treatment from a physician. The following section outlines some of the potential questions a CFS patient may ask a family physician, an internist, or a neurologist, as well as explaining why such questions must be asked by a patient.

### "What Causes CFS?"

According to a study of 1,000 participants, about 8.5 percent had unbearable fatigue for at least six months without any clear justification.[29] Thus, it's essential for the patient to ask the specific cause of his syndrome to identify why he's affected by CFS. Some of the common viruses presumed to initiate CFS are Epstein-Barr, varicella-zoster, hepatitis B, and *mycoplasma pneumoniae*.[30] A patient with CFS may ask his physician if any of these viruses caused his syndrome. Another question that can be raised to a physician is in regard to the potential ways of acquiring viruses that cause CFS. Aside from viruses, an uncharacteristic immune system and hormonal problems may also be factors related to chronic fatigue.[31] Discovering the possible reasons behind CFS is also important for a patient to prevent such disease in the future.

### "Is CFS Inherited?"

Since a family physician usually tracks the medical history of a patient and his family record, this physician is the most appropriate doctor to ask this. A family doctor can access a CFS patient's medical archives to determine if the patient's CFS is hereditary. This question is also crucial in diagnosing the immediate family members of the patient. In this way, the syndrome can be immediately eliminated.[32]

## "What Are the Symptoms and Consequences of Having CFS?"

The most common symptom of CFS is, of course, fatigue, which can't be cured with bed rest and continues for a minimum of six months.[33] Depending on the severity of the syndrome, the symptoms from one patient to another vary, yet another reason why the CFS patient should ask his doctor about them. Further consequences of CFS include headache, muscle pain, inability to concentrate, enlarged lymph nodes in the neck or armpit, sore throat, memory loss, difficulty in sleeping, and joint pain.[34] A CFS patient may also be angry, frustrated, and depressed.[35] If a CFS sufferer is made aware of these symptoms, he'll be prepared should they materialize.

## "What Other Diseases Are Related to CFS?"

Chronic fatigue syndrome can also occur together with other illnesses.[36] Other than fatigue, a patient with CFS should also ask about illnesses related to the syndrome. This information is quintessential in preventing other health issues in a CFS patient. Based on a study, CFS might be related to blood-brain barrier permeability (BBBP).[37] A CFS patient may ask a neurologist if his syndrome has a connection to BBBP and if it can cause another neurological quagmire.

This enables the patient to manage or prevent other potential health concerns regarding his nervous system health. CFS is also associated with fibromyalgia and Gulf War syndrome, which are both related to long-term fatigue.[38] A CFS patient may also ask a physician if he has a risk of having those disorders. Another purpose of this question is for the physician to treat not only the syndrome, but also the patient's other health problems at the same time.[39]

## "What Are the Possible Ways to Treat CFS?"

Some of the common treatments for CFS are cognitive behavior therapy, exercise programs, and pharmacological therapy.[40] A CFS patient must know which specific medical plan suits him. The patient may also ask a family physician, an internist, or a neurologist about the appropriate person to provide such treatment. It's always better to seek a physician's advice regarding the treatment instead of using alternative therapies, such as an exclusion diet and aromatherapy.[41] Such alternative therapies pose a higher risk and the potential for harm. Recommendations from healthcare professionals like family doctors, internists, and neurologists are more trustworthy and reliable.

A patient can also ask his healthcare provider about possible medications. Since a CFS patient often suffers from unbearable pain, he may ask for pain relievers for immediate and temporary relief. Based on the patient's treatment plan, a physician knows if temporary medication is necessary. If medicine is prohibited, a patient may solicit advice from the physician about other methods of reducing pain. Preparing a treatment plan may take days, thus it's important for a patient to have a reprieve when necessary. Exhausting all the suitable CFS treatments also gives the patients better alternatives to choose from. In addition, a patient can set his schedule in accordance to the medical treatment once a treatment regimen has been established.[42]

## "How Is the Improvement of the CFS Patient Measured?"

There isn't any blood test or recognizable physical condition that determines the improvement of a CFS patient.[43] Thus, the patient should ask the physician for a tangible way to measure the progress of his treatment. Questionnaires, roundtables with the patient, and a patient's self-records are some of the tools that can be used to assess the CFS sufferer's response to medical treatment.[44] A CFS patient may also inquire about the frequency of conducting these assessments. Identifying the right tool and its occurrence enables the CFS patient to prepare for his recovery, and questions about health progress also help the patient to understand the goal of the medication schemata.

## "Are Support Groups Necessary?"

Depending on the CFS patient's situation, a physician may recommend a support group, which is a valuable resource for all.[45] It's best to ask if this pack of friends is mandated for a specific patient. Just as symptoms vary from one patient to another, so does the sine qua non for a support group. For a child with CFS, a family physician who's also well-rounded in pediatrics can offer emotional support. According to a study, constant pediatric support lessens symptoms during the child's recovery period.[46]

## "Is a CFS Patient Considered a Fully Disabled Person?"

In medico-legal terms, a CFS patient who is disabled for years and who shows less than 10 to 20 percent improvement over the course of ten years is considered to be permanently disabled.[47] In some cases, CFS isn't qualified as an unending disability when a patient shows progressive improvement.[48] A CFS patient should know if his condition can be considered as a disability. It's important for a patient to be aware of his eligibility for medical disability benefits. If necessary, a client may also ask the attending physician to issue the required clinical papers to validate the degree of injury.

## QUESTIONS FOR THE PATIENT

A patient with CFS should also be prepared for the questions that a physician may ask. The following sections outline topics that may arise during the consultation with a family physician, an internist, or a neurologist. These are the questions necessary for an in-depth exploration of a patient's CFS. It's useful for the CFS sufferer to be aware of these inquiries prior to the appointment with the physician. Preparation leads to a more productive medical consultation for both the patient and doctor.[49]

## "What Are the Symptoms Currently Experienced?"

Even if a client is already diagnosed with CFS, a physician may still ask this question to monitor the patient's condition. This question covers all of the patient's unusual and unbearable symptoms. Since CFS shares similar medical signs with other illnesses, a physician may ask the CFS patient to divulge such information to immediately eliminate other related diseases or to confirm a CFS diagnosis.[50]

## "For How Long and How Often Are the Symptoms Experienced?"

Intolerable fatigue is considered "chronic" only when it lasts more than six months.[51] This means that tiredness over the course of a month or two may not be classified as chronic fatigue syndrome. It also proves that the duration of the symptom is crucial for evaluating the extent of CFS. Aside from identifying the nature of the symptoms experienced by the patient, the time period and frequency of the patient's CFS symptoms are also the physician's concern when analyzing the syndrome.[52]

A family physician or an internist also asks this question in order to monitor the development of a patient. By asking this question, the doctor expects the CFS patient to be able to identify how long or how frequently the symptoms occur. As a follow-up question, a physician may also ask when the patient experienced the symptom. This information determines not only the duration and frequency, but also the time of the day of the symptom's occurrence.[53]

## "Does the Patient Also Have a Family Member with CFS?"

This question may arise during the initial consultation when attending doctor isn't the patient's regular family physician. Chronic fatigue syndrome can be genetically inherited by a person, so knowing the family's medical history enables the physician to confirm the probable cause of the syndrome. In addition, the doctor may also ask how the patient's relative recovered from CFS.[54]

He may opt to follow the same procedure adopted by the patient's relative who successfully recovered. If the treatment for the patient's relative doesn't work, the healthcare professional may amend the treatment that was proposed in the past. This question helps the physician formulate possible ways to manage the sufferer's condition. The inquiry is unnecessary when the attending physician is the family's longtime doctor, since that ensures the patient's medical history is known.[55]

## "Was Trauma Experienced in the Past?"

Traumatic situations such as medical operations or severe accidents are identified to cause CFS.[56] A physician needs to ask this question to determine whether traumatic events led to a patient's syndrome. The physician presents this question not only to the patient, but also to the patient's family, since a patient may not remember or be aware of some traumatic events if they occurred long ago or while the patient was still a juvenile. In this situation, the physician's only resource is the patient's family members, specifically the parents who witnessed the growth of the patient.[57]

This question helps the physician to figure out the cause of the client's syndrome. Another purpose of the question is to record such traumatic events that may help in the recovery process. For an exhaustive analysis, the physician may also ask follow-up questions to learn more about his patient's health status. The doctor may study the patient's tragic experience and analyze how to minimize its effect on the life situation of the patient.[58]

## "Does the Medical Treatment Suit the Patient's Schedule?"

The treatment plan is arranged and set by the doctor, but he generally asks this question to be considerate. If a physician organized a treatment schedule without consulting the patient, it is possible that the allotted time of the physician may not complement the patient's daily schedule. Identifying the availability of the patient assists the physician in constructing an attainable medical plan for the CFS sufferer.[59]

## "Is Treatment Affordable for the Patient?"

The medical treatments for CFS are usually expensive.[60] This question ensures that the physician builds a treatment plan that's affordable for the CFS patient. Financial status should be considered prior to treatment planning. It's possible that the money prepared by the patient for his consultation is much less than the amount later realized. For improved fee arrangements, the physician might ask his patient to identify the specific amount of money dedicated for treating the CFS. This question also resolves the possible problem regarding money matters between the patient and the physician.[61]

## ANALYSIS

When all is said and done, the roles of a family physician, an internist, and a neurologist are vital to an individual with CFS. These physicians have commonalities in terms of conventional functions but still make distinct contributions to the patient's medical development. There are cases where patients who have severe symptoms of CFS become so dependent on other people that they become housebound or bed-bound. Access to healthcare services may be laden if the professionals involved such as internists, family physicians, and neurologists aren't well-informed about the possible attitudes of their patients toward them. Unfortunately, the skeptical attitudes of these caregivers may cause further suffering to CFS patients.

# 7

# ROLE OF THE HOSPITAL IN CHRONIC FATIGUE SYNDROME

Due to its persistent recurrence of symptoms, chronic fatigue syndrome (CFS) requires delicate, continual, and appropriate treatment by the hospital. Besides the support received from the patient's family, hospitals with professional staff and the proper facilities also play a big role in the physical and psychological treatment of people who deal with this disorder. The hospital is often responsible for the diagnosis of the patient's condition.[1]

Chronic fatigue syndrome patients don't usually look as sick as they may feel. That's why friends, family members, and others may not always take a CFS patient's complaints seriously. During these times, *hospitalists*, who try to properly understand the patient's experience and provide an accurate diagnosis and the proper care required for their condition, can become a lifeline for the CFS patient. Hospitalists also provide a sense of hope for the CFS sufferer.[2]

## HOSPITALS AND PATIENT-DOCTOR INTERACTION

Hospitals provide treatment such as cognitive behavioral therapy (CBT) and psychiatric consultations. This kind of medical treatment involves a series of one-hour sessions that focuses on discussing the nature of the patient's illness and the behaviors that may get in the way of the recovery.[3] Although CBT can only prevent the occurrence of some of the symptoms, studies have shown that the cognitive behavioral therapy performed in hospitals greatly influences a patient's improvement in terms of self-esteem and social interaction. Besides CBT, graded exercise therapy—a course of action often found in hospitals—and medications also contribute to diminishing the symptoms of CFS.[4]

Personal medical treatment aside, hospital care environments also contribute a great deal to the well-being of CFS sufferers along with other patients who experience different kinds of illnesses. A 2008 survey revealed the importance of a proper hospital environment for the betterment of its patients.[5] In their studies, researchers noted the effects of factors such as the number of educated staff and the quality of the hospital's facilities on the mortality rate and well-being of the patients residing on hospital grounds. Not surprisingly, data showed higher mortality rates in the hospitals with lesser staff and facilities.[6]

Research proves that better healthcare ambience enhances patient self-improvement, which is needed by CFS patients who are confused by their current state and troubled by the fact that the origin of the disease can't be precisely verified. This applies not only to CFS patients, but to others, too, such as cancer patients. Being in an environment where people share similar experiences helps CFS patients to understand how to deal with what they're experiencing and to realize that they're not alone.[7]

Hospitals and their staff—notwithstanding the medical services that they provide to their patients (like those who suffer from CFS)—also offer social interaction and reassurance to their clients. That's not always easy to do, as the patient is often in a threadbare state of mind in such a setting, but even the slightest encouragement can lead to positive changes.[8] At this point, the CFS patient learns to trust the hospital. If not, there won't be much progress. The healthcare professional at the hospital stands as a reflection of a friend who a patient can rely on and take advice from, thereby meaningfully boosting the patient's level of social interaction.[9]

In general, a hospital's contribution to its CFS patients and others includes not only the medical treatment for their disorders or diseases, but also a certain level of emotional and social support. The patient-doctor interface helps boost the sufferer's outlook on his condition. This psychological stimulation, delivered by various counseling and physical and psychological treatments, improves the patient's quality of life despite his disorder. Also, the hospital provides a secure environment where CFS clients can interact without being worried about their condition or about being criticized by others, as well as a complete facility to ensure the proper amount of determination required for an individual to improve both physically and mentally.[10]

## CFS SETTINGS: INPATIENT VS. OUTPATIENT

In brief, an inpatient is someone who receives treatment requiring him to stay on hospital premises, whereas an outpatient obtains medical assistance beyond hospitals, whether at his home or in a doctor's office. Because there isn't a cure for CFS at present, both inpatient and outpatient methods are used to ease the symptoms caused by this disorder.[11]

In an inpatient setting, the CFS patient's medical condition is continually monitored and treated. Outpatient care, on the other hand, can integrate diverse forms of treatment such as family sessions, graded activities, and exercise programs that involve trainers or physiotherapists whose goal is to reestablish the client's self-esteem. Since CFS is to some degree both a physical and a psychological disorder (since factors such as stress are also involved), the inpatient setting relies more on the patient-doctor interaction represented by firsthand counseling by medical specialists. The outpatient setting ferries more of the approach outside of the hospital.[12]

### Inpatient Setting

The severity of the patient's condition determines whether an inpatient setting is appropriate for a CFS patient. Most likely, people with moderate to very severe levels of fatigue will be subjected to intensive monitoring and care. The different clinical strata of fatigue are described in many works of research.[13]

Moderate fatigue is the level at which the patient has reduced mobility and is restricted from some activities in his daily life. Most likely, people with moderate fatigue would have to stop work and are required to have many rest periods. Patients with severe cases have the ability to carry out only the minimal tasks of daily living, such as washing their faces, and they rely on wheelchairs for mobility. In very severe cases, individuals are bedridden and immobilized due to fatigue. The hospital then would need to admit the patient, who would undergo unremitting monitoring.[14]

Inpatient settings are abundant in larger urban hospitals and fewer in smaller, rural hospitals.[15] A CFS patient in an inpatient setting commonly receives medication to help ease the effects of the symptoms. A comprehensive care package, such as one that includes treatment as well as follow-up rehabilitation, would be appropriate to describe this setting. In an event where the person can no longer perform daily tasks, the hospital rehabilitates him to regain strength and to recover by providing counseling and by prescribing treatments such as graded exercises accompanied by workout management strategies, sleep supervision, or relaxation techniques, as well as proper medications for relieving the pain caused by other conditions such as fibromyalgia.[16]

Among the various hospital treatments, stress and sleep management as well as psychological healing and exercise regimens are beneficial among CFS patients. In a hospital setting for CFS patients, it's first determined if stress management is applicable for the patient. This goes for the rest of the possible treatments considered. Chronic fatigue syndrome naturally manifests immobility and sudden fatigue, although in an inpatient setting, treatments promoting physical movements are often endorsed. The reason for this is that the significant decrease in muscular strength and agility results from the patient's moderate amount of physical activity.[17]

## Outpatient Setting

Outpatient settings could also be termed *home health care*. In the past, home health care, or the outpatient setting, was a treatment normally associated with family members taking care of their ill, along with nurses assisting the family and providing for the proper medical care required by the patient, in their own homes. Delivering professional nursing services to patients' homes has now become more in demand, wider in range, and complex as manifested by the conditions of CFS. Some factors have greatly contributed to the changes in the home care trend:[18]

- Rising costs of medical care;

- A growing population of elderly people;
- A continually rising need to manage chronic disorders;
- Preventing illnesses; and
- Enhancing patients' quality of life.

In the past, home health care began when the client was discharged by the hospital. Nowadays, outpatient care has morphed into a way to avoid hospitalization.[19] Outpatient settings most likely involve the intervention of physical therapists for nonhospital activities as well as the family members. The hourly sessions provided by cognitive behavioral therapy also endure in this type of setting since the patient doesn't require admission to the hospital. He's given counseling to regain confidence that may have been affected by the lack of social involvement due to the symptoms of fatigue brought about by CFS.[20]

Family sessions also count as outpatient resolutions. With this approach, the patient is counseled along with his family. The CFS patient's current condition is explained to the whole family in order to introduce them to lifestyle changes he might require. The sessions are concerned with task management issues such as organizing schoolwork, reintegrating exercise into daily life, reestablishing the patient's normal sleeping routines, helping relatives with social issues, and assisting the family in restoring some sense of normalcy to their family life.[21]

Graded activities and exercise programs are also used in outpatient settings. These activities focus on bridging the gap between the patient's current physical condition and the physical ability required to accomplish the basic tasks of daily living. The kinds of programs initiated in these treatments are also decided by the patient and his family at the same time. Patients and caregivers should also take note of which setting (inpatient vs. outpatient) has a more positive effect on the patient's lifestyle, the kind of medical disorder he's experiencing, and primary factors affecting the occurrence of his symptoms.[22]

## QUALITY OF HOSPITAL CARE VS. OUTCOME OF TREATMENT

The quality of hospital care hinges on health care delivery and how the staff manages the patients. Since CFS patients aren't the only population in the hospital warranting medical assistance, other clients must also be accounted for. The elderly, most especially, are high priorities in a hospital setting. It's estimated that by 2020 the number of U.S. adults over the age of sixty-five will be more than 53 million, with many of those being CFS sufferers.[23]

This means that there'll be a higher occurrence of other kinds of illnesses that a hospital must prioritize. Just as with CFS patients, older people require monitoring and psychological support because they too need to feel as if they're still a part of the community.[24] This affects the quality of health care that CFS patients are subjected to. Since their condition also requires continual monitoring, psychological assistance, and care as well as rehabilitation, a hospital must be able to provide appropriate services for all patients regardless of the medical condition in question.

Uneven distribution of amenities can also be a serious problem in terms of quality health care for individuals who have CFS. Two facets of this problem are (a) unequal distribution of care, and (b) increasing specialization. In some areas, particularly remote and rural locations, there are insufficient healthcare professionals and services available to meet the needs of individuals. Ruralized CFS clients may need to drive sizable distances for the services they require. Furthermore, an increasing number of healthcare personnel provide specialized services.[25]

Specialization can lead to fragmentation of care and often to increased cost, which can be a problem for CFS patients who aren't financially stable or capable, considering their disorder may have reduced greatly their economic support. To patients, this may mean receiving care from anywhere from five to thirty people during a hospital stay. This seemingly endless stream of personnel is often confusing and frightening and may greatly affect the hospital care of CFS sufferers.[26]

Another problem concerning the quality of health care that CFS patients receive is access to health care itself. This concerns not being able to have health insurance. Absence of health insurance is connected to low income, which has a great effect on CFS sufferers incapable of sufficient mobility. Low income has been associated with (a) relatively higher rates of infectious diseases such as tuberculosis and AIDS, (b) problems such as substance abuse, rape, and violence, and (c) chronic diseases or disorders like chronic fatigue syndrome.[27]

The use of healthcare services is also largely sprung by unemployment and increasing rate of poverty. Even though some government programs and assistance is available, benefits vary considerably from place to place and are continually being reevaluated.[28] A person who is unemployed due to CFS is affected by this type of problem. Although unforeseen circumstances arise, there are also admirable changes that are improving hospital care around the world, such as advanced technologies that allow for more accurate diagnosis and more appropriate treatment.[29] For CFS patients to receive proper and adequate treatment, a hospital must increase the quality of its health care primarily by responding to and rectifying organizational problems. Quality health care equates to the apt management of hospital patients, together with properly educated staff who can respond to miscellaneous cases. As a general conclusion, of course, the proper management of these issues leads to better treatment of the patients, especially CFS sufferers, in a hospital system.[30]

In a study in 2001, scientists determined that there were a significant number of CFS patients unsatisfied not only with the quality of health care delivery, but also with the interpersonal skills possessed by their attending physician.[31] In the research that they conducted, sixty-eight patients completed a survey about their overall satisfaction with the medical assistance that they received since the onset of their condition and their perspective on certain aspects of health care. Two-thirds of the patients were disappointed in the quality of medical care that they received. Those patients who were dissatisfied significantly (a) were more likely to protest about the delay, contradictions, or misunderstandings regarding their diagnosis, (b) received and simultaneously rejected a psychiatric diagnosis, or (c) saw doctors as indifferent, doubtful, or uninformed about CFS. They also distrusted the advice given to them since they saw it as both insufficient and conflicting in nature.[32]

Those patients who were satisfied were pointedly more likely to distinguish their doctors as considerate, supportive, and committed to uncovering their illness. These patients also claimed that they didn't expect their doctors to cure CFS and perceived their general physicians as the source of their greatest help in the course of their illness. Many patients were also critical of the small number of treatments employed, although this matter wasn't a great factor affecting their general satisfaction.[33] This study revealed that a doctor who has more information about the illness is preferred. Since the patient is already knowledge-able that his illness has no particular cure, he prefers someone with whom he can talk informatively and communicate on a much more personal level.

The findings of this study then alluded that hospital care was evaluated by CFS patients less on the doctor's ability to cure their illness but rather on his interpersonal skills and knowledge about the illness.[34] This then would be greatly affected by the uneven distribution of the health workforce around the world, such as in Africa, where thirty-six out of fifty-seven countries are currently facing a shortage in human resources, leaving fewer adequately informed health personnel to address the needs of CFS patients.[35] The authors and their study have advocated better communication and better education for hospital physicians in the diagnosis and management of CFS. Generally, the outcome of CFS patients' treatment has its foundation in the ability of healthcare personnel to cater to their physical, psychological, and interpersonal needs.

## Doctor Involvement in CFS Hospital Care

The physician is responsible for the medical diagnosis and for shaping the therapy required by a person suffering with chronic fatigue syndrome. The physician's role has traditionally been the treatment of disease and trauma; however, many hospital doctors are now including health promotion as well as disease prevention in their repertoire.[36]

In the hospital care of CFS patients, doctors carry on with diagnosis, treatment, and proper communication with their patients. Their primary obligation is to correctly diagnose the patient's health situation as well as to provide them proper information on what to do, what they should expect, and what they may experience throughout the course of their illness. Although CFS patients prefer a more personal relationship with their doctor, hospital-based healthcare professionals must also be straightforward and precise with the information they share, even if it's bad news for the client.[37]

The attending physician is adequately informed about the disorder and is capable of giving the proper treatment to the patient suffering from CFS. Most likely, physicians who treat chronic fatigue must focus on treating multiple symptoms that prevail during the course of the condition. These two primary symptoms are sleep abnormalities and chronic pain. The treatment of both greatly helps the recovery of the patient. Proper sleep management helps the CFS patient regain strength and makes him more relaxed despite the cyclical stints of fatigue. Healing the chronic pain also helps improve the CFS client's living situation at the hospital, and the reduction of the pain provides more comfort and thus enhanced health.[38]

Hospital physicians are responsible for monitoring the patient's daily activities and for finding suitable treatments. At times, patients misinterpret the meaning of exercise and physical activity, but for a physician attending a CFS patient, minimal exercise is required, depending on the severity of the case. The goal is to help the hospital patient regain mobility gradually by practicing normal bodily movements. Of course, the severity of the condition must be accurately diagnosed in order for the hospital to determine the extent of appropriate activities for the patient. Basically, the physician is there to guide and instruct the patient and to ensure that he systematically follows advices for his recovery.[39]

Psychologically, physicians aid in the recovery of CFS through interpersonal communication, since CFS patients may suffer mental disarray due to the loss of their jobs, their inability to perform daily tasks, and the like. Physicians become more of a trusted friend than a doctor. Knowing that there's someone else who can properly empathize with this condition and who can give credible advice can help frustrated individuals who are suffering from CFS.[40]

## ANALYSIS

Undoubtedly, the involvement of a physician in the hospital care of a CFS patient is vital. Since a one-stop cure for this disorder is yet to be found, treatments can only manage the patient's symptoms. The hospital's help in determining the appropriate course of treatment for the patient is paramount. Whether it's the management of stress, sleep, or daily activities or prescribing medications, the role of the hospital has always been to give proper diagnosis and to ensure that the patient recovers from the symptoms of CFS.

# Part III

# Many Faces

# 8

# FATIGUE AND THE HUMAN BODY

**F**atigue, generally expressed as the deterioration of physical performance, is a complex physical phenomenon that affects both the physiological and psychological disposition and functioning of the human body.[1] It's likened to a feeling of tiredness and exhaustion, a state wherein the individual lacks vitality, alertness, and motivation (subjective fatigue); is unable to accomplish tasks with expected quality and timeliness (objective fatigue); and exhibits significant changes in physiological processes, such as sustained muscular contractions (physiological fatigue).[2]

It can be caused by (a) motor units, such as muscle contractions (peripheral fatigue) or (b) bustles in the brain or the spine (central fatigue). Fatigue may be the result of overwork, lack of curative sleep, anxiety, boredom, or lack of exercise. It can also be a symptom caused by illness, medication, medical treatment, anxiety, and depression. It can be an accumulation of fatigue-causing stress or an acute application of significant stress that leads to a *failing point*, thereby triggering the brain to take impulsive action such as daytime dozing.[3]

Fresh developments in understanding fatigue have also led to decryption of CFS occurrences, also known as myalgic encephalomyelitis, which has proven to be as serious as other common chronic illnesses. Fatigue is even considered to be more blighting, such that patients with those illnesses associated with CFS (usually heart failure, suicide, and cancer) die relatively younger. Fatigue weighs on significant anatomical perturbations (i.e., nervous, endocrine, circulatory), but exhibits external symptoms that may not always indicate serious health concerns. A disadvantage, however, is the perception of CFS: whether it deserves the same attention as those with other common chronic ailments like heart disease and cancer. The disadvantage affects the societal construct and perception of CFS, where the possibilities of patient recovery lie: patients report poor experiences with healthcare providers, some of whom doubt the validity of CFS as a real medical problem.[4]

While the signals of fatigue on the organs can be identified by specific archetypes such as respiration, heartbeat, skin temperature, sweating, and pulse rate, the effect of fatigue can be observed from how the CFS patient's vital organs react to the stress stimulus that causes it, aside from the perceived disposition of the individual (i.e., psychological bearing of fatigue).[5]

Based on various studies that have pointed out the different effects of fatigue on the human body, the influence of fatigue can be focused on six anatomical systems: the nervous system, the endocrine system, the respiratory system, the circulatory system, the musculoskeletal system, and the digestive system.[6] Each system has its own story about how tiredness becomes a threat to the normal functions of the body, as well as how these threats are treated to prevent possible dangers. That said, the rest of this chapter describes the effects of fatigue on these six human body systems based on contemporary findings from various fields.

## FATIGUE AND THE NERVOUS AND ENDOCRINE SYSTEMS

### Nervous System

Although fatigue is usually associated with the exertion of muscular effort, it's possible to experience fatigue without physical activity, that is, while performing normal daily activities, during postoperative recovery, and when confronting sleep disturbances or deprivation. Fatigue that occurs in this way may be attributed to mechanisms in the central nervous system (CNS), which may later be expressed physically as the following:

- Underperformance;
- Decreased motivation;
- Lethargy;
- Tiredness;
- Loss of motor coordination;
- Obvious confusion and disorientation;
- Loss of concentration;
- Difficulty in processing and categorizing information;
- Hardship in remembering words or phrases; and
- Sensory disorientation.

A person suffering from fatigue may also experience sensory overload, such as hypersensitivity to light and sound, and emotional overload, which may cause anxiety attacks. This is known as CNS fatigue or neuromuscular fatigue. Unlike muscular fatigue, CNS fatigue is triggered by activities in the brain and the spinal column, which can occur even without immediate observable stress. [7]

Understanding CNS fatigue entails knowing how the central nervous system works. Studies in 1997 and 2001 explain that full fatigue occurs during increased levels of serotonin (also known as hydroxytryptamine [5-HT]) and lower levels of dopamine in the brain. [8] The mushrooming levels of serotonin are caused by an increase in free tryptophan (TRP) in the brain, which is later synthesized into serotonin.

The TRP is usually connected with albumin in the blood and is transported to the brain via specific receptors, which the TRP shares with branched-chain amino acid (BCAA). However, during exercise, fatty acids separate the TRP from their connection with the albumin, while the BCAA is molded into energy, thus leaving the TRP free to connect with the receptors and cross through the blood-brain barrier. This causes the increase of TRP in the brain, and eventually an elevation in serotonin levels. Given this process, serotonin levels may swell in the brain when fatty acids are abundant and the BCAA is low; this will subsequently increase fatigue. [9]

Although this usually occurs during exercise, there is evidence that the level of serotonin can climb even during a sedentary state, when experiencing immobilizing stress (caused by the redoubled movement of TRP to the brain), or when consuming food rich in carbohydrates without exercising. High levels of serotonin are also observed in elderly people, individuals who are depressed, and those with liver failure, renal disease, and appetite disorders.[10]

Several theories of CNS fatigue have been conjectured throughout the years. These may be categorized into physiological and psychological treatments: physiological implications are nutrition, medication, and hormonal supplements. Some studies have found that the introduction of BCAA can reduce the potential for CNS fatigue, especially for those doing exercises. Psychological treatments include rest and meditation. However, the most common advice in addressing CNS fatigue is moderation in activities: avoiding both a sedentary lifestyle and the overexertion of muscles.[11]

## Endocrine System

Endocrine-related fatigue is a reduction in physiological and psychological capacity, usually associated with an ailment of the endocrine system. This is difficult to diagnose because oftentimes it is overshadowed by some other ailment or dismissed as psychological in nature. Tests, unless directed to determine fatigue, don't necessarily point in this direction; endocrine tests tend to show normal results. As a consequence, fatigue remains untreated.[12]

Endocrine-provoked fatigue differs from other causes because in addition to fatigue indicators (i.e., retardation of movement, confusion, and weakness or tiredness), patients experience a variety of symptoms. They can include the following:

- Irregular menstrual period;
- Abnormal body hair growth (for women);
- Carbohydrate craving;
- Sleep disturbances or deprivation;
- Depression;
- Dizziness when standing;
- Concentration problems;
- Unexplained weight loss or weight gain;
- Osteoporosis;
- Breast discharge;
- Memory loss;
- Decreased sex drive; and

- Erectile problems.

This is expected in endocrine-related fatigue and is connected with marked disorders such as the following:

- Thyroid disease;
- Growth hormone deficiency;
- Adrenal insufficiency;
- Metabolic syndrome (also known as insulin resistance);
- Diabetes;
- Low glucose sugar;
- Cushing's syndrome;
- Deficiencies in androgen;
- Vitamin D; and
- Estrogen.

If the fatigue symptoms persist and recur for more than six months and notably affect the patient's performance, a CFS diagnosis is strongly considered, which requires a different set of protocols for treatment. Treatment of endocrine-caused fatigue requires two important points. First is diagnosis. As stated earlier, fatigue caused by dysfunctions in the endocrine system is diagnosed only in consultation with an endocrinologist who administers tests specifically to identify the cause of the fatigue.[13]

Proper diagnosis enables medical practitioners as well as affected persons to determine proper treatment. Treatment occurring in unison with comorbid illness comes second. Fatigue, if associated with an existing ailment, such as diabetes and adult growth hormone deficiency, needs to be addressed as soon as possible. Hence, treatment of the fatigue as a symptom calls for the treatment of the whole ailment as well.[14]

# FATIGUE AND THE RESPIRATORY AND CIRCULATORY SYSTEMS

## Respiratory System

Respiratory muscle fatigue is the inability of the respiratory muscles to generate enough pressure to maintain proper ventilation during respiration, which can eventually result in *ventilatory failure*. This is usually caused by lung diseases, wherein the respiratory system suffers from added stress from an ailment.[15]

The mechanisms for respiratory muscular fatigue and muscle fatigue are similar: that is, the brain signals the muscles to exert effort (or contract) in order to undertake a target action. What differs about normal muscle fatigue and respiratory muscle fatigue is the unmistakeable interaction between central and peripheral fatigue. Both central and peripheral fatigue is observed in respiratory muscular fatigue. Studies have shown an equal decrease in effort from the brain and respiratory muscles during episodes of fatigue.[16]

The relationships among the body's systems are interdependent, such that an emergency mechanism is engaged when extreme fatigue occurs. To illustrate, imagine that a CFS patient's lung muscles are already fatigued, meaning that they can no longer sustain the pressure or load they bear. In order to protect the lung muscles from totally collapsing, the brain ceases sending activation signals to the muscles, which in turn disables the respiratory muscles from exerting further stress to the already fatigued area. This will therefore delay respiratory fatigue from occurring, and respiratory failure is stalled. This happens as a protective mechanism of the CNS, adapting against possible damages to the respiratory muscles. Otherwise, the unceasing signal from the brain for muscles to exert more effort could lead to irreparable respiratory failure and eventually significantly compromise the person's health.[17]

Respiratory muscular fatigue can be treated in two ways: (1) decreasing the demand on the lung muscles and (2) improving the endurance of lung muscles. Regarding the first note, it's logical that respiratory muscular fatigue can be addressed by reducing the need for lung muscles to exert energy. This can be done by reducing the resistance in the lung muscles. As for the second point, improving the strength of lung muscles is necessary to ensure the endurance of the lungs. This can be done through medication, training, rest, and proper nutrition.[18]

## Circulatory System

As the brain is important in delivering instruction for action to the different parts of the body, so too is the circulatory system, which serves as a pathway for oxygen, vital nutrients, and hormones to ensure the efficient functioning of the CFS sufferer's organs. Persons with cardio-vascular fatigue exhibit symptoms of orthostatic intolerance (i.e., the inability to stay upright). Simply put, when a CFS sufferer experiences poor blood circulation, the different organs of the body have a hard time carrying out their regular functions and duties. The circulatory system, constituting the heart, blood, arteries, and veins, functions as the oxygen and nutrient carrier to the different organs of the body.[19]

If the circulatory system is unable to deliver the essentials for normal body function, the inability is probably due to a malfunctioning auto-nomic nervous system, and therefore the CFS patient starts to experi-ence muscle cramping. *Hypotension* is accompanied by dizziness and light-headedness, visual disturbances, and slow response to stimuli. Postural orthostatic tachycardia syndrome (an increase in heart rate and a drop in pulse upon standing) or delayed postural hypotension (symp-toms of hypotension occurring minutes after standing up) can also strike.[20]

To determine the presence of stress or fatigue in the circulatory system and specifically in the heart, a tilt test is usually administered to patients who exhibit a fleeting increase in heart rate together with a brusque decrease in blood pressure when standing up (that quickly improves after sitting or lying down). Monitoring for *arrhythmia* is also undertaken to determine regularity of heartbeat.[21] First-line treatment for a person experiencing cardiovascular fatigue would be to drink much water and take in a bit more salt. Movement (avoiding a seden-tary state) is necessary to assist blood circulation. Patients are also ad-vised to wear medical stockings that'll help in blood circulation.[22]

# FATIGUE AND THE MUSCULOSKELETAL AND DIGESTIVE SYSTEMS

## Musculoskeletal System

Musculoskeletal fatigue occurs when muscles or joints have limited function. This occurs when muscles are unable to generate sufficient force for and velocity of the contractions needed to achieve an activity.[23] Muscular fatigue originates in either the muscles or joints. Either way, such a form of fatigue is usually exhibited by hindrance in movement, inability to exert normal levels of strength for a task, and an overall collapse while performing a task. The musculoskeletal system can normally recover from fatigue after sufficient rest, in contrast to CFS-related fatigue wherein the muscle is unable to recuperate even with rest.

The delivery of a message from the brain to the muscle can be summarized in three stages: (1) the central motor unit delivers the message to the target muscle, (2) enzymes are metabolized to produce energy for the action, and (3) the muscles are excited, which leads to contraction or application of force. The message contains what sort of activity is to be conducted and how much energy is needed.[24]

Muscle fatigue occurs when the amount of energy required is greater than the amount of energy the body can provide and when there are disruptions in the transmission from the neuromuscular transmission to the *actin-myosin cross bridging*. The energy requirement, however, is determined not only at the peripheral level (the degree to which a muscle group can contract), but also on the neural level. Based on that, it can be noted that muscle fatigue can happen at any time during the process of determining the required physical effort (central fatigue) to the actual exertion of effort or contraction of muscles to complete the activity (peripheral fatigue).[25]

## Digestive System

Digestive system fatigue is caused by the overuse of energy to digest food. In the digestive system, whose operations are affected by the autonomic nervous system, fatigue in the generally happens when there's food intolerance or when the person is suffering from Hirschprung disease, *achalasia cardia, cancer cachexia*, and sphincter abnormalities. Essentially, digestion-related fatigue is caused by issues in food processing: when the routine of digesting food is disrupted due to other issues, the body exerts more energy to cope with the digestion requirements.[26]

This overexertion of effort comes with gastrointestinal discomforts such as diarrhea, constipation, or alternating diarrhea and constipation, abdominal cramps, bloating, nausea, and anorexia. If digestive troubles persist, the absorption of essential nutrients may not take place, affecting the rest of the organs, consequently causing more fatigue. Suggestions to address digestion-related fatigue include avoiding foods that exacerbate the CFS patient's condition, abstaining from processed foods, and thoroughly chewing food.[27]

## ANALYSIS

Although fatigue might appear to be a mere symptom signaling the need for rest, the concept of fatigue has garnered significant interest from various fields due to its impact on a person's well-being. In surgery, for instance, a high rate of errors in medical treatment that may be attributed to fatigue and sleep deprivation has led to calls for change in healthcare protocols.[28]

The sports industry has invested significant funds in the development of training programs to help to prevent muscular fatigue and its effects on athletic performance. Automobile regulatory boards have undertaken tremendous efforts to institutionalize road safety measures to counter possible effects of fatigued driving. Even long-term treatments such as those for cancer have established protocols for addressing fatigue-related reactions to ailments and treatments. Studies on treating fatigue, medical or otherwise, became a running objective for various professional turfs, but fatigue still eludes complete understanding.

# 9

# VIRAL, NEUROPSYCHIATRIC, AND NEUROENDOCRINE HYPOTHESES

**V**iruses' structures and reproduction strategies are diverse. The virus is usually rather small and it replicates in many ways. Even a small quantity of virus particles can affect a person's heath. Still, viruses don't carry out metabolic processes, and there are restricted *intracellular* parasites that are inanimate. Viruses represent the class of capsid-encoding organisms, or CEOs.

## VIRAL HYPOTHESIS FOR CHRONIC FATIGUE SYNDROME

There are three primary hypotheses for chronic fatigue syndrome (CFS): the progressive hypothesis, the regressive hypothesis, and the virus-first hypothesis. The progressive or escape hypothesis posits that viruses originate from genetic elements that obtained the capacity to progress between cells. Regressive or reductive hypotheses declare that a virus is a remnant of cellular organisms, and the virus-first hypothesis claims that viruses predate and coevolved with current cellular hosts.[1]

Retroviruses are viruses that through progressive biological processes become infectious agents. Large DNA viruses take a regressive course, by which a once-independent body lost its key genes over a point of time and took up a parasitic reproduction strategy. Viruses may arise several times through several bodily processes. Continuous research in areas like genomics, structural biology, and microbiology may supply answers yet to be discovered, but until now no precise explanation about the origin of viruses exists.[2]

Using the aforesaid pathways, an active viral infection that's often bracketed with the symptoms of CFS has guided researchers to hypothesize that viruses stimulate the syndrome. The hormone, immune, and central nervous systems and the possibility that stress, reproduction, or reactivation of latent viruses could adjust to the immune system to cause CFS should be explored.[3]

## Vagus Nerve Infection

The vagus nerve infection hypothesis (VNIH), suggests that nerve-loving viruses cause an immune response that's difficult to detect, sparking fatigue and other prognostic symptoms of CFS.[4] This hypothesis suggests that infections cause CFS and that the most significant thing about the infection is its source, which is the vagus nerve, the largest in the body. This wandering nerve stretches over the human trunk, conveying its roots into most organs of the body. An infection doesn't need to be powerful; it need only be present in the vagus nerve to generate havoc in the brain.[5]

As the vagus nerve winds through the body, it approaches viral havens that harbor herpesviruses such as the cytomegalovirus and Epstein-Barr virus. Nearly all humans bear some of these herpesviruses in latent form; biological events or stressors permit reactivation. Upon recrudescence, it's thought that these viruses leave the nerves and run into glial cells that try to gobble them up. The glial cells put out all manner of nerve-exciting and pro-inflammatory compounds in the presence of viruses. The vagus nerve receptors sniff out the alarm signals and inform the brain that an infection exists, and it'll send out signals to shut off or slow down the movements of the CFS patient's torso.[6]

## New Model of Fatigue

Studies on animals show that fatigue and flulike symptoms thrive when the vagus nerve is infected.[7] Flulike symptoms that are attendant with infections may not survive without the vagus nerve, because rodents infected with pathogens don't act sick after having their vagus nerves cut. The symptoms of a sickness would be intense and uncontrollable if the vagus nerve receptors were endlessly attacked with these cytokines. A raging infection can have a similar allergic response in the vagus nerve when glial cells encircle the nerve. Researchers propose that CFS could in fact be a hodgepodge of glial cell diseases.[8]

## Infections That Don't Appear in the Blood

Researchers aren't able to detect these groups of viruses through biopsy of the vagus nerve and in the blood because the viruses may be expanding their path of destruction onto different tissues. Studies have been performed using HIV protein to mimic a certain nervous system infection.[9] Researchers discovered that glial cells stack up and begin to raise pro-inflammatory cytokines to handle the intruder. However, cytokines couldn't be found in the rodents' bloodstreams even though the animal acted sick, isolated, and despondent. Proof of growth in cytokine levels was attainable only when the rodent's spinal cord was sampled near the infected region.[10]

Cytokines may be found in the spinal fluid when the vagus nerve is infected close to the brain stem but they wouldn't be traceable in the blood. However, cytokines reside in the blood and not in the spinal fluid when the vagus nerve is infected in the abdominal region. Cytokines, for example, are revealed if the lungs of the mice with lung infections were sampled. It's therefore believed that cytokines can't be distinguished at all, wherever the infection may be.[11]

Animal studies have been proposed to improve the understanding of vagus nerve infections. Magnetic resonance imaging might have the capacity to identify viral lesions in the cardinal nervous system tissues, and special PET scans may be used to evaluate microglial activation. Moreover, reports on seriously ill patients and cadaver studies should be carried out in the future to discover viral infections, activated glia, and inflammation.[12]

## Neuropsychiatric Hypothesis for Chronic Fatigue Syndrome

Neuropsychiatric problems are far-flung in chronic fatigue syndrome and are connected to disorders of behavior and mood. Depression and major depressive disorder (MDD) are often experienced by CFS patients. The exact causal link between CFS and MDD is still not understood, despite much research, resulting in the development of polarized hypotheses concerning the true clinical causes of CFS.[13]

A number of intriguing immunological and inflammatory clarifications have recently been revealed, proposing that CFS and MDD are recognizably different yet have related conditions. The overlap between CFS and MDD is the shared inflammatory, oxidative, and nitrosative stress (IO&NS) pathways. Chronic fatigue syndrome is also linked to neuropsychological symptoms such as impaired memory, attention, and response time. The syndrome is a systemic, severe, obtained illness of extreme fatigue that can't be moderated by rest and might even be worsened by neuropsychiatric and physical activity.[14]

## Neuropsychiatric Features

Chronic fatigue syndrome sufferers often describe a variety of neuropsychiatric symptoms, typically marked by a decrease in cognitive functions. Until now, neuropsychological research in chronic fatigue syndrome has strived to envision the exact identity of cognitive complaints in CFS. Objective proof of cognitive distraction has been connected to a deficiency in reaction time, with memory and attention being the most knotty for patients who have CFS.[15]

Written reports have revealed a substantial connection between depressive, somatoform, anxiety, and personality-associated disorders and CFS. Many CFS patients are whispered to be suffering from psychiatric disorders, particularly depressive illness, and studies indicate remarkable comorbidity between depression and CFS. Fifteen to 40 percent of its patients were judged to be suffering from major depression, 5 to 15 percent of patients were estimated to have somatization disorders, and 20 percent of its patients have been found with anxiety disorders. Nevertheless, the huge majority of neuropsychiatric information is committed to depression because depression is one of the most important clinical obstacles faced in CFS.[16]

## Depressive Illness

Depression shares several remarkable overlapping symptoms with CFS, and some of its eminent characteristics are poor concentration, memory difficulties, sleep disturbance, and overwhelming fatigue. The exact relationship between depression and CFS remains unknown, and this is still an area of intense disagreement. The chief arenas that the debate centers on are: (a) disabilities inflicted by the disease activity, (b) that depression and CFS share sources, and (c) that CFS is actually considered a configuration of depression.[17]

Although absence of a confirmed cause of CFS has created a rift in the debate and steered several researchers to claim that CFS has psychiatric roots, CFS is recognized as a disabling disorder with astronomical rates of depression. The magnitude of depression in CFS is significantly more conspicuous than those revealed in other chronic maladies.[18]

## Investigating Major Depressive Disorder

Major depressive disorder is a neuropsychiatric disorder characterized by pathologically impaired sleep, depressed mood, tiredness, and ephemeral motivation. Major depressive disorder (MDD) and CFS symptoms overlap astonishingly, thus CFS literature specifies that MDD is the single most prevalent psychiatric illness linked with CFS. Yet, not all CFS patients encounter psychiatric symptoms, therefore it's sensible to state that even though MDD is an important characteristic of CFS, it affects some but not all, CFS sufferers.[19]

In terms of symptom grouping, major depressive disorder and CFS are categorized differently. The Beck depression inventory (BDI) differentiates patients with CFS from those with MDD, and this study discloses that MDD patients are recognized by symptoms such as self-reproach and disturbed mood, while CFS patients had BDI scores associated particularly with symptoms of fatigue and physical complaints.[20]

Compared with MDD patients, CFS patients show less difficulty with guilt, suicidal ideation, and self-esteem. The MDD patients also have "inward attribution" of their symptoms, whereas CFS clients were prone to blame their symptoms on physical sources. Recently, it's been discovered that in order to successfully distinguish between those suffering from MDD and CFS, one needs to consider the severity of shortness of breath, unrefreshing sleep, impaired concentration, and post-exercise malaise.[21]

These analyses illustrate that even though CFS and MDD share numerous similar symptoms, such as poor concentration, pain, sleep disruption, and profound fatigue, CFS and MDD are distinct ill-nesses.[22] The analyses also emphasize that the kind of symptoms indi-cated by CFS patients are dissimilar. By observing their reaction to physical exertion, CFS patients could be differentiated from depressive patients.[23] After exertion, CFS patients experience increased fatigue, whereas the depressed patients enjoy a rise in positive mood. In short, experts determined that typical CFS symptoms like sore throat, painful lymph nodes, and post-exertional malaise aren't commonly noticed in MDD, because the latter disorder points to a separate underpinning of disease.[24]

## Biological Foundation of Major Depressive Disorder

The connection between CFS and MDD is multifarious, yet, in spite of the complexities, there's visible proof that the connection between the two may be distinguished through the IO&NS pathways. This pathway introduces a complex series of biochemical responses that results in the destruction of free radicals and nitric oxide outcomes at a cellular lev-el.[25] In research, IO&NS was discovered to be accountable for destroy-ing fatty acids, proteins, and DNA and was remarkably connected to patients' complaints of flulike malaise, fatigue, and muscle pain.[26]

The stimulation of IO&NS pathways is recognized to increase fa-tigue and body symptoms, and it could be triggered by immune disor-ders, infections, and psychosocial stress.[27] This shows that CFS and MDD might share clinical symptoms of a shared IO&NS pathway, but it's also been claimed that CFS and MDD could be differentiated from each other by concentrating on research that appears from other biolog-ical systems.[28] For instance, MDD is traditionally linked with elevated cortisol levels and increased hypothalamus-pituitary-adrenal (HPA) axis process.[29]

Raised cortisol in MDD produces difficulties in executive thought functioning, visuo-spatial memory, and verbal memory, but HPA ex-periments on CFS patients discovered lesser, not higher, cortisol lev-els.[30] The damaged HPA axis operation is believed to be accountable for the symptoms of headaches, post-exertional malaise, and tiredness in CFS sufferers, unlike for MDD.[31]

Currently the *adrenal androgens dehydroepiandrosterone (DHEA)* and *dehydroepiandrosterone-sulphate (DHEA-S)* are the center of attention, though less intensively studied in reference to CFS. The metabolic connection between DHEA and cortisol is an intense area of interest because in order to preserve homeostasis, the production of androgens transfer to glucocorticoids throughout physical and psychological stress.[32] Nevertheless, in an initial research of DHEA in CFS, scientists found that the predicted metabolic transfer from HDEA to cortisol didn't occur in CFS patients.[33]

The research also emphasized that CFS patients displayed lower levels of DHEA and remarkably lesser DHEA-S in contrast to MDD patients and healthy controls. Furthermore, patients reacted positively to DHEA replacement treatment in a small uncontrolled test.[34]

## Depression and Illness Limitations

Since CFS is linked with serious illness-imposed limitations, it has caused some researchers to declare that depressive illness in CFS is merely a natural reaction to the debilitating symptoms encountered by its sufferers. There was no cogent proof that patients with CFS are really *hypochondriacal*, hence psychiatric illness is concluded to be an outcome of CFS rather than something that caused the development of the syndrome.[35]

In research comparing patients with CFS and patients with MDD and multiple sclerosis (MS), it was discovered that patients with CFS resembled the MS patients more closely than the MDD group, and the study also noted that the CFS group encountered fewer *axis 1 disorders* than MDD patients.[36]

## Generalized Anxiety Disorder

Anxiety disorder involves reactive stress due to medical conditions or substances, post-traumatic stress disorder, agoraphobia, social anxiety, generalized anxiety, panic disorder, and other trauma-related reactions. The primary characteristic of anxiety disorder is mental or physical anxiety that is out of proportion with the recent condition and that particularly affects the quality or functioning of life. People with CFS were found to have higher rates of generalized anxiety disorder (GAD), which was placed by an earlier beginning and high rates of psychiatric comorbidity that specifies a tendency to develop CFS.[37]

Nevertheless, there's no clear understanding about the specific neurobiological changes that lead to this condition, although generalized anxiety disorder is a regular and significant disorder. Even though some research to date has been performed on neurobiological function in GAD patients, only limited qualified data is available for depression. The bridges between CFS and GAD, such as sleep abnormalities, sympathetic hyperactivity, and vegetated cerebral blood flow, still require more analysis.[38]

## Somatoform Disorder

Somatization is described as the tendency to convert psychological distress into physical symptoms and obtain medical assistance to reduce them.[39] Somatization encompasses a wide scope of patients' perceptions and experiences, which results in patients reporting symptoms that are completely physical.[40] It's usual to assume that clinically unknown patient complaints are the result of underlying emotional distress among these three groups of somatization behavior.

In that respect, somatization disorder is also a recognized psychiatric barrier in the *Diagnostic and Statistical Manual of Mental Disorders 3 (DSM-III)*. Somatization disorder is diagnosed when an individual suffers at least thirteen of its thirty-five recognized symptoms over a period of years, with onset before the age of thirty.[41] Surveys of psychiatric illness in CFS have demonstrated extremely high rates of somatization disorders, and in other analyses, investigators discovered that patients displayed a higher rate of somatization disorder symptoms than in clients with multiple sclerosis.[42] The research, however, specifies that few of the patients with CFS represent the precise DSM-III-R standard for somatization disorder.

Further research disclosed that changing how somatization symptoms were categorized also changed the likelihood of diagnosis of somatization disorder.[43] An example of changing the attribution of somatization symptoms would be to code the CFS symptoms as psychiatric. It was discovered that six of thirty patients exhibited a lifetime history of major depression when symptoms attributed to CFS were abolished.[44]

However, twelve of thirty patients described a lifetime history of major depressive illness as diagnostic protocols of all symptoms were used. These studies thus displayed that the recognition of CFS relies upon a patient's account of physical symptoms and the researcher's conclusion that there's no physical cause for the symptoms. Lastly, if CFS patients were covering up their psychological sufferings with physical symptoms, then there should be a reverse connection between anxiety and depression symptoms and the reported numbers of physical symptoms.[45] Yet CFS patients haven't detailed anxiety-related, depressive, and physical symptoms simultaneously.[46]

## Personality Disorder

Evidence from research specifies that personality disorder—mainly obsessive-compulsive disorder (OCD)—exists in approximately 40 percent of CFS patients.[47] In research, 37 percent of CFS cases met the criterion for at least one personality disorder such as borderline or histrionic personality disorder.[48] Among CFS patients, there are higher rates of personality disorder compared to nonpatients. Furthermore, a few of the measures applied could increase the probability of finding personality disorder in patients who are chronically ill. In one study, comorbid depression was reported as personality pathologies.[49]

## Reaction Time

Numerous neuropsychological inquiries have evaluated and analyzed the reaction time of patients with CFS, based on easy and complex information-processing assignments. The most noted cognitive difficulty discovered in CFS relates to an abnormality in patient information-processing efficiency and speed.[50] Countless research indicates that patients with CFS don't perform well on coursework that requires swift handling of information and on time-limited and complex assignments.[51] Currently, in a population-based analysis of neuropsychological performance, it was learned that in contrast to controls, patients with CFS displayed a remarkable decrease in motor speed.[52]

Furthermore, CFS patients with higher levels of cognitive difficulties also displayed more immune abnormalities, which suggests that cognitive difficulties in CFS can be described independently of those that generally exist with depression.[53] Lastly, the cognitive dysfunction seen in CFS patients is unlikely to be explained by anxiety and depression.[54] These analyses specify that CFS patients display moderate to significant abnormalities in reaction times, and the information-processing difficulties of CFS patients contribute to abnormalities in reaction-time assignments.[55] Fine motor speed was not lost in individuals with CFS. Thus, it's unlikely that motor performance is primarily connected to slower reaction times.[56]

## Memory

Scientific opinion about links between memory problems and CFS is split; some research found proof of memory deficits in CFS while others didn't.[57] This conflict is linked to nonverbal and verbal memory problems in CFS sufferers.[58] Most neuropsychological research on memory in CFS utilized visual and verbal memory tests. Specifically, some trials evaluated memory utilizing word lists, and in terms of verbal memory, some analyses indicate minimal "word list" learning.[59] Recognition, delayed recall, and immediate recollection were abnormal in CFS cases. Patients with CFS have trouble with obtaining verbal information and require greater effort in memorizing a word list compared to healthy controls.[60] The conclusion was that the memory burdens encountered by CFS patients are connected to compromises in their ability to recall verbal information. These memory difficulties may be a result of poor initial learning.[61] An analysis of patients with MDD and CFS and healthy controls discovered that patients with CFS show deviant brain physiology.[62]

## Attention

The scientific research models about working memory and attention span maintain that they're both essential cognitive functions for productive learning and reasoning. In a functional MRI study of the working memory, significant differences were discovered in the brain activation between control subjects and CFS patients, especially as demands were increased on the working memory.[63] The inquiry concluded that patients with CFS didn't engage working memory in a similar manner as healthy subjects, and the outcome specifies that the CFS patients had to use additional approaches to neutralize their underlying cognitive difficulties. In research with patients focusing over extended periods of time, CFS sufferers also showed consistent difficulty with working memory.[64]

## NEUROENDOCRINE HYPOTHESIS FOR CHRONIC FATIGUE SYNDROME

The neuroendocrine system consists of the nervous and the endocrine systems, which work together to keep the body functioning regularly. The nervous system and the endocrine system consist of neuroendocrine cells, which are situated throughout the body and release hormones transmitting messages to cells. The interactions between the brain and the glands that produce hormones could assist in explaining the neuroendocrine symptoms of CFS. Thought-provoking studies have proposed a neuroendocrine context for CFS, but the true vices these symptoms carry out are still enigmas. Scientists have discovered that several patients with CFS have low levels of cortisol, which is a hormone processed by the HPA axis that holds the potential key to fatigue and sleep disorders. Neuroendocrine participation in CFS and its treatment strategies to enhance a patient's daily life still require further research from quite a few fields of study.[65]

### Disturbed Neuroendocrine-Immune Interactions

The symptomatology in CFS was hypothesized to be an effect from abnormalities in inter-organ transmission rather than from oddities in a specific organ system. A feature of inter-organ transmission is the reactivity of certain receptors in the target organs as well as the production and secretion of mediator chemicals by other organ systems. Hence, variations in the way target organs react to the mediators and changes in the actual level of neuroendocrine mediators might result in poor transmission. Poor transmission could lead to the pathophysiology of CFS and might explain the mixed outcomes cited in many works that concentrate on a specific organ system. Currently, the neuroendocrine system and the immune system have been well proven to closely interact with each other.[66]

Psychological stress is applied to modulate immune reactivity through complex interactions that utilize the autonomic nervous system as well as the HPA axis while the immune system cells express receptors for neurotransmitters and hormones. Activating these receptors results in modulation of immune responsiveness. The immune system cells that are easily attainable in the peripheral blood and that could be examined *ex vivo* are used to inspect the integrity of neuroendocrine regulation. To date, the pathophysiology of CFS is still poorly understood, and analysis performed over the past ten years indicates that the syndrome can't be identified by a deficiency in one specific organ system. Current perspectives are therefore not meant to define changes in a single system, but to inspect the integrity of inter-organ transmission in CFS patients.[67]

In a study of inter-organ transmission, the interaction between the neuroendocrine system and the immune system was chosen as a model system. The outcome reveals that the transmission between the neuroendocrine system and the immune system is different for adolescents than it is for adults. It was also hypothesized that neuroendocrine-immune transmission abnormalities in chronic fatigue syndrome are a result of preexisting psychological distress and precipitating events such as viral infections. In summary, the recent analysis reveals that chemical exchange between neuroendocrine mediators and the immune system is disturbed in CFS.[68]

## Critical Issues of the Neuroendocrine System

The basic HPA role in CFS still requires clarification, and there's proof that the HPA axis malfunctions in patients with CFS, even though experimentation has produced inconsistent outcomes. Neuroendocrine faults, CFS, cytokine abnormalities, and orthostatic intolerance may be interconnected. Cytokines, which are chemical messengers, activate the HPA axis each time a body is experiencing an infection or is under stress. Interleukin-6 (IL-6), tumor necrosis factor (TNF), and a few others have been implicated in CFS.[69]

Research has revealed that corticotrophin-releasing hormone (CRH) levels in a human's cerebrospinal fluid is normal or low in patients with CFS but might increase in depressed patients.[70] Patients with CFS also display a decreased cortisol reaction when compared to patients with depression. Even though there was no correlation between CFS and stress, stressors such as automobile accidents, traumatic life events, physical abuse, and viral infections might generate CFS symptoms. To date, there's still not enough evidence to determine a connection between neuroendocrine abnormalities and specific stressors in CFS.[71]

Sleep abnormalities and sleep disturbances might also lead to CFS symptoms and have been shown to produce an increased production of TNF and IL-6.[72] However, research on the connection between sleep abnormalities, cytokine secretion patterns, and HPA axis alteration hasn't been conducted thus far in patients with CFS. Further probing is required to describe the neuroendocrine features of the syndrome, which calls for studies to identify neuroendocrine activity in larger populations of patients with CFS, including sufferers that fit specific subtypes of the syndrome, test strategies that involve prescription drugs to affect the HPA axis, and evaluation of stress that was previously hypothesized to generate CFS.[73]

Possible human experimental models, which can temporarily recreate the symptoms of CFS to help in identifying biological markers for the ailment, might be brewing sometime in the near future. Long-term research to capture the fluctuations in symptom severity that most CFS patients encounter may assist in bypassing common research obstacles. A CFS symposium series produced by the CFIDS Association of America was designed to analyze the task of the endocrine, immune, circulatory, and neurological systems in CFS. The symposium assembled research collaboration teams and summoned experts to assess findings, shed light on research and funding priorities, and highlighted the most positive next steps for research.[74]

## ANALYSIS

When a viral CFS patient coughs, anyone can get infected by breathing in the particles expelled. Several days after the viruses procreate within human bodies, people become sick. Since viruses change and develop over time, CFS patients are advised to get vaccinated yearly. Moreover, caregivers should note that the immune system and autonomic nervous system are two of the primary players in CFS, which focus on the herpesviruses, comprise sensory nerves, and pursue an established model of related disorders such as fibromyalgia.

# Part IV


# Resolutions

# 10

# NATURAL APPROACHES TO CHRONIC FATIGUE SYNDROME

Chronic fatigue syndrome (CFS) is a medical condition for which there isn't yet a fully refined, conventional drug. Both pharmacological and natural treatments aim at improving the symptoms such as fatigue, anxiety, muscle pains, and depression. Natural treatment, as the name implies, requires acumen for nonchemical intervention for CFS. It's often considered a more "unadulterated" approach that doesn't involve prescription drugs. Ongoing research examines a broad variety of natural treatment methods and introduces new interventions for managing symptoms.[1]

Complementary and alternative medicine (CAM) is the common name used for herbal and homeopathic medicines. These medicines are often administered by a complementary medicine practitioner. Homeopathy is a system of complementary and alternative medicines based on the belief that a distinct disease or syndrome like CFS can be treated by something other than standard medication. Homeopathic remedies are concoctions of substances often so diluted that the main ingredients are barely detectable. Herbal medicines can be administered to patients by drinking a particular plant in powdered or brewed form. Herbal medications use the power of nature to be effective.[2]

## SIGNIFICANCE OF APPROACHING CFS NATURALLY: BENEFITS

Discourses are circulating surrounding the different natural approaches to chronic fatigue syndrome. The benefits and drawbacks of addressing CFS naturally are diverse, and the results of experiments and studies fickle. However, a significant number of medical researchers and health advocates favor natural approaches for treating and managing CFS, because these methods can be tested with little or no adverse effects.[3]

### Easily Attainable and Less Expensive Treatments

Natural therapies such as herbal and homeopathic remedies are less expensive than chemically processed drugs. Some popular natural herbs such as ginseng, which is known to ward off fatigue, can be bought from the nearest market and can in fact grow at home. Implementing a healthy diet is a natural approach to CFS that compels patients to remove unhealthy and sometimes expensive foods from their diet.[4]

Some oral supplements are easily located at drugstores and in health food stores, as is the case with natural herbs. Supplements are usually less expensive than commercial drugs, since they're widely processed and don't require a prescription. Some methods for improving physical, social, and psychological health, which are proven to be of substantial importance in the treatment of chronic fatigue syndrome, are free: CFS sufferers can exercise and meditate at home.[5]

### Less Adverse Effects

Drug dependency is common in CFS patients who take pharmacological medications. Since CFS doesn't have an orthodox prescription, patients tend to self-medicate with over-the-counter (OTC) drugs such as painkillers to reduce discomfort. Erroneous dosage may result in drug abuse or other dire aftershocks. Both OTC and prescription medicines that aren't administered cautiously can cause substance abuse and addiction. Consequently, people suffering from medical conditions sometimes resort to natural approaches, regarding them as safer alternatives to contentious pharmacological drugs.[6]

Natural approaches to CFS are widely used, with or without prescription, as they have fewer adverse side effects than pharmacological drugs. Alternative and supplementary medicines, cognitive behavioral therapy, change in diet, and other natural approaches could easily be subjected to research and clinical trials without diminishing the condition of the patients involved.[7]

## Medical Attention to Patients with Allergic Reactions to Drugs

It's not uncommon for CFS clients to be sensitive to some medications such as antidepressants, sedatives, and anticholinergic drugs. The patient instead could ask for supervision and take alternative drugs in order to manage pain and improve symptoms. Individuals with mild CFS can also make use of the recuperative effects of meditation, exercise, and a salubrious diet without the use of any medicinal intervention.[8]

## SIGNIFICANCE OF APPROACHING CFS NATURALLY: DRAWBACKS

Although research reports have flooded scientific journals recently, investigators still can't offer a sure answer about the effectiveness of natural approaches in treating CFS. Due to the limited number of randomized controlled trial (RCT) samples, a majority of studies still have the possibility of bias. Some patients respond well to natural approaches but others don't.[9]

Studies have been replicated but the results are typically sparse and inconclusive. The main reasons for bias include inconsistent dosage of an unorthodox medicine, different intervals for physical and psychological therapies, and failure to address the diverse factors of CFS in patients. The studies made on the different interventions have divergent outcomes, thus, further studies and stricter methodologies are encouraged.[10]

## Anecdotal Theories

Being termed "natural" doesn't automatically mean that using natural remedies is without risk. People with CFS might self-medicate with natural herbs or homeopathic medicines that they believe would cure their symptoms. However, rigorous studies haven't been conducted. The utility of herbal and homeopathic medicines is primarily based on ancient traditions. Some herbal supplements aren't subjected to research but are still regularly prescribed by alternative medicine practitioners.[11]

## Tendency for Self-medication

Patients with chronic fatigue might be swindled by advertisements on the Internet and social media sites about OTC supplements and homeopathic remedies, which allow them to treat themselves without seeking qualified guidance. There's a high risk for side effects of medications in the absence of clinical evidence or at least a few nominal scientific studies. Some advertised medicines are unacknowledged by medical authorities and their manufacturers could be unregulated to a certain extent.[12]

## Effects Are Relative to the Patient

Another reason why there's no single, conventional medicine prescribed for CFS is that patients have capricious symptoms and severity levels. The effect of a particular approach can be very beneficial to one patient but tremendously detrimental to the other. For instance, support groups might be able to help CFS patients to cope with their illness through enrichment of social involvement. However, some patients still consider therapy unhelpful and stressful, especially if the support group is comprised of people they're not comfortable with. Drugs sometimes offer the same mixed response. Individual patients have their own level of drug resistance and sensitivity. Thus, they interact with medications differently.[13]

## CHANGING THE SOCIAL AND LIVING ENVIRONMENT OF THE PATIENT

The social determinants of a particular medical disorder include the level of education, employment, social status, social support connections, healthy child development, the living environment, and health services available for the patient.[14] These factors can influence the prevalence of a medical disorder in a given population, as well as increase the probability of suffering from a disorder later in life. These factors also help to provide medical researchers and practitioners with a better understanding of how CFS originated and how severely it disturbs the patient. The sufferer's social and living environment can be deeply improved through the implementation of *psychosocial* management techniques.

### Improving the Social Environment of the Patient

The CFS patient's social milieu—his home, workplace, and community—proves to be a significant factor affecting his ailment. Only a few studies have sought to ascertain the social determinants of CFS. In one research, it was found out that most CFS patients carry a heavy psychosocial burden.[15] Chronic fatigue sufferers might call themselves "busy people." They often have tedious high-profile or low-paying jobs, as well as unhealthy relationships with other members of society. For example, parents who work outside the home throughout the workday arrive home to cook, care for children, and perform errands for the family. This can be stressful and dreadfully fatiguing by midnight.[16]

People who are very busy with work and frequently put in overtime hours are often stressed due to the expectations they set for themselves. Ignoring rest until they've completed their work, being perfectionists, and setting unrealistic goals may deprive them of sleep and may cause stress and fatigue, which diminishes their energy. Unfortunately, patients with severe cases of CFS are usually those with the fewest health and social support services.[17]

That's because (a) the usual therapies given to medical clients who don't have unyielding CFS have different medication dosage or (b) the method of delivery to those with a less severe form of the syndrome. The results of research on chronic fatigue syndrome are highly variable.

CFS patients with different levels of clinical severity react differently to a particular approach. Repercussions vary from patient to patient, but tweaking the lifestyle of a CFS sufferer in a natural way can jam the symptoms at the very least. Some methods to improve social health in the CFS sufferer are as follows:[18]

- Managing family-related problems;
- Joining a support group;
- Building a healthy relationship with one's doctor; and
- Integrating cognitive behavioral therapy into the patient's lifestyle.

## Family Problems

It can become exhausting for people to return to an unhealthy home environment after an interminable day of work. The reasons for this can include altercations with a disloyal spouse or dealing with a problematic teenager, and this can precipitate a CFS patient's depression. Management of patients' relationships with others, especially those who are close to them, such as their own family or relatives, has been shown to minimize the symptoms of CFS. One study found out that patients who have a designated person to care for them, such as a best friend or a spouse, are likely to heal.[19]

## Support Groups

Although there are drawbacks to support groups as explained earlier, these groups can also help a person with CFS. The daily activities of a support group can favorably improve CFS patients' conditions. Through the supervision of doctors, a patient becomes active socially, mentally, and physically without overexerting his mental and physical capacities. However, as mentioned, not all patients respond well to support groups.[20]

Some of them are either uncomfortable with the other patients or with their doctors; others prefer isolation. People suffering from a disorder argue that they often can't maintain the physical activity level that's required each day. For example, support groups employ a standard exercise routine based on the physical capacity of its members.

Some may be unable to perform the prescribed activity well, so those patients may be better cured away from others.[21]

## Doctor-patient Relationship as a Natural Approach

In one study, 84 percent of 126 children with chronic fatigue syndrome alleged that they felt bullied by authorities such as medical and educational professionals.[22] Eighty-seven percent of them asserted that they lacked support and recognition of their needs. Physicians can help patients meet their sociological and psychological needs through empathic support, which consequently improves patient recovery in a natural manner. A person with CFS won't improve greatly if there's discord between the patient and his doctor. Although it's true that doctors should properly care for their CFS patients, the latter should also believe in their professional caregivers. The two parties should respect one another by communicating in ethical and benevolent ways.[23]

## Exercise as a Natural Approach

Generally, inactive patients are considered unhealthy—even those without any diagnosis of disease. Lack of physical activity can be either the cause or effect of CFS, but due to the syndrome, patients tend to exercise less since they become easily fatigued. Exercise is indirectly related to the physiological health of individuals with CFS. As the severity of the condition snowballs, the physical activity of the patient might also decline. Patients who can't participate normally in gym workouts might be left in isolation. Some clients fear post-exertional malaise (PEM), which may lead to setbacks.[24] Therefore, exercising with someone who supports them and matters to them could naturally accelerate healing. There's a vast multitude of research regarding the positive effects of exercise in CFS patients. There are two kinds of physical activities currently examined with effective results for most patients—graded exercise therapy (GET) and pacing.[25]

GET is a form of physical therapy wherein a person exercises at a gentle pace and gradually increases intensity over time. Normally it all starts with simple stretching. The frequency of the activity is increased depending on the CFS patient's ability to cope. In one study, gradual treatment of clients has been shown to produce positive effects. After six months, however, about 30 to 50 percent of the patients who received GET weren't significantly healthier than those who hadn't.[26]

Pacing is another form of physical activity wherein the patient exercises for a certain period of time for as long as he can manage without exacerbating symptoms and triggering post-exertional malaise. Pacing is generally better than graded exercise therapy. About 96 percent of 828 patients who participated in a study in 2008 evaluated pacing as exceedingly helpful.[27]

## Psychological Health

People who manage stress using cognitive behavioral therapy (CBT) claim that they effectively reduced symptoms brought on by chronic fatigue syndrome. They also have healthier social lives and respond well to social groups. Cognitive behavioral therapies such as daily meditation and hypnotic therapy could improve the CFS patient's condition. The practice of CBT is effective not only in managing diseases, but also for a better lifestyle.[28]

One study evaluated fifty-three patients who received cognitive behavioral therapy. After treatments, the majority improved their social adjustments (such as exposure to new acquaintances), their outlook on longtime goals, and their fatigue three months later compared to the treatment on the first interval of the study. A six-month follow-up also showed an increase in improvement.[29]

## Physical Environment of the CFS Patient

A CFS patient's health is massively influenced by the environment in which he lives. Where the patient resides, where he works, and where he gets treatment also play a seminal role in CFS. It's common advice for people and disease sufferers to live in a place that's comfortable. Clean air and a clean home in an ambient area are weighty considerations when choosing where to live. Although there's been overwhelming research on immunological, nutritional, and sociological factors in the study of CFS, there are relatively few studies on the effects of the environment in which the patient lives and works.[30]

The living environment of an individual could have a mammoth effect on health. For example, in 1990 a study found that poor people living in a neighborhood with wealthy residents are generally healthier than poor people who lived in a neighborhood with poor residents.[31] This is called the "neighborhood effect." The study was based on the mortality rates and incidence of heart disease among the families.[32]

## Exposure to Harsh Environments

One study searched for evidence of environmental exposure to CFS.[33] A few patients were found to have environmental and food toxicity before they showed symptoms of CFS. The clients examined had a history of either chemical or food poisoning, such as exposure to pesticides, fish poisoning, sick building syndrome (SBS), Gulf War syndrome (GWS), and many more.[34]

A recent study divulged that exposure to moldy environments such as water-damaged homes or workplaces cause CFS-like illness.[35] It's still unclear whether it's a CFS-related problem or unrelated periphery. The pediatric diagnosis of the illness matched the symptoms of CFS. Further studies on environmental toxicity could provide valuable knowledge about the pathophysiology of chronic fatigue syndrome. Reducing these toxic exposures could act as a natural preventive measure and might also improve the conditions of the individuals suffering from CFS.[36]

## NATURAL DRUGS AND SUPPLEMENTS

Natural drugs such as herbal medicines and homeopathic medicines are generally termed safe and effective. Although the majority of these natural remedies do have fewer negative effects, some are not recommended. These alternative drugs usually aren't subjected to research, and most are used in accordance with ancient, traditional practice without proof that they really cure CFS.

Studies have found homeopathy to be effective in CFS. One study found improved reduction in functional limitations and fatigue, and others unearthed symptomatic improvement of CFS.[37]

## Ginseng

Ginseng is often marketed to help patients with chronic fatigue syndrome. However, one study found that incorporating ginseng into one's medication had little discernible effect on patients and it failed to show effectively on the Rand vitality index scale.[38]

## Mechanism of Action

The hypothesized mechanism of action of complementary medicines describes how the substance is scientifically practical. The benefits of using complementary medications in the treatment of chronic fatigue syndrome are often anecdotal. These experiments are also often judged as biased, so more studies need to be commissioned.[39] Likewise, only trace amounts of the active ingredients are found in alternative medicines. This is often criticized by researchers and doctors, as the dose-response relationship of these medications—which is often incorporated in surveys on therapeutic drugs—can't be gauged. Complementary medicine researchers, however, claim that the more an alternative drug is diluted, the greater it stimulates health. This paradox is still scientifically unexplained.[40]

## Side Effects

Homeopathic medicines are diluted in such a way that the main component can be traced in very small amounts. In this way, practitioners argue that side effects and incorrect dosage are prevented. This is often termed as a paradoxical effect similar to placebo but more effective. Homeopathic treatments are considered nontoxic and are made from all-natural herbs and other compounds. The primary drawbacks or adverse effects that a patient feels are symptoms of healing crisis, wherein the CFS patient may feel poor during the initial stages of treatment, but later, as the homeopathic drug is sustained, he gets better.[41]

## DIET AND ITS ROLE IN CFS

People who maintain a healthy diet have a better response to diseases including CFS. In terms of natural health, diet—hand in hand with mild exercise—can deeply improve CFS. Compared to homeopathy and other alternative medical treatments, supplements have been far more accepted in the treatment of CFS. Diet management includes drinking supplementary medicines, eating the right food, and pursuing hale habits in order to supply essential nutrients, to enjoy a happier life, and to live a healthier lifestyle. Some scholars postulate that CFS is inflamed by nutritional deficiency, and current research is examining the effects of integrating vitamin and mineral supplements into one's diet.[42]

It's advised that an individual shouldn't skip meals. Multiple smaller meals should be eaten daily and include nutritious foods from all the food groups, which not only maintains a balanced diet, but also regulates the CFS patient's blood glucose at a healthy level. This also inhibits excess insulin production and regulates cortisol levels, which then helps to maintain a healthy weight and appetite.[43]

Processed foods may contain high levels of sodium and sugar, which tends to increase the body's insulin level. That in turn makes the person feel hungry and increases the cortisol levels in the person's blood. Whole grains such as cereals, oat cookies, or multigrain biscuits better balance insulin levels and control the level of glucose in blood. These types of foods are better choices when considering daily snacks rather than those high in salt, calories, and sugar.[44]

Supplements are regarded as far safer than herbal medicines. They are for the prevention and treatment of chronic fatigue syndrome, because researchers have hypothesized that CFS is also set off by an imbalance of nutrients. Essential body nutrients may not be successfully incorporated into a patient's diet, thus a doctor may prescribe supplements to normalize this imbalance.[45]

By extension, some medical disorders such as CFS also deplete important vitamins and minerals, as well as drain *phytochemicals* from the organs. Ingestion of vitamins and supplements would also be strategic, especially when combined with proper diet. Dietary change is a key to being healthy. Not only does it require dedication, but it also helps one to live healthfully using a natural approach.[46]

## L-carnitine

L-carnitine is an amino acid that's vital to cell, brain, heart, and muscular function by infusing the human organism with energy. It prevents fatty acids from accumulating in the *mitochondria*, which helps in the metabolism of energy. It occurs naturally in the body. However, some people have naturally low levels of L-carnitine. Because of its significance to the CFS sufferer's metabolism, low levels of L-carnitine in the organs may lead to symptoms such as general fatigue, physical weakness, and muscular pain. Those suffering from insufficiency are thus required to have L-carnitine supplementation.[47]

Evidence has been found that patients with CFS also have L-carnitine deficiency, but research results are mixed.[48] A third of the samples in one trial responded well to L-carnitine supplements, drastically improving their well-being, even when they previously had been severely affected by CFS. The other two-thirds, however, didn't respond positively.[49]

New reviews, however, prove the effectiveness of L-carnitine in CFS patients. A systematic assessment of two studies in 2006 found that L-carnitine improved the overall health of patients, although there was no placebo control.[50] L-carnitine is vital and has been often used as a supplement for a variety of heart conditions such as diabetes, heart attack, rheumatic heart disease, and more. It's also used as supplementary medicine for thyroid disease and even for AIDS medications.

## Magnesium

Patients with CFS are more likely to suffer magnesium deficiency as well. Stress hormones, which increase in those who suffer from CFS, slash the magnesium levels of the red blood cells in the body.[51] The many studies conducted on the effects of magnesium in the patient have had mixed results. Some studies reported favorable effects but were unable to provide rock-solid conclusions. A recent review in 2008 asserted that magnesium supplements still can't be deemed an official treatment for chronic fatigue syndrome.[52]

## Essential Fatty Acids

Patients with CFS are also found to have low essential fatty acid levels. It is postulated that the low levels of essential fatty acids (EFA) caused CFS symptoms and other dysfunctions in the immune, endocrine, and sympathetic nervous systems. One study examined the effect of EFA intervention on post-viral fatigue by using evening primrose oil and fish oil. The patients showed significant improvement in their symptoms such as fatigue and depression.[53]

Researchers tried to replicate the study for chronic fatigue syndrome, using sunflower oil as their medium rather than paraffin, as in the first study. Research, however, arrived at a different outcome. A possible explanation can be deduced from the difference of symptomatic criteria and the medium used to supply EFAs.[54]

Positive effects were shown in another study, where almost thirty patients who were ill for about six years were subjected to trial. They were given EFA supplements along with cognitive behavioral therapy and graded exercise therapy. After three months, the condition of twenty-seven patients improved.[55]

## Vitamin B12

Vitamin B12, or cobalamin, is vital for DNA synthesis and normal functioning of the brain and the nervous system. It helps the tissues to tender more red blood cells. A deficiency in vitamin B12 makes an individual lethargic and leads to the development of anemia. Although fatigue and depression are typical symptoms of CFS and vitamin B12 deficiency, there's little scientific data to prove that they're directly related. Like most research, one way to find out is to examine whether incorporating vitamin B12 supplements could help CFS.[56]

Studies over the years have shown that vitamin B12 supplements offer therapeutic and pharmacological effects for CFS. A total of four studies examined vitamin B12 effects on patients suffering with chronic fatigue syndrome. Three of the studies exhibited desirable results.[57] It was concluded that as the dosage is increased above the amount needed to correct vitamin B12 deficiency, the effectiveness also increases. Fifty to 80 percent of the patients experienced less fatigue and improved stamina. In the fourth study, however, vitamin B12 was administered at very low doses and didn't prove effective.[58]

Evidence was found that 40 to 100 percent of CFS patients have eccentric red blood cells called *nondiscocytes*.[59] It was postulated that these abnormal erythrocytes impair proper cellular respiration and oxidation in the CFS patient's body. In an open trial, vitamin B12 was administered to CFS patients. Half responded well, evincing enhanced well-being within twenty-four hours. Researchers observed decreased deformation and a significant reduction of the nondiscocytes in their blood. However, the remaining participants weren't affected at all and the structure of their red blood cells never transmuted.[60]

It was settled in the study that supplementation with vitamin B12 lessens fatigue, reduces physical pain, and also improves blood circulation, thus signifying vitamin B12 as a future treatment for CFS. However, an experiment in 2010 revealed that incorporating vitamin B12 into patients' diets didn't have any significant effects on fatigue or other CFS symptoms.[61] The contrasting outcomes suggest the need for further research.

### Candida albicans

*Candida albicans* are the microorganisms that cause yeast infection and *thrush*. They normally thrive in the large intestines, genitals, mouth, and even on the skin. *Candida* overgrown has been suggested as one cause of CFS. People who suffer from candidiasis are known to exhibit symptoms of CFS. One clinical study identified *candida albicans* as a causal agent of CFS by triggering immune dysfunction caused by yeast overgrowth.[62]

The study also showed a beneficial effect of the *candida* diet on a significant number of patients. Many health experts and CFS patients practiced supervised, independent *candida* diets. In response, a new study placed CFS patients on either a low-sugar, low-yeast diet (LSLY) or healthy eating (HE) program. It was found out that the two interventions were not as efficacious in terms of fatigue levels. One bias could be that the LSLY diet was too complicated and not practical.[63]

## Balanced Nutrition

Nutritional balancing is extremely gentle and safe, which can't be said of other treatments used today. Vegetarianism, fasting, and other extreme diets worsen the problems in many instances.[64] A specific three-step program in eliminating fatigue through natural approaches is advisable. First, a patient should incorporate pacing. Second, an individual with CFS is instructed to take cognitive behavioral therapy. Lastly, one should also eat nutritious foods.[65] Experts often advise others to eat about five times a day but in small amounts. Low-carbohydrate, high-protein foods are recommended in the morning and in between meals to help stabilize blood sugar and to replenish energy.

According to studies, mornings are the best part of the day to consume food.[66] Upon waking up, blood glucose levels decline and cortisol levels rise. Eating in the morning balances blood sugar and reduces cortisol levels in the blood. Balanced blood glucose replenishes energy, and the reduction in cortisol leads to a lower appetite. Moreover, the levels of cortisol and blood sugar are retained throughout the day, thus making an individual energized and satiated.[67]

According to scientists, in order to suppress fatigue, one should begin by replenishing the body by eating the right foods.[68] The consumption of fresh fruits, uncooked vegetables, nuts, and freshly milled cereals are recommended. Drinking supplements alone is highly unadvisable. Supplements or alternative medications cannot take the place of well-balanced nutrition. Before taking a supplement or alternative medicine, one should discuss it with a well-qualified health professional first.

## SLEEP IS A NATURAL APPROACH

It's sensible to strictly observe bedtimes in order to set one's body clock properly. Should there be changes in sleeping patterns, it's recommended that healthcare professionals be involved with the monitoring. Patients may experience sleep disturbances like insomnia and sleep-wake reversals.[69]

Lack of sleep would then distress an individual's mood and energy level, which are essential for cognitive and other physical functions.

Sleep can determine a CFS patient's performance level at work. "Recharging" sleep helps to prevent or lessen the person's feelings of exhaustion, or worse, fatigue. Patients must remain conscientious with their sleep schedules.[70]

## ANALYSIS

Although the pathophysiology of CFS remains a mystery, different treatment trials have been advanced to improve the patient's symptoms. Many researchers and sufferers unceasingly seek ways to cure CFS and its symptoms in a manner that makes the patients feel safe and comfortable. When considering safe methods of tackling CFS, natural approaches immediately come to mind.

# 11

# PHARMACOLOGICAL APPROACHES TO CHRONIC FATIGUE SYNDROME

The pharmacological management of chronic fatigue syndrome (CFS) is geared toward alleviating the most debilitating and disruptive symptoms of the disorder as prioritized by the client. This view is also shared by the Centers for Disease Control, since each individual experiences varying manifestations, degrees of severity, and responses to medication. The term "management" is an appropriate term to use because there's no single drug or line of prescription medication that can completely cure the complex nature of CFS. Rather, a highly individualized approach is more effective, since one drug may work for one client but not for another.[1]

Frequently used medications to relieve symptoms can range from over-the-counter products to some controlled substances, for which the cost and availability differs, too. The efficacy of these medications is on a case-by-case basis, so it's best to consult with a physician and a reliable healthcare team. Clients must always keep in mind that managing this disorder by using prescribed medications is only effective when taken as instructed by a physician. This includes the timely consumption of the drug and taking it only for the specific length of time prescribed by a physician in order to maximize the benefits, prevent long-term adverse reactions, and avoid drug-to-drug interactions that can further harm the individual. Hence, cooperation between the client and the health team provides the best chance for successful CFS management.[2]

# ANTIPYRETICS, ANALGESICS, AND ANTI-INFLAMMATORY MEDICATIONS

Chronic fatigue syndrome was once called the "yuppie flu," with the flulike symptoms including fever and muscular pain among apparent CFS sufferers. Antipyretics for fever, analgesics for pain, and anti-inflammatories for inflammation were commonly prescribed at the time. Medications that can relieve these symptoms include nonsteroidal anti-inflammatory drugs (NSAIDs) such as ibuprofen, aspirin, naprosensodium, and feldene.[3]

## Indications and Mechanisms of Action

Inhibition of the prostaglandin synthesis, mainly of the *cyclooxygenase 2* type of prostaglandin responsible for smooth muscle contraction and relaxation results in reduced fever, pain, and inflammation—all symptoms of which CFS patients complain. These should be taken an hour before or two hours after a meal, but if adverse reactions follow, the drugs may be taken with milk.[4]

## Benefits, Drawbacks, and Side Effects

NSAIDs are prescribed because they work with the same potency as—but without the ravaging side effects of—steroids or narcotics. Adverse effects include tinnitus or ringing in the ear, *pharyngitis*, prolonged bleeding time, hepatitis, and increased potassium (also known as hyperkalemia). Chronic fatigue syndrome sufferers are also advised not to take alcohol and to avoid hazardous activities while on medication. It's also important to talk to the physician when combining drugs in this class to avert kidney damage and gastrointestinal bleeding, especially when using the drug on a long-term basis. It's important to schedule an appointment for kidney and liver function tests regularly, so that health care providers can monitor the dose or to refashion the prescription.[5]

## ANTIDEPRESSANTS

Mild doses of antidepressants are prescribed to clients with CFS because they help manage mood swings and are believed to improve the quality of sleep and sometimes decrease pain. There are however, different types of antidepressants and their use is controversial. Selective serotonin reuptake inhibitors, or SSRIs, and selective norepinephrine reuptake inhibitors, or SNRIs, include fluoxetine, sertraline, paroxetine, venlafaxine, trazodone, and bupropion. Another type commonly used is the tricyclic antidepressant, or TCA, named for its molecular structure containing three atom rings. Examples of TCA include doxepin, amitriptyline, desipramine, and nortriptyline.[6]

Patients diagnosed with CFS tend to respond promisingly to lower doses of antidepressant drugs than the average doses typically used for depression in patients without the syndrome. In some cases, CFS sufferers can't tolerate the usual doses used for patients without CFS. Since it may take several weeks before the drugs have the desired effect, it's best to work with closely with a professional caregiver regarding pharmacologic therapy for depression.[7]

### Indications and Mechanisms of Action

SSRI, SNRI, and TCA act on neurotransmitters such as serotonin and norepinephrine. These neurotransmitters, which are comparatively lower in CFS clients, are responsible for sleep and wake cycles and for bursts of energy. Only the smallest doses of these drugs are prescribed in order to prevent addiction and dependency.[8]

### Benefits, Drawbacks, and Side Effects

Depression is believed not to originate from the disorder itself, but as a by-product of the continual fatigue that hinders the individual from participating in the normal social activities that one is accustomed to do. The use of SSRI, SNRI, and TCA is applicable but may take several weeks to enrich mood. The important thing is to remind the client to continue taking the medication as prescribed even when the desired effects aren't yet felt. However, there's an arsenal of side effects from antidepressant drugs, such as the following:[9]

- Drowsiness;
- Constipation;
- Hyperglycemia;
- Dry mouth;
- Orthostatic hypotension;
- Palpitations;
- Blurred vision;
- Urine retention;
- Rashes;
- Weight gain;
- Abdominal pain;
- Increased salivation;
- Decreased immune function;
- Decreased sexual desire; and
- Congestive heart failure.

These reactions need to be taken into serious consideration, and a complete clinical history must be completed before these drugs are prescribed in order to avoid contraindications for other past or present conditions. There are also specific instructions to be taken to heart, for instance, abstaining from all forms of alcoholic beverages, avoiding excessive sun exposure, and discontinuing the use of certain herbs that affect the potency of antidepressants such as St. John's wort and evening primrose. Consultation with a doctor is vital, as these medications must be taken at specific times during the day to maintain the drug blood level, and they can't be discontinued abruptly, as this can lead to bewildering thoughts, contemplation of suicide, or psychosis.[10]

## ANXIOLYTICS

Some CFS clients may report anxiety or panic attacks. However, the value of anti-anxiety medications is questionable and they must be used only when the alms outweigh the adverse effects. Benzodiazepines, a class of anxiolytic commonly used, include alprazolam, diazepam, lorazepam, midazolam hydrochloride, and oxazepam.[11]

## Indications and Mechanism of Action

The specific action of benzodiazepines is unknown, but it's believed to affect a neurotransmitter called *gamma-aminobutyric acid* or GABA, which is responsible for the excitability of the central nervous system (CNS). Benzodiazepines are also known to depress the CNS at the brain level.[12]

## Benefits, Drawbacks, and Side Effects

The efficacy of benzodiazepines is based on both the client's responsiveness to the drug and his commitment to adhere to the treatment plan. It's also important to inform prescribers about all the medications one is currently taking to avoid drug-to-drug interactions. Anxiolytics are available in different forms, such as oral gels, injectable solutions, and tablets, so it's important that the CFS patient asks the physician about the best option for his condition. Side effects are closely similar to those of an antidepressant but they can also vary among individuals. Drowsiness, hypotension, visual disturbances, abdominal discomfort, nausea, and hepatic dysfunction can occur. Chronic fatigue sufferers with sensitivity to soy protein should avoid soy, since it can affect liver function tests.[13]

## SLEEPING PILLS

Insomnia is one of the most reported symptoms of CFS and probably the most debilitating, since lack of sleep aggravates the client's fatigue. Some of the popular sleeping pills prescribed are sedative hypnotics like zolpidem tartrate, eszopiclone, orphenadrine, melatonin, and zopiclone. These are usually given in low doses to provide a peaceful and restful sleep. When larger doses are necessary, they are used with meticulous care.[14]

## Indications and Mechanisms of Action

Sleeping pills are a combination of different classes of drugs ranging from antihistamines, antidepressants, or sedative-hypnotics. The main mechanism of action is to decrease the ability of neurons to fire signals and excite neighboring neurons located within the *limbic system* and the CNS, thereby allowing for a restful sleep. However, sleeping pills may also be required, as well. Antihistamines are mainly respiratory tract drugs used to treat certain allergies, but the side effects include sedation. Therefore, these drugs are also used to manage insomnia, especially for newly diagnosed clients, while antidepressants reportedly improve sleep patterns.[15]

## Benefits, Drawbacks, and Side Effects

Sedatives are effective to help curb sleep deprivation when used correctly. Sedatives are beneficial, but like any medication, the CFS sufferer must be evaluated first to determine what drug is appropriate and how long it should be used. The adverse effects of sleeping pills are the same as for antidepressants: hallucinations, vertigo, peripheral edema, ear discomfort, conjunctivitis, bronchitis, and fever. Ironically, too many sedatives can lead to insomnia. Adverse reactions are mostly dose related, so a dose reduction might be merited if the reactions become too bothersome for the clients. It's essential to check with a sleep specialist because nonrestorative sleep may be present even while taking the medications. A careful sleep study should be urged if that happens.[16]

## ANTIVIRALS

Antivirals such as acyclovir, valacyclovir, and valganciclovir are commonly used for CFS, since it is thought that viral infection may be one cause of the disorder. This relates to several reported cases of Epstein-Barr virus, herpesviruses, and human cytomegalovirus (HCMV) in CFS clients and the success of antivirals in significantly reducing overall fatigue.[17]

### Indications and Mechanisms of Actions

The mechanism of action of antiviral drugs differs depending on their subclasses, yet the goal remains to prohibit the virus from reproducing by attacking the viral DNA chain. This can be achieved by attacking the virus's nucleus, thus preventing synthesis. Clients are advised to take these drugs on an empty stomach or to consume them with liquids such as skim milk, juice, coffee, or tea. It should also be noted that eating a high-calorie, high-fat meal might hinder the absorption process of the gut.[18]

## Benefits, Drawbacks, and Side Effects

Studies confirm the effects of using antiviral medications to improve CFS. However, this may not be true for all CFS clients. The use of these drugs is largely dependent upon the symptoms and client's response to the treatment. Antivirals should be used cautiously because inappropriate use can lead to overdose and resistant viruses. Adverse reactions may include the following:[19]

- Agitation;
- Amnesia;
- Confusion;
- Hallucinations;
- Bronchitis;
- Lung edema;
- Muscle pain;
- Anorexia;
- Diarrhea;
- Nausea and vomiting;
- Kidney stones;
- Hematuria; and
- *Stevens-Johnson syndrome.*

Abdominal pain must be reported immediately to the prescriber because this may mean gastro-intestinal bleeding. Clients must also note that drug-to-drug interactions may influence efficacy of medications. For instance, using antidepressants and antivirals together can cause respiratory depression, thus they cannot be taken simultaneously. Chronic fatigue syndrome patients who are also on oral contraceptives must be warned about their decreased effectiveness when other medicines are being taken, and an alternate method of contraception should be used.[20]

## ANTIBIOTICS

Some clients report chronic fatigue soon after being infected with a respiratory disorder called mononucleosis, which is treated with anti-biotics. However, antibiotics are composed of a wide array of medica-tions, so a single class or a combination from distinct classes can be prescribed based on the client's medical history. Some of the antibiotic groups commonly used are aminoglycosides, gentamycin, streptomycin sulfate, and neomycin. Penicillins that also work include the following:[21]

- Ampicillin;
- Amoxicillin;
- Cloxacillin;
- Oxacillin; and
- Penicillin G.

Other effective medications are as follows:

- Cefaclor;
- Cefixime;
- Ceftazadine;
- Ceftriaxone;
- Cephalexin;
- Doxycyline;
- Tetracycline;
- Hydrochloride;
- Ciprofloxacin;
- Levofloxacin;
- Norfloxacin; and
- Sparfloxacin.

## Indications and Mechanisms of Action

Antibiotics act by killing bacteria. Cell wall manufacture is prevented during bacterial multiplication. Most antibiotics are taken as a five- to seven-day continuous treatment, as clients are advised to take the drug at specific times, every twelve or eight hours, to stabilize the drug blood level. This makes the drug more effective in combating the bacteria that's causing infection. Antibiotic administration is more effective when a bacteria culture and sensitivity test identifies the specific microorganism causing the problem. Although this may take time, the first dose can be given while awaiting test results.[22]

## Benefits, Drawbacks, and Side Effects

Like antiviral medications, antibiotics should be taken cautiously because unsupervised use results in resistant bacteria, a more serious medical condition to treat. If taken correctly, the rate of effectiveness is high and symptoms of the infection usually abate after three days. Patients must be warned to take the drug for the entire course of treatment for complete healing. Adverse effects, such as oral lesion, *enterocolitis*, nephropathy, and *agranulocytosis* must be reported to the physician. Moreover, hypersensitivity reactions are common, thus testing and asking about any allergies before dispensation is essential.[23]

## ANTIPROTOZOALS

A protozoal infection such as pneumocystis carinii pneumonia (PCP) isn't very common, occurring only when one's immune system is severely compromised. This is undeniably true among CFS clients, so the use of antiprotozoal medications could be compulsory. These drugs include atovaquone and pentamidine.[24]

## Indications and Mechanisms of Action

Antiprotozoals must be used carefully in patients with impaired liver and kidney function as they may further damage said organs. Patients should take the medication with food, which enhances absorption. The

exact mechanism of action of antiprotozoals is unknown, but it's believed that they interfere with the reproduction of susceptible organisms by blocking the DNA and RNA. Drugs must be used with extreme
caution in clients with preexisting disorders such as hypertension, hypotension, hypoglycemia, hypocalcemia, diabetes, and pancreatitis.[25]

### Benefits, Drawbacks, and Side Effects

The whole point of antimicrobials such as antiprotozoals is to treat the
principal cause of infection that may be the cradle for CFS. Thus clients
need to be monitored closely during therapy due to the high risk of
concurrent respiratory infection. This is a concern that needs to be
addressed immediately by the doctor and the entire health care team.[26]

Adverse effects include vertigo, headache, dizziness, seizures, darkened urine, increased urination, metallic taste in the mouth, vaginal
candidiasis, joint pains, and rashes. This drug can also escalate liver
enzymes and lessen sodium and glucose levels, so CFS clients with
preexisting conditions upsetting these blood serums must be monitored
closely. Antiprotozoals are also protein bound, so they must be used
thoughtfully with other protein-bound medications and checked for
toxicity when combined.[27]

## NEW ADVANCES IN PHARMACOLOGICAL TREATMENT

Vagus nerve stimulation, antivirals to attack pathogens, glial cell inhibitors to cease immune activations, and surgical adjustment of the vagus
nerve are possible treatments of the future. A drug called Ibudilast was
used in Japan to inhibit glial cell activation by discouraging the production of proflammatory cytokine, and its blood vessel–dilating and
neuron-protecting effects prove beneficial in the treatment of stroke
and asthma.[28]

Ibudilast is also appropriate for nerve pain because it regulates glial
cell activation and is capable of stopping replication of viruses. The
National Institutes of Health have been funding experiments in the
United States to determine the drug's effectiveness in treating addiction so that it could be used in the future for CFS patients suffering
from substance addiction. Since herpesviruses residing in the sensory

nerve complexes might be shielded from antiviral drugs and antibodies, it may be easier to stop glial cell activation. Moreover, other types of viruses might be causing the malady.[29]

## Rintatolimod

Rintatolimod is a new drug that's designed to target viruses at the molecular level. Rintatolimod contains nucleic acid components believed to serve two purposes at the same time: it acts as an immune system inducer and an antiviral. However, in 2009, the FDA rejected rintatolimod as a treatment of CFS and vetoed its sale in U.S. markets, asserting that it wasn't proven be to be safe or effective. At present, the pharmaceutical company developing the drug is still performing tests and analyses on rintatolimod in order to gain approval.[30]

## Interferons

Interferons, or IFNs, belong to a class of glycoproteins responsible for antiviral activity. These proteins inhibit virus production by propagating white blood cells (called leucocytes and fibroblasts), which engulf invading pathogens. There are two types: type I (alpha and beta interferon) and type II (gamma interferon), the former being more of an antiviral component than the latter. Type II is voided by CD8 T cells and the helper T subset of CD4 cells that are used to stimulate various antigens. It's also distinctively different because it's used to patch up chronic *granulomatous disease*.[31]

## Cortisones

Evidence indicates that the reactivity of the HPA axis decreases in adult CFS patients when compared with control subjects. Hydrocortisone treatment produced minimum development, whereas oral administration of low doses of hydrocortisone showed improvement in the clinical condition of about 30 percent of a select group of CFS patients.[32] An oral hydrocortisone deployed in other research also shows some improvement when measured through fluctuations in wellness scores. Still, there weren't any substantial changes in fatigue and activity in this study. The search for a specific cause in regard to the generalized symptomology of CFS doesn't seem to be the most appropriate approach to use.

## Immunotherapy

The immune system is thought to be one of the culprits for acquiring CFS, so physicians and patients are looking into the possibility of boosting the immune system to improve symptoms. Immunoglobulins are a group of plasma proteins that help protect the body by fighting infection. Immunoglobulin G, or IgG, is the primary immunoglobulin in human serum. It can move through the placental barrier, thereby allowing the mother to pass on immunity to the fetus before birth. Immunoglobulin G is the major antibody for viruses, bacteria, and toxins. The efficacy among CFS sufferers is still individualized; therefore more research needs to be done before the administration of immunoglobulins.[33]

Rituximab is an antineoplastic drug that's used to treat Hodgkin's lymphoma, a form of blood cancer. The direct correlation between CFS and rituximab isn't well established but clinical trials have been done, with some clients reported improvement after taking rituximab. However, the drug is still open for trials to further develop the ultimate remedial plan (curing CFS completely) and to prove its efficacy for CFS. Patients on this medication are encouraged to avoid tyramine-rich foods and drinks such as smoked meats, wine, cheese, coffee, bananas, cola, and tea, because these may cause further tumors. Likewise, the use of antineoplastic agents for patients without cancer is controversial because the drug can also injure healthy cells, which may further aggravate the client's condition. Clients on rituximab are susceptible to irregular heart rhythms and fatal low blood pressure, hence strict cardiac monitoring is essential.[34]

## Hormones

Other drug classes for CFS hormonal therapy include steroid, cortisol, and thyroid hormone replacement. Clinical trials continue to prove the success of these medications in treating CFS. Although some CFS clients may find relief with these drugs, it's best to consult a doctor before taking hormones to avoid dangerous side effects. Long-term effects of hormonal medications such as steroids can result in heart failure, seizures, blood clots, inflammation of the pancreas, susceptibility to infections, acute adrenal insufficiency, and a *cushingoid* state of the body due to toxicity. Hormones must be used carefully, especially in conjunction with other medications, to prevent adverse reactions due to drug interaction.[35]

## IMPORTANCE OF TAKING ALL POTENTIAL SIDE EFFECTS SERIOUSLY

The dangers of side effects from medications are real and should be taken to heart. Medications that enter the CFS patient's body are digested in the stomach, metabolized and synthesized by the liver metabolites and other drug particles, and filtered by the kidneys. These organs are affected when medications aren't used correctly or when used for prolonged periods without the oversight of a physician. There's also a risk of severe, life-threatening allergies, so it's wise not to take side effects lightly. The following paragraphs explain medication side effects that pose a great danger to overall health.

### Systemic Anaphylaxis

Among the major effects of drugs are mild to severe allergies. Mild allergies may present minor symptoms such as rashes and itchy skin. Severe allergic reactions, however, can lead to anaphylaxis and anaphylactic shock. Responses include hives, wheezing, flushing, nausea and vomiting, *dyspnea*, increased mucus production, and feelings of generalized anxiety. The respiratory, cardiovascular and gastrointestinal systems are greatly affected. The most dangerous symptoms are wheezing and dyspnea, which indicates that the airway is swelling. If air passage is blocked for a while, it can result to death.[36]

The aim of anaphylaxis management is prevention. Before a drug is prescribed, clients are asked about any allergies such as egg, fish, specific drugs, or contrast media. Patients are taught which symptoms to watch out for, as well as those that need to be managed immediately, like dyspnea and wheezing. However, prevention isn't a foolproof plan when it comes to drug allergies because some clients may be allergic to a medication without exhibiting symptoms the first time it was administered.[37]

### Increased Cholesterol, Fatty Liver, and Liver Damage

The liver is a processer of nutrients and medications. This organ works diligently to ensure that drugs are metabolized in a way that delivers them to the parts of the body where they are needed. Most drugs can cause increases in cholesterol, leading to fatty liver, which can progress to liver damage. The best treatment is of course prevention; CFS clients must have their liver function tested and cholesterol levels checked regularly, especially when taking drugs for prolonged periods of time. It's essential to help the liver manage lipids and cholesterol by practicing a balanced, low-fat diet.[38]

### Kidney Failure

Kidney failure is a tricky side effect of the medications that may be offered to CFS sufferers. The kidney, responsible for sifting out waste products including excessive drug residues, is a steadfast organ. The problem is that a person won't experience major symptoms of kidney failure until the kidneys fail. The kidneys try to compensate for loss of function over time until they can no longer cope. Clients with CFS should be warned about the prolonged usage of pain relievers such as NSAIDs because this is the usual cause of kidney damage. Medications, especially NSAIDs, shouldn't be abused. Clients should have their *creatinine* and blood urea nitrogen (BUN) routinely checked for signs of kidney damage in order to halt its progression.[39]

If kidney damage isn't managed, it can lead to end-stage kidney failure, or ESRD, wherein dialysis is required, which is expensive and has many complications. Other options include kidney transplantation, but the waiting list is long and it can take years to find a suitable kidney. People with CFS should be monitored to preserve their kidney function while still possible.[40]

Many substances have been used in an attempt to cure CFS. Antivirals, anticholinergics, hormones, nicotinamide adenine dinucleotide (NAD), and antidepressants have been tried without conclusive, positive results thus far. On the flip side, steroid treatments show evidence of decreased fatigue.[41] Low doses of nortriptylin at bedtime suggest improved sleep and diminished pain in the patient. For musculoskeletal complaints, nonsteroidal anti-inflammatory agents and acetaminophen might be effective.[42] Also, reports indicate that fibromyalgia, introduced earlier in this book, is improved using antidepressant medications.[43]

## ANALYSIS

Pharmacological CFS medications should be used in moderation. Too much of anything, when taken incorrectly, does more harm than good—no matter how good it makes a person feel or how much it improves one's symptoms. It's vital that physicians oversee the prescription of medications and that patients follow their instructions exactly. CFS patients must report any new symptoms or side effects that they experience to their doctors. The treatment plan for CFS is individualized for every sufferer, and pharmacological approaches may not work depending on the individual and other factors. Therefore, individuals with CFS should take medications with extra caution and "listen to their body."[44]

# 12

# ADDRESSING THE MIND

It's inevitable that chronic fatigue syndrome (CFS) patients undergo mental and psychological issues brought about by the syndrome. The following chapter focuses on how to deal with psychological matters that weren't already covered in chapter 9, as well as how to deal with CFS-related stress in the comfort of one's home.

## MENTAL ISSUES

### How Chronic Fatigue Syndrome Affects Memory

CFS is shown to be associated with deficits in verbal and nonverbal memory tasks.[1] Patients may find it tiring to recall things that require rapid cognition of short-term or working memory. Fatigue brought on by CFS affects the retrospective memory of patients. Retrospective memory includes the memory of what's known: the informational content, such as people of acquaintance, events that happened previously, and other existing information that folks have about themselves and others.[2]

However, fatigue doesn't affect *prospective* memory—remembering *when* to act.[3] This is a pattern of memory that involves "remembering to do planned or intended actions" or activities at an appropriate time.[4] Retrospective memory is important in order for the CFS patient to function effectively in everyday life. It even encompasses daily, routine activities. Patients would then need a daily plan of activities and to remember to cross out what's already been done. However, to avoid overwhelming the patient with his tasks, a long list isn't effective.

In order to avoid creating anxiety and agitation in the patient, the list should break down the tasks, for example, by listing only the first three priorities. After that, patients can reward themselves with some rest or a small incentive for finishing the tasks as a kind of mini-celebration. This activity employs the method of pacing—tackling tasks in increments of time or effort. Pacing is a strategy that encourages CFS patients to find a balance between rest and activity and to live with the physical limitations imposed by CFS. Pacing also helps the patients avoid the detrimental effects of deconditioning, should they fall into drawn-out periods of inactivity.

## Self-efficacy and CFS

Psychological factors are found to predict health outcomes—a person's feelings of self-efficacy were associated with CFS.[5] Self-efficacy is defined as the extent or strength of an individual's belief in his own ability to complete tasks and reach goals.[6] Fatigue, depression, and overall self-efficacy are undeniably related to cognitive failures. People with CFS tend to be more depressed than those with many other illnesses. In effect, the lack of motivation associated with depression may lead to low self-efficacy, which in turn leads to cognitive failures.[7] People should not minimize, or much worse, overlook chronic fatigue syndrome. Patients can't treat the mind without treating the health of the whole body and vice versa. People with this disorder have to press on with motivation and perseverance.

## Financial Pressures Related to Chronic Fatigue Syndrome

CFS pervasively affects many areas of the patient's life and may even cause financial hardship. The majority of families with little ones face increased expenditures, indicating that some families might experience financial problems caused by caring for a child while also suffering from CFS.[8] Higher expenditures can result in more debt, which only increases the guilt that CFS patients experience when their illness prevents them from working.[9]

## STAYING HAPPY AS A CFS PATIENT

It is difficult to believe in one's own ability to prevent or relieve ill-ness—more so when one faces a chronic, seemingly irrepressible ill-ness.[10] However, the mind is powerful, so if patients with CFS can't stop themselves from feeling fatigued, their only recourse is to turn their minds toward positivity and optimism. Thus, CFS patients must accept every new day as a challenge.

### Coping Strategies and Their Effects

Individuals with CFS often have to rework their coping mechanisms in order to deal with this disabling chronic syndrome. Cognitive function-ing deficits may impair the patient's ability to employ a wide variety of coping strategies, and changing those strategies could refresh the mind again and again.[11] Pursuing viable ways to recover from the syndrome requires creativity and drive.

### Optimism

Some people with CFS view the disorder as uncontrollable, which may lead to pessimism and emotion-focused coping. In turn, these coping styles and pessimistic attitudes may lead to poorer health outcomes.[12] CFS inevitably affects emotional well-being. Research suggests that maintaining social activities and a sense of optimism correspond to more positive mental composite scores. This means that the more a patient feels destitute, the more he's drawn to poor outcomes.

Maintaining activities and remaining positive both appear to be re-lated to heightened functionality.[13] Day by day, CFS patients need to "maintain altitude" of their emotions, energy levels, patience, accep-tance, and understanding of their condition. Each new day necessitates a positive mind-set among patients with CFS, and the people around them must try fiercely to understand and get along with them, because no one's to blame. No one chooses such an illness. Coping with CFS is about making joy more contagious than it already is.

## Acceptance

Embracing the mind means accepting oneself, physically linking oneself to the biological chemicals one is born with, and accepting one's effects on human behavior. This is connected to how recovery or alleviation of symptoms may hinge on the sufferers' perception that they're in control of their syndrome. Psychosocial disturbances are of course linked to one's happiness, despite being a CFS patient.[14]

The key is acceptance, as well as happiness, when managing CFS, and this requires effort from the patient and the people around him. Accepting the disorder is a major step in dealing with CFS in a more effective manner. Since the malady exists, the patient is best served by focusing on solutions rather than negative emotions like sadness or depression, which can lead to immobility.[15]

Acceptance is a great challenge the patient and the people around him must face bravely. Surely no one would ever want to have CFS; however, having CFS is not a choice nor is it within one's control. Friends may recommend health professionals who can take care of him.[16]

## Social Disengagement or Isolation

Some people who suffer from CFS isolate themselves because of physical limitations: perhaps in order to preserve their energy, or on the negative side, perhaps they feel inadequate. Other patients eliminate socialization and time spent with their friends because of very low energy levels. CFS sufferers likely prefer staying home and resting rather than attending parties.[17]

By disengaging themselves from the people in their lives, patients conceivably risk losing them in the long run. Humans are social beings—it's only natural to mingle with others outside the immediate family. It's also the right of every child to play and be happy. As people get older and mature further, play becomes different and they reestablish themselves in a more complex manner. Patients with CFS must continue interacting with others rather than staying at home, which may even result in oversleeping and overeating. CFS is always a balance between managing time and energy. Chronic fatigue syndrome sufferers could enjoy some "alone time" while ambling in the park with a pet.[18]

Patients could also maximize family interaction without overexerting themselves simply by watching their children play at the park; if the patient feels like dozing off, he could place a mat on the grass and sleep there. At safe levels, sunlight is actually a great source of energy. If a patient is too tired to function at the office, a fifteen-minute nap should help, whereupon the sufferer can resume work again. Surely all employees know that an eight-hour job isn't really a cakewalk, because everyone, even a nation's president, needs time to relax.[19]

Among CFS patients, behavioral disengagement is related to worsening mental composite scores.[20] Social disengagement is clearly a maladaptive coping style for people with CFS. Much like the rest and proper nutrition required to get through the day, CFS patients also need motivation to stay positive while living with CFS. As everyone knows, it's not as easy as simply reading motivational quotes, but with effort, people can ditch chronic fatigue.

## Social Support

CFS patients often encounter poor understanding and inadequate awareness of CFS by healthcare professionals and the public. This compounds the problems faced by CFS patients, including children. Moreover, others lose support from family and friends due to the popular misperception that CFS "isn't real."[21] Professional caregivers must then broaden their services to include briefing the people close to the patient about the need for understanding.

Studies have found that improvement in people with CFS was associated with social support.[22] They also found that during the year before the onset of CFS, people acknowledged less social support than healthy controls.[23] This is in line with the detrimental effects of social disengagement, but this time, the disconnection was on the part of people around the patient. Moreover, CFS is linked with an individual's overall happiness, including his relationships with loved ones and coworkers, as well as other social aspects outside the family.

People around the patient must fathom the CFS patient's circumstances when interacting with him. All of this is key to maintaining good collaborative relationships aimed at improving the patient's health.

# HOW TO DEAL WITH CFS-RELATED STRESS

One common indicator of life-threatening stress is post-traumatic stress disorder (PTSD). Somatic complaints of CFS were thought to enhance the stress disorder. Experts have asserted that CFS might have been triggered by deployment-related stress. The study involves 15,000 former Gulf War soldiers and 15,000 other veterans who completed questionnaires evaluating their exposure to possible risks, potential variables, their functional impairments, and their medical past. The questionnaire included the somatic symptoms prevalent in previous patients.[24]

From the data collected, researchers found that the level of stress varies based on the deployment of the veterans. Those who aren't utilized in warfare have minimal stress; reservists deployed to a location away from the Persian Gulf possess moderate stress; and those deployed to the Gulf have the highest levels of stress. The demographics were analyzed, and the groups that had post-traumatic stress disorder or CFS-like illnesses were compared. The veterans demonstrating positivity in spite of post-traumatic stress are mainly older nonwhite females in the enlisted ranks in the Army and National Guard. Soldiers who are positive for CFS-like illness tend to be younger, single, and enlisted in the reserves. The prevalence of traumatic stress was found to range from 3.3 to 22.6 percent.[25]

The correlation between post-traumatic stress or CFS-like illness and the development of full-blown diagnosed CFS has been proven. Stressor intensity affects the rate of post-traumatic stress. From here, it's argued that post-traumatic stress leads to the stress-related behavioral problems in chronic fatigue syndrome. The rate is substantially higher in conflicts where stressor intensity is greater. When related to combat, the rate of CFS-like illness didn't change significantly for Gulf War veterans. Deployment stress relates to the onset of CFS in a veteran population. However, scientists can't be assured that other elements specific to serving in the Gulf might have contributed to the accelerated rates of CFS among Gulf War veterans. Aside from this, there are no other studies that relate the occurrence of CFS with stress, though the latter is an established indicator of the former. Stressor intensity is pertinent when studying the medical aftermath of stress, which plays a relatively minor role in CFS in the Gulf environment.[26]

In the workplace, employers need to make adjustments for workers with CFS; to do otherwise, they risk compromising work quality. The symptoms brought about by CFS may also affect employee evaluations. Employers and superiors must be patient with workers suffering with CFS. Moreover, society ought to be cognizant of such a syndrome in order to employ psychiatric maneuvers that can often impose on the physical well-being of the patient. Someone who cannot work because of a disorder is at risk for depression, which is needless when solutions for dealing with CFS are available. Lastly, solidarity and camaraderie among coworkers are needed to address the occupation-related effects of CFS.[27]

### Positive Mood

As in the case of office culture, work efficiency and effectiveness is reliant upon how well people work with tiredness, and having a positive mood only makes things better. This is where drive and motivation comes in—drive and motivation should be as pervasive as the illness. When organs deteriorate, all that's left is the mind fervently believing that the body still can go on. It means striving for happiness through optimism—unless the person prefers rotting away with the illness. If a patient is already sick, expelling negative thoughts can only help.[28]

A low mood can result in further exhaustion. When a CFS patient feels downcast to the point of moroseness around others, mood regulation should be employed with care. Asking others to try to understand him might be a form of straightforward communication that assists everyone in adjusting to interactions with him.

### ANALYSIS

Mental state has been found to predict health outcomes, and the mind and body form a fascinating and indeed powerful link. It's amazing how serenity or doom can spring from a material organ such as the brain.

# 13

# COLLECTIVE EFFORTS

**A**s this comprehensive discussion about chronic fatigue syndrome (CFS) nears its end, patients and caregivers should know that CFS has a huge impact on the community and society in general, since it largely affects the productivity and the ability of an individual to work and fully function, as well as to execute routines of daily life. The disorder also causes financial hardship to those afflicted, which is all related to the decreased productivity of the affected population.[1] In recent years, governments have played a substantial role in the advocacy and treatment of CFS.[2]

## WHY THE GOVERNMENT NEEDS TO GET MORE INVOLVED

Millions of people are affected by CFS in the United States, and documents have stated that affected individuals endure long-term, chronic, debilitating, and incapacitating mental and physical pain, as well as aftereffects of fatigue that don't respond to rest. The fatigue is worsened by physical and mental stress or exertion, which diminishes the individual's capability to concentrate and causes impaired memory, tiredness and lethargy, and sleep disturbances. CFS patients must also deal with extensive diagnostic tests and clinical assessments that bear on their productivity at work and cause additional healthcare-related expenses. Again, all the above is why chronic fatigue syndrome can't be eradicated without a collective effort.[3]

Some patients with CFS might ask what their healthcare professional can do to help them. Even though the cause of chronic fatigue syndrome hasn't been identified, healthcare professionals can offer palliative treatment or treat the symptoms stemming from the disorder.[4] Informing the healthcare professional about the specific symptoms the patient experiences is an important step, since many of these symptoms can be treated. The healthcare professional can also recommend support groups and other therapies tailored to the CFS sufferer that can help him cope with the condition.

Another question that frequently comes to mind is why the symptoms of CFS seem to come and go. Although CFS can persist for years at a time, studies (some are funded by governments) indicate that chronic fatigue syndrome isn't classified as a progressive condition due to its cognitive symptoms.[5] The worst symptoms tend to occur during the first two years, after which the symptoms stabilize but persist chronically, wax and wane, or finally improve. Symptoms are unique to each patient involved, and the course of chronic fatigue syndrome can't be predicted. Yet another reason why government needs to get involved.[6]

Healthcare professionals diagnose CFS based on the client's symptoms and medical history, as well as through diagnostic tests used to rule out other clinical anomalies. At present, there's no known cure for chronic fatigue syndrome and there is not a surefire treatment for the disorder itself; amelioration of the individual symptoms is the treatment. Most CFS patients fully recover from the disorder, and a few partially recover yet still experience symptoms, since clinical indicators may persist for years. Some CFS sufferers may experience periodic relapse, and since little is known regarding the actual cause of the disorder, the course of the disorder can't be determined in large-scale populations. Governments can assist in that regard.[7]

Chronic fatigue syndrome isn't contagious, and there's no known data indicating that it can be transferred from one individual to another. Barring viral implications, it can't be transmitted by contact, airborne droplet, blood transfusion, or other modes of diffusion, so there's no need to isolate patients diagnosed with chronic fatigue syndrome. Should governments get involved in the effort to find a cure, the need for emergency quarantine will not be of concern.

Chronic fatigue syndrome limits the individual's ability to work and stay productive in both home and the workplace, and it impairs the person's ability to participate fully in their daily activities. Hence, this condition tends to cause absenteeism from work, which may then lead to lost hours or even unemployment. Governments should take that into consideration. With fewer productive work periods, an individual's earnings would also decrease, resulting in less spending power or decreased earnings with which to support himself. This also causes a burden on the employers as well as family members due to unresolved conflicts that can arise because of the condition.[8]

CFS affects not only the diagnosed individuals and their families, but also their workplace, relationships, community, and society in general. Fewer productive employees means a decline in the labor force, which causes a decline in work that tends to have a negative impact on both employer and employee. A healthier population is more efficient, performing tasks on time, delivering positive work performance, generating more revenue for businesses and corporations, and ensuring the success of their companies. Ultimately, with the government receiving more taxpayer funds, improvements in the care of CFS would commence.[9]

## HOW CORPORATIONS CAN HELP

### Support Groups

The importance of support groups for chronic fatigue syndrome can't be overemphasized. No one is alone with the affliction, and recuperation is a collective effort: first, by ensuring the full cooperation of the individual and the desire to get well and to overcome the disorder, and second through the collective efforts of corporations, including nonprofits, and public awareness regarding the implications of CFS. Managing the symptoms of CFS is a struggle, but the cooperation and participation of companies helps significantly.

## Agencies and Nonprofit Organizations Aimed at Eradicating CFS

Today, there's no known cure for CFS, although palliative options can help alleviate its symptoms. Treatments for CFS depend on the person's symptoms, as well as the prognosis and early detection of the disease. Research has been done in the United States and abroad to develop advanced treatments for chronic fatigue syndrome, as well as to document the neurological, immunological, cardiovascular, and respiratory effects on CFS patients. Such experiments have been funded by various nonprofit agencies such as those mentioned in the following paragraphs.

### National Fibromyalgia Association (NFA)

Established in 1997, the NFA supports people diagnosed with fibromyalgia as well as other disorders related to pain symptoms, such as CFS. Its mission is to develop programs dedicated to improving the quality of life of the patients suffering from these diseases.[10]

### National Fibromyalgia Research Association

National Fibromyalgia Research Association is an organization that funds research and continuing education for physicians and other healthcare workers. It organizes efforts in raising public awareness about the causes, early detection, prevention, and treatment of fibromyalgia. It has also produced a fibromyalgia exercise and fitness video, as well as fibromyalgia bracelets to raise awareness and garner support from the general public.[11]

### International Association for CFS/ME

International Association for CFS/ME is a private organization that primarily aims to boost research and awareness for CFS. The group also advocates education regarding patient care, early discernment, and treatment. It conducts regular conferences with other groups to promote and evaluate research regarding the disorder and to strengthen efforts to decode it. This organization also runs seminars to educate doctors and other healthcare workers about treatment for patients.[12]

## HHV-6 Foundation

HHV-6 Foundation is an entity that encourages research and the exchange of information among researchers and scientists in order to acquire grants to uphold research. One of its first advocacies was to determine the difference between an active and latent infection, as well as biological ciphers in the individuals diagnosed with CFS. The name HHV-6 stands for human herpesvirus 6, which many believe to be linked to chronic fatigue syndrome and pain-related symptoms.[13]

## National Institute for Health and Care Excellence

National Institute for Health and Care Excellence is a British agency that advises individual treatment programs that prioritize maintaining optimum physical functions and abilities of the individual as well as strengthening emotional support, managing the symptoms of the condition, and raising public awareness of CFS.[14]

## Organizations for CFS Education

### PANDORA

PANDORA is an advocacy group that's one of the most active in fighting chronic fatigue syndrome through education and awareness regarding the prevention of CFS. This organization is located in Miami and was founded in 2007.[15]

### Rocky Mountain CFIDS and FMS Association

Rocky Mountain CFIDS and FMS Association is an institute that maintains a website and online forums that provide education regarding CFS. They also offer practicums on its prevention and treatment.[16]

### Wisconsin Chronic Fatigue Syndrome Association

Wisconsin Chronic Fatigue Syndrome Association is one of the first organizations supporting CFS education. They publish newsletters that offer information and updates about the disorder. They also host discussion forums as well as support services via phone, where people can talk to someone regarding their concerns about the syndrome.[17]

## HOW CFS PATIENTS CAN HELP EACH OTHER

Since CFS itself is a formidable enemy, the CFS patient community should possess a strong community support network. Patient-to-patient groups provide information, research, encouragement, and support services to people suffering from the condition. They rally around relevant issues, such as the social and medical implications of labeling CFS as a medical and psychiatric form of disorder. They're the ones who push through studies in order to gain untarnished understanding of the medical condition. There are countless sites in the Internet promoting self-help and patient advocacy for this syndrome. After all, who can better help CFS patients than those who have suffered CFS themselves?[18]

Individuals diagnosed with chronic fatigue syndrome help each other by offering encouragement in promoting lifestyle changes.[19] Lifestyle changes are an most important aspect for a good prognosis since CFS hinders most patients in ways that cause both physical and emotional burdens. Through encouragement and patronage from fellow CFS patients, they can make their lives more enjoyable. Promoting rest as well as learning different stress-relieving techniques also helps the patient, because most suffer from extreme fatigue and nonrevitalizing sleep. Dietary modification—eating healthy foods in appropriate amounts—is also important, greatly improving the overall nutrition and well-being of the patient. Taking cooking classes or joining diet or weight-loss groups with other CFS sufferers is a good activity to support others and to promote companionship. People with CFS can also attend counseling sessions together, where healthcare professionals provide activities that help CFS patients to express their emotions and to share stories and experiences. Attending counseling sessions with other CFS patients allows one to explore sound coping strategies and also to learn how other people are surviving their disorder.[20]

Another way CFS patients can support each other is through use of an "energy diary" or journal. Logging activities as well as noting thoughts and feelings help identify the times of the day and activities that trigger stress or fatigue. This also helps to confirm the CFS patient's activities during the day and documents certain patterns of the disorder as well as the factors contributing to increased fatigue and other symptoms such as headaches and muscle weakness. Through the use of an energy diary, a CFS patient is also able to effectively schedule his activities—such as taking naps at predetermined times—and to identify stressors to eradicate from his daily routine.[21]

Individuals with CFS can also support each other by attending relaxation and meditation classes. Through relaxation and meditation, patients learn to scope out the situations that they find psychologically and physically stressful, as well as the activities that help them to handle these different stressors. A healthcare provider may create an exercise plan for the group. Most CFS patients experience fatigue easily, even as a result of moderate exercise, so the healthcare professional should start with light exercises and gradually increase the intensity according to each patient's ability. Group moderators can also provide patients evaluations at each week's end to identify areas of improvement.[22]

Support among patients with CFS, such as meetings and discussion groups, helps lessen the possibility of developing depression or other mental health–related disorders. Since CFS is a debilitating, long-term condition, CFS sufferers in some cases may develop depression due to decreased physical activity, inability to work, and lack of support from friends or family members. Although there are certain medications for treating depression, such as SSRIs, being able to express and communicate feelings and to articulate emotions and stressful experiences to someone else decreases the chances of developing depression, especially in patients with CFS.[23] Another way CFS sufferers can support each other is to encourage each other to follow the course of treatment advocated by their physician and other healthcare professionals.[24]

## CFS Patients Helping Each Other to Deal with Stress

People have their own ways of shoring up against stress. Some studies show that stress can cause excessive eating or other unhealthy habits. Research demonstrates that a healthier way to deal with stress is through exercise, healthier eating habits, and more effective ways in dealing with stressful situations, coupled with support from family and friends.[25]

CFS patients can help each other identify potential stressors and consider ways to cope with the disorder effectively. Group exercises are a fun way of supporting each other. Not only does exercise burn calories, but it also produces biochemicals known to counter the negative effect of cortisol, a stress hormone mentioned in an earlier chapter of this book. Exercise also helps control the blood's insulin and glucose levels. A minimum of twenty to thirty minutes of exercise each day, two or three times a week is recommended. Collaborative exercise is indispensible, but it's important to be careful not to overexert, since this may lead to increased cortisol levels, which is harmful to one's health.[26]

Classes that CFS patients could attend together include relaxation exercises, such as meditation sessions or yoga, deep-breathing courses, or guided imagery classes, wherein the patient would learn about ways to relax body and mind—a healthy way to deal with all types of stress. Some of these classes, often moderated by a CFS patient, teach participants to possess a sea of calmness wherein the body and mind are free from external stressors. This helps the patient develop his own relaxation and meditation techniques.[27]

Baking and cooking sessions are also activities in which CFS patients can enroll together, since from-scratch, homemade foods are healthier than processed foods, which are known to contain harmful chemicals that aren't the best for the patient's health. CFS patients could also collectively help each other by encouraging each other in breaking bad habits, such as smoking and alcohol consumption, which are known to increase cortisol levels and subsequently increase feelings of stress, lethargy, tiredness, and muscle weakness.[28]

## ANALYSIS

Much like other chronic disorders and debilitating conditions, CFS accounts for a large portion of personal, medical, as well as healthcare-related economic costs. That's partially why the dilemma of CFS should be addressed collectively. As is the case with other conditions such as cardiovascular diseases, diabetes mellitus, and cancer, government agencies have spearheaded funding and organized advocacy groups to raise public awareness and support.

# 14

# CONCLUSION

Time and again, humanity is pushed to the brink of its limits. Here comes another complex disorder with devastating ramifications, the origins of which remain shadowy. Despite the efforts of healthcare professionals, definitive treatment of chronic fatigue syndrome (CFS) remains elusive.[1] By now, the reader should understand that what makes CFS even more difficult is the diagnosis—it's almost impossible to self-diagnose, and help from experts is uncertain, as its symptoms are rampant in many other medical disorders. Studies revealed that in the United States, less than 20 percent of the estimated four million people with CFS have been diagnosed.[2]

## HOPE DESPITE THE DAMAGING NATURE OF CFS

So, what more is there to do? Will it be to despair over one's current helplessness or to continue working harder? There's nothing wrong in hoping for better. Hope is what keeps individuals moving forward. Continuing studies and clinical surveys will provide the most accurate test for the diagnosis of CFS, as well as the most effective treatment. As experts note, there has been progress in understanding the nature and management of CFS over the years as more countries, researchers, and clinicians have become involved. Therefore, there's much reason for hope, which is perhaps the most beautiful thing in this world. Indeed, recovery starts with hope.[3]

**It All Starts Here**

Nowadays, many advancements have been made. In fact, progress is a never-ending process. Humans have an insatiable hunger for unraveling mysteries and making discoveries. They seek infinite answers from their inestimable questions. However, there are still many things beyond clear understanding, just like CFS. Looking back, where does anything really start? Long before Neil Armstrong landed on the moon, he may have struggled first learning to balance on his bike.

Surely, this is similar to understanding CFS. The disorder began hobbling people without their least knowledge of it. It's no wonder it was years before this condition was identified. Nonetheless, because of its continual recurrence, it was finally given a clear-cut definition by the Centers for Disease Control in 1994 as an unexplained, persistent, or relapsing fatigue of six months duration that can't be explained by other medical conditions. [4]

This was a major breakthrough, and since then, research followed suit. Currently, it can be said that scientists are attempting to fully decipher the nature of CFS and provide the definitive medication for it. That's why there's no place for anxiety. Everything will fall into position as long as hope and courage are in the driver's seat. [5]

**Mystery of the Day: What's Really There to Hope For?**

Chronic fatigue syndrome poses four major challenges. First, it's a major disorder. Second, it's not well known or understood by the general public. Although unfamiliar, it's not uncommon. [6] Third, its cause is still unknown, so prevention isn't foolproof. Fourth, there's still no official therapy, medicines, or treatment used today by healthcare professionals. Perhaps the greatest challenge posed by CFS is that it's very difficult to diagnose in a person without professional assistance.

The good news is that it's not as bad as it sounds. There's no standard treatment, but the medical community has developed several strategies based on the severity of a patient's CFS. Addressing the challenge in diagnosis, numerous different studies are simultaneously working on providing better case definitions and encouraging professional caregivers from around the world to take up the challenge that CFS brings to the table. Raising awareness may be challenging at this point, but as long as there are different organizations and companies that continue to nurture concern, worldwide awareness of CFS may be achieved.[7]

The cause of CFS is still undetermined but several theories are already in line. Persistence and patience link the doctors specializing in CFS, and it's almost certain that the exact cause will be discovered eventually. Also, cures are elusive for many disorders, although their causes may have long been identified. The point being that pinpointing the source of CFS won't automatically eradicate it. Right now, the process of interpreting the mystery of CFS is already underway.

## It's All There

When does consistent and sincere hard work really end? Today, it's apparent that there's still a lot of light to be shed on the gloom of CFS but all that's to be done is to keep moving forward. CFS is a disorder about to be cracked wide open.

## IMPORTANCE OF SEEKING PROFESSIONAL HELP

Every patient needs the courage to stand up and take on the challenges of his disorder. However, he also needs the help of a healthcare professional to diagnose and prescribe a course of treatment. Self-examination is one of the best things a patient can do for himself, but self-examination is only the start. It's usually ineffective to examine oneself without consulting a doctor, leaving the management of the disorder to hearsay.[8]

It's like playing darts with a blindfold; the target is there, but it can't be seen. Nothing beats proper diagnosis from professionals. Medical-based approaches offer more accurate diagnoses and treatments. From there, the patient is poised to get healthier.[9]

## Better to Be Safe than Sorry

With one's health at stake, CFS patients should never take symptoms for granted. A mild fever could be the result of malaria, while a simple string of infections can indicate bone cancer. Alternative and substandard medication can lessen or perhaps resolve an ailment but not in the long run. What's even worse: as people keep relying on these short-term remedies, eventually they lose effectiveness. It's therefore highly recommended that prescribers oversee treatments for patients with CFS. Investment in health is the best wager of all.[10]

## When Darkness Gets Darker

Many questions still surround chronic fatigue syndrome in the medical world. As stated by experts, CFS patients have great variability in their reactions to treatments.[11] Finding treatments and dosages that help is by trial and error. Since even experts have yet to arrive at a definitive treatment, CFS patients must rely on their expertise all the more. The concept is simple: don't swing a hammer at a rock that even a backhoe can't break. Taking matters into one's own hands comes into play after getting guidelines from the doctor. Treatment doesn't end inside the hospital or clinic; it continues into the patient's day-to-day life.

## THE IMPORTANCE OF PATIENCE AND CONFIDENCE

Optimism and consistency are important for patients with any type of disability. Before one can do something, he first has to *believe* that he can do it. Moreover, he has to maintain his belief that he can do it. These characteristics, together with the wonders of science, ensure a bright outlook for patients. But without a clear understanding of the disorder, patients diagnosed with CFS should seek appropriate professional medical help. The bigger the impediment, the more help and belief one must possess in order to overcome it.[12]

## Getting Better through Patience

In a strange way, simply knowing that one has CFS is something for which to be thankful. A patient diagnosed with CFS has already overcome one hurdle: the diagnosis of the disorder remains difficult even among professionals. With a firm diagnosis, the CFS patient can obtain appropriate therapy and medication. However, how long recovery takes remains uncertain. CFS symptoms vary in degree, and although there are many cases in which improvement was reported, no single definitive therapy or treatment has been uncovered by medical experts. One can only bear with it and trust that the condition will be subdued sooner or later.[13]

### Having the Confidence to Cope

It's not impossible for people with CFS to improve their health and quality of life. Several self-care strategies have been laid out for them. Physically, one must live a healthy lifestyle that includes exercise, a balanced diet, and restful sleep. He must pay attention to and take action for his health. The paradox is that strenuous exercise often makes CFS symptoms worse, but people with the syndrome must exercise in order to feel more energetic. So what should be done? Several studies proved that activities such as aerobic exercise and other low-impact activities can improve the nervous system function of people with CFS.[14]

Generally, the key is to balance and pace the workouts: they should never be beyond one's capacity but beneficial enough to improve one's physical condition. Healthcare professionals can suggest specific therapies based on the degree of the patient's CFS, which should give the patient confidence in coping with CFS.[15]

## ANALYSIS

In the final analysis, denying CFS of its wrathful onslaughts truly depends on the willpower of the sufferer. Patience and confidence are important characteristics, but the reader should also remember that it's not impossible for people with CFS to improve the health and quality of their lives. After all, only amid darkness is the brightest lamp sought.

# GLOSSARY

**acetylcholinesterase:** An enzyme that carries out the process of breakdown of acetylcholine (a neurotransmitter) in the region between two nerve cells (the synaptic cleft) in order to transmit impulses from one neuron to another.

**achalasiacardia:** Also called cardiospasm. In this case, it's the neuro-muscular failure of esophagus relaxation, especially at its lower end.

**actin-myosin cross bridging:** Responsible for the force generation and contraction of skeletal muscle. Certain myosin-binding sites present on actin that bond with myosin, forming cross bridges, which is an important step in skeletal muscle contraction.

**adenine:** One of the four nucleic acid bases derived from purine. It combines with thymine to form the double-stranded DNA.

**adenosinediphosphate (ADP):** An organic compound that is essential for the process of metabolism. One molecule of ADP is composed of one molecule of adenine combined with two molecules of phosphate on a sugar base.

**adenosine triphosphate:** A nucleotide with three phosphate groups that is regarded as the currency unit of energy in a cell.

**adrenal androgens dehydroepiandrosterone (DHEA):** A steroid hormone produced by the adrenal cortex that in females is responsible for control of processes like growth of pubic or axillary hair and mainte-nance of female sex drive.

**agranulocytosis:** A condition in which granulocyte counts decrease. The granulocytes are neutrophils, basophils, and eosinophils.

**alpha-intrusion:** Alpha waves are a kind of brain wave that originate from the occipital lobe primarily when a person is awake and relaxing but has closed his eyes. Alpha-intrusion occurs when a person generates alpha waves during non-REM sleep.

**anemia:** A condition in which the number of the red blood cells or the amount of hemoglobin decreases. It can also be explained as the reduced capacity of oxygen transport.

**arrhythmia:** Irregular heartbeat.

**arthralgias:** Joint pain.

**autoantibodies:** Antibodies produced by one's body as an immune response to destroy one's own specific proteins.

**autonomic nervous system:** A part of the peripheral nervous system that is responsible for involuntary responses like digestion, salivation, heart rate, and breathing.

**axis 1 disorders:** These disorders fall under the category of psychiatric disorders and include anxiety disorders, mood disorders, eating and psychotic disorders, as well as dissociative and substance use disorders.

**biomarker:** A biological indicator—a molecule, gene, or simply a characteristic trait—that primarily is used to study various aspects of a disease or a biological condition like the onset of disease and its progress, how well it is responding to treatment measures, and so on.

**bursae:** A closed, fluid-filled sac lined with a synovial membrane that is usually found in regions of friction, such as in an area where the tendon rubs against the bone.

**cancer cachexia:** A multifactorial syndrome that has characteristic features like anorexia and loss of appetite resulting in wasting of body tissues, atrophy of skeletal muscles, and immunity-related problems.

**catalysis:** The process altering (increasing or decreasing) the velocity of a chemical reaction in the presence of a compound (catalyst) that doesn't get used up during the process.

**cavernosal arteries:** These are deep blood vessels in the penis that supply blood to the corpora cavernosa and aid in erection.

**chromosomes:** Chromosomes are present within the nucleus of a cell and carry the genetic information that is passed on from parents to their children.

**ciliary beating:** Cilia are thin extensions that line various body parts like the trachea and fallopian tubes. They move in a beating manner to thrust out dirt and dust (as in the case of the trachea) and transport ovum to ovary (in the case of Fallopian tubes).

**creatinine:** A chemical waste product of muscles that's used for measuring kidney health.

**cushingoid:** Describes the features of a Cushing's syndrome or Cushing's disease, such as excessive facial hair, striations on the trunk, and pads of fat on face and upper part of back.

**cytomegalovirus:** A group of herpesviruses that have mild or no significant effects on a normal healthy person but that can create serious complications in fetuses, patients who have undergone organ transplantation, and those with HIV.

**dysautonomia:** When the autonomic nervous system isn't functioning properly.

**dysmenorrhea:** Painful menstruation.

**dysphoria:** Diffuse uneasiness with life.

**dyspnea:** Shortness of breath or difficulty breathing due to lung or heart problems.

**endergonic:** Any reaction that requires external energy to progress.

**endocrine system:** The system of glands that are responsible for controlling metabolism and other physiological processes through the secretion of hormones into blood circulation.

**enterocolitis:** Inflammation of the colon and small intestine.

**epidemiology:** The science in which various aspects of a disease process like the incidence and pattern of distribution is dealt with.

**ergosterol:** A sterol produced by yeasts that undergoes conversion to form vitamin D12 under ultraviolet rays.

**exergonic:** Any reaction that causes the release of energy into the external environment.

**ex-vivo:** That which happens outside the organism's body.

**gastroesophageal junction:** Also known as cardia, this is the junction between the distal part of the esophagus and the proximal part of the stomach.

**gastrointestinal mucosa:** The innermost layer of the gastrointestinal tract, which that has three layers: epithelium, lamina propria, and muscularis mucosa.

**glial cell:** A cell that forms the neuroglia like astrocutes and microglia.

**granulomatous disease:** Any disease in which the growth of minute blood vessels and connective tissue can be observed.

**hematopoiesis:** The creation and development of blood cells inside the body.

**homeoregulatory:** Involving the regulation of body temperature.

**homeostasis:** The tendency of the body to maintain a state of equilibrium by regulating various physiological processes within the body.

**hospitalists:** Medical professionals or physicians who take care of the medical needs of hospitalized patients.

**hypochondriacal:** Related to hypochondria, or phobia or anxiety regarding one's health in which an individual suspects or fears that he is suffering from a grave illness.

**hypocortisolism:** Also known as adrenal insufficiency, a condition in which the adrenal glands fail to produce enough steroid hormones.

**hypoperfusion:** The reduced flow of blood through any organ.

**hypotension:** Blood pressure lower than the normal range.

**interferons:** Glycoproteins that are released from animal cells as an immune response and can inhibit the replication process in viruses.

**interleukins:** Cytokines produced by leukocytes for immune response regulation.

**intracellular:** That which occurs within a cell.

**mitochondria:** Cytoplasmic organelles that are spherical or rod shaped and are referred to as the powerhouses of a cell, as they are concerned with ATP synthesis.

**mycoplasmapneumonia:** An infectious disease that occurs in children and adults and is caused by mycoplasma pneumonia. Since the disease affects the lungs, the symptoms generally include fever, cough, and upper respiratory infection.

**nondiscocytes:** Abnormal and less flexible red blood cells that lack the typical disc shape of a red blood cell and that occur due to magnesium deficiency.

**non-REM sleep:** Of the five stages of sleep, non-REM sleep comprises stages one through four and is characterized by reduced heart and breathing rates, decreased metabolic activity, and an absence of dreaming.

**osteoporosis:** A disease that causes the formation of porous bones due to excessive loss of proteins as well as minerals like calcium.

**pathophysiology:** The study of the ways that the normal functions of the body get disrupted due to disease process.

**perfusion:** The process of fluid passage through any organ, such as the heart.

**peripheral nervous system:** One of the two major nervous systems of the body that forms a link between the central nervous system and the sensory organs.

**pharyngitis:** Inflammation of the pharynx characterized by symptoms like sore throat.

**phonasthenia:** Difficulty experienced during voice production due to factors like fatigue.

**photosynthesis:** A chemical process occurring in green plants in which carbon dioxide and water in the presence of sunlight are converted into carbohydrates.

**physiological:** Related to the physiology or the normal functioning of any living organism.

**phytochemicals:** A class of chemicals naturally found in plants.

**postural orthostatic tachycardia syndrome (POTS):** The condition in which the heart rate shoots up abnormally when a person stands in an upright position.

**psychosocial:** Psychological and social.

**psychosomatic:** Anything pertaining to the interaction of the body and mind.

**school avoidance behavior:** A type of anxiety diorder seen in children when they refuse to go to school due to various reasons like separation anxiety or depression.

**somatic nervous system:** A division of the peripheral nervous system responsible for all the body's voluntary movements by conveying impulses from central nervous system to skeletal muscles and vice versa.

**Stevens-Johnson syndrome:** A form of erythema multiforme that occurs as an allergic reaction to certain drugs. It is a fatal condition in which the person has symptoms like flu and red rash all over the body that become painful blisters.

**temporomandibular joint (TMJ) disorder:** A disorder affecting the temporomandibular joint, which is located between the mandible and the skull, with symptoms that include jaw pain and pain in the adjoining muscles.

**tonsiliar:** Related to tonsils, a collection of lymphatic tissues present at various sites of the body and named accordingly. For instance, palatine tonsils are at the back of the mouth.

**urticaria:** An allergic response of the body to some food or medicines that is represented by the presence of itchy skin at various places on the body.

**ventilatory failure:** Type II respiratory failure in which the ventilator process is hampered and the carbon dioxide produced by the body isn't excreted adequately.

# APPENDIX A

## Chronic Fatigue Syndrome–Related Links

- www.betterhealth.vic.gov.au/bhcv2/bhcarticles.nsf/pages/Chronic_fatigue_syndrome
- www.bupa.co.uk/individuals/health-information/directory/c/hi-chronic-fatigue-syndrome
- www.cdc.gov/cfs/
- www.cfids-cab.org/MESA/ccpccd.pdf
- http://chealth.canoe.ca/condition_info_details.asp?disease_id=32
- www.co-cure.org/MEICC.pdf
- www.dailymail.co.uk/health/article-2006038/Myalgic-encephalomyelitis-caused-virus.html
- www.fm-cfs.ca/
- http://guidance.nice.org.uk/CG53
- www.hfme.org/whatisme.htm
- www.hhs.gov/advcomcfs/
- http://jnm.snmjournals.org/content/early/2014/03/21/jnumed.113.131045.abstract
- http://kidshealth.org/parent/system/ill/cfs.html
- www.mayoclinic.org/diseases-conditions/chronic-fatigue-syndrome/
- www.meassociation.org.uk
- www.mecfs.org.au/what-is-meorcfs
- http://medical-dictionary.thefreedictionary.com/Myalgic+encephalitis

- www.medscape.com/viewarticle/773334
- www.name-us.org/
- www.ncbi.nlm.nih.gov/books/NBK53577/
- www.netdoctor.co.uk/diseases/facts/cfs_managing_003805.htm
- www.nhs.uk/conditions/Chronic-fatigue-syndrome
- www.nlm.nih.gov/medlineplus/chronicfatiguesyndrome.html
- http://onlinelibrary.wiley.com/doi/10.1111/j.1365-2796.2011.02428.x/full
- www.patient.co.uk/doctor/chronic-fatigue-syndrome
- www.sciencedaily.com/news/health_medicine/chronic_fatigue_syndrome/
- www.thegracecharityforme.org/what.asp

# APPENDIX B

## Chronic Fatigue Syndrome Research and Training

Alison Hunter Memorial
Foundation
PO Box 6132
North Sydney NSW 2059
Australia
+61 2 9958 6285
www.ahmf.org

Associated New Zealand ME
Society
PO Box 36-307, Northcote
Auckland, New Zealand
+64 (09) 269 6374
www.anzmes.org.nz

Autoimmunity Research
Foundation
3423 Hill Canyon Ave.
Thousand Oaks, CA 91360
(818) 584-1201
foundation@
autoimmunityresearch.org

www.autoimmunityresearch.org

California Capital CFIDS
Association
PO Box 660362
Sacramento, CA 95866
(916) 484-3788
CalcapitalCFIDS@bigfoot.com
http://ottem.org/ccca

CFIDS Association of America
6827 Colony on Fairview Dr.
Charlotte, NC 28210
(704) 364-0016
http://solvecfs.org

CFS Research Foundation
2 The Briars
Sarratt, Rickmansworth
Hertfordshire WD3 6AU, United
Kingdom
+44 (0)192 326 8641

http://cfsrf.org.uk/

Chronic Fatigue Research and
Treatment Unit at King's College
London
Mapother House, 1st Floor
De Crespigny Park
Denmark Hill
London, United Kingdom SE5
8AZ
+44 (0)203 228 5075
Fax: +44 (0)203 228 5074
www.kcl.ac.uk/innovation/groups/
projects/cfs/index.aspx

Chronic Fatigue Syndrome,
Fibromyalgia & Chemical
Sensitivity Coalition of Chicago
PO Box 277
Wilmette, IL 60091
(773) 650-1332
www.cfccc.net

Chronic Pain and Fatigue
Research Center at University of
Michigan Health System
24 Frank Lloyd Wright Dr.
Ann Arbor, MI 48106
(734) 998-6939
Fax: (734) 998-6900
www.med.umich.edu/painre-
search

The Connecticut CFIDS & FM
Association, Inc.
PO Box 3010
Milford, CT 06460
(800) 952-2037

www.ct-cfids-fm.org

FM-CFS Canada
310-1500 Bank Street
Ottawa, Ontario K1H 1B8
(877) 437-4673
office@fm-cfs.ca
http://fm-cfs.ca

International Association for
Chronic Fatigue Syndrome/ Myalgic Encephalomyelitis
27 N. Wacker Dr., Suite 416
Chicago, IL 60606
(847) 258-7248
Fax: (847) 579-0975
admin@iacfsme.org
www.iacfsme.org

Invest in ME
PO Box 561
Eastleigh SO50 0GQ
Hampshire
United Kingdom
+44 (0) 238 025 1719
Fax: +44 (0) 238 000 0040
www.investinme.org

Irish ME Trust
Carmichael House
North Brunswick Street
Dublin 7
00 353 1 401 3629
Fax: 00 353 1 401 3736
info@imet.ie
www.imet.ie

Massachusetts CFIDS/ME & FM
Association
PO Box 690305
Quincy, MA 02269
(617) 471-5559
www.masscfids.org

ME Association
7 Apollo Office Court
Radclive Road
Gawcott, Bucks MK18 4DF
United Kingdom
+44 (0)128 081 8964
admin@meassociation.org.uk
www.meassociation.org.uk

ME Research UK
The Gateway, North Methven St.
Perth PH1 5PP, United Kingdom
+44 (0)173 845 1234
editor@meresearch.org.uk

ME/CFS Australia Ltd.
2/240 Chapel Street
PRAHAN VIC 3181
+61 (03) 9529 1344
www.mecfs.org.au

ME/CFS Foreningen
Radhustorvet 1, 1
Sal 3520 Farum
44 95 97 00
mail@me-cfs.dk
www.me-cfs.dk

ME/CFS Society WA
The Centre for Neurological
Support

The Niche, 11 Aberdare Road
Nedlands, Perth
Western Australia 6009
+61 (08) 9346 7477
Fax: +61 (08) 9346 7534
www.mecfswa.org.au

ME/CFS/FM Support Association
Qld Inc.
St. Vincents Hospital
Scott Street, Toowoomba
Queensland 4350, Australia
+61 (07) 4632 8173
Fax: +61 (07) 4632 8173
www.mecfsfmq.org.au/

The National CFIDS Foundation
103 Aletha Rd.
Needham, MA 02492
(781) 449-3535
Fax: (781) 449-8606
info@ncf-net.org
www.ncf-net.org

New Jersey Chronic Fatigue
Syndrome Association, Inc.
PO Box 477
Florham Park, NJ 07932
(888) 835-3677
www.njcfsa.org

Nightingale Research Foundation
121 Iona St.
Ottawa Ontario K1Y 3M1
Canada
www.nigthingale.ca

Partnership for Research in CFS
and ME (PRIME)
Minervation Ltd.
Salter's Boat Yard
Folly Bridge
Oxford OX1 4LB
www.prime-cfs.org

Simmaron Research Foundation
948 Incline Way
Incline Village, NV 89451
(775) 298-0030
Fax: (775) 298-0031
redefiningmecfs@gmail.com
http://simmaronresearch.org

Stanford Myalgic Encephalomye-
litis/Chronic Fatigue Syndrome
(ME/CFS) Initiative at Stanford
University of Medicine
291 Campus Drive Rm LK3C02

Li Ka Shing Building, 3rd floor
Stanford, CA 94305
(650) 725-3900
http://chronicfatigue.stanford.edu/

Whitmore Peterson Institute for
Neuro-Immune Disease at
University of Nevada
1664 N. Virginia St.
Reno, NV 89557
(775) 682-8250
Fax: +1 (775) 682-8258
info@wpinstitute.org
www.wpinstitute.org

Wisconsin ME/CFS Association,
Inc.
733 Lois Dr.
Sun Prairie, WI 53590
(608) 834-1001
www.wicfs-me.org

# APPENDIX C

## Chronic Fatigue Syndrome–Related Organizations

California Capital CFIDS
Association (CCCA)
PO Box 660362
Sacramento, CA 95866
(916) 484-3788
CalCapitalCFIDS@bigfoot.com
www.ottem.org

Central Virginia Chronic Fatigue
Syndrome and Fibromyalgia
Association
PO Box 5733
Charlottesville, VA 22905
(434) 984-3419
cfsfma@avenue.org
www.cfsfma.avenue.org

CFIDS Association of America
6827 Colony Fairview Dr.
Charlotte, NC 28210
(704) 364-0016
CFIDS@CFIDS.ORG

www.cfids.org

Chronic Fatigue Syndrome/
Fibromyalgia Organization
of Georgia, Inc.
1210 Wooten Lake Rd. NW
Kennesaw, GA 30144
(770) 974-0157
www.cfog.us

Chronic Syndrome Support
Association, Inc.
801 Riverside Drive
Lumberton, NC 28358
www.cssa-inc.org

Connecticut CFIDS & FM
Association, Inc.
PO Box 3010
Milford, CT 06460
(800) 952-2037
www.ct-cfids-fm.org

Fibromyalgia Network
PO Box 31750
Tucson, AZ 85751
(520) 290-5508
www.fmnetnews.com

International Association for CFS/
ME
27 N. Wacker Dr., Suite 416
Chicago, IL 60606
(847) 258-7248
Fax: (847) 579-0975
admin@iacfsme.org
www.iacfsme.org

Las Vegas Fibromyalgia/Chronic
Fatigue Syndrome Support Group
4308 Rosebank Circle
Las Vegas, NV 89108
(702) 647-4791
shebrews@yahoo.com

Massachusetts CFIDS/ME & FM
Association
PO Box 690305
Quincy, MA 02269
(617) 471-5559
www.masscfids.org

National CFIDS Foundation, Inc.
103 Aletha Rd.
Needham, MA 02492
(781) 449-3535
Fax: (781) 449-8606
info@ncf-net.org
www.ncf-net.org

National Fibromyalgia
Partnership, Inc.
140 Zinn Way
Linden, VA 22642
www.fmpartnership.org

New Jersey Chronic Fatigue
Syndrome Association, Inc.
PO Box 477
Florham Park, NJ 07932
( 888) 835-3677
pegwalk@aol.com
www.njcfsa.org

Open Medicine Institute
2500 Hospital Dr., Bldg. 2
Mountain View, CA 94040
(650) 691-8633
Fax: (650) 644-3223
info@openmedicineinstitute.org
www.openmedicineinstitute.org

Organization for Fatigue &
Fibromyalgia Education & Research
1002 E. South Temple, Suite 408
Salt Lake City, UT 84102
support@OfferUtah.org
www.offerutah.org

Rocky Mountain CFS/ME & FM
Association
7020 E Girard Ave., Suite 207
Denver, CO 80224
(303) 423-7367
link@rmcfa.org
www.rmcfa.org

Wisconsin Myalgic Encephalom-
yelitis/Chronic Fatigue Syndrome
Association, Inc.
733 Lois Dr.

Sun Prairie, WI 53590
(608) 834-1001
www.wicfs-me.org

# APPENDIX D

## Nationally Recognized Chronic Fatigue Syndrome Clinics

Alternatives: A Center for
Conscious Health
11036 Oak St.
Rockbrook Village
Omaha, NE 68144
(402) 827-9450
Fax: (402) 827-9471
info@alternativesomaha.com
www.centerforconscioushealth
.com

Amen Clinic
1000 Marina Blvd.
Brisbane, CA, 94005
(650) 416-7830
Fax: (650) 871-8874
www.amenclinics.com

Annapolis Integrative Medicine
1819 Bay Ridge Ave., Suite 200
Annapolis, MD 21403

(410) 266-3613
Fax: (410) 266-6104
www.annapolisintegrative
medicine.com

Austin Family Practice
11410 Jolleyville Rd.
Austin, TX 78759
(512) 346-3637
www.robertthoresondo.com

Barrow Neurological Institute
350 West Thomas Rd.
Phoenix, AZ 85013
(602) 406-6281
www.thebarrow.org

Black Bear Naturopathic Clinic
2831 Fort Missoula Rd, Suite 105
Missoula, MT 59804
(406) 542-2147

Fax: (406) 728-0978
www.blackbearnaturopaths.com

Boston Medical Center
840 Harrison Ave.
Boston, MA 02118
(617) 638-8000
www.bmc.org

Caring Counselor
Boulder, CO 80304
(303) 413-8091
pat@caringcounselor.com
www.caringcounselor.com

Celebration of Health Association
122 Thurman St.
Bluffton, OH 45817
(800) 788-4627
Fax: (419) 358-1855
mail@healthcelebration.com
www.healthcelebration.com

Center for Integrative Medicine
81 Hall St., Suite 1
Concord, NH 03301
(603) 228-7600
www.cfim.org

Charles R. Meyers, LAC
Acupuncture and Traditional
Chinese Medicine
2 West Park St.
Lebanon, NH 03766
(603) 442-9535
chas@charlesmeyerstcm.com
www.charlesmeyerstcm.com

Cheney Clinic
80 Peachtree Rd., Suite 208
Asheville, NC 28803
(828) 274-6665
Fax: (828) 274-6917
ddamron@cheneyclinic.com
www.cheneyclinic.com

Choices Integrative Healthcare
95 Soldiers Pass Rd., Suite B
Sedona, AZ 86336
(928) 203-4844
www.choiceshealthcare.com

Chronic Fatigue Clinic
Stanford School of Medicine
300 Pasteur Dr.
Stanford, CA 94305
(650) 723-6961
Fax: (650) 725-8418
www.chronicfatigue.stanford.edu

Chronic Fatigue Clinic at
Harborview
Harborview Medical Center
325 Ninth Ave., 7th Floor, Maleng
Building
Seattle, WA 98104
(206) 520-5000
www.uwmedicine.org

Cleveland Clinic
9500 Euclid Ave.
Cleveland, OH 44195
(216) 444–2200
www.clevelandclinic.org

Combined Health Care

Professionals
5140 NE Antioch Rd.
Kansas City, MO 64119
(816) 453-5545
www.drnancy.com

Connecticut Center for Health
87 Bernie O'Rourke Dr.
Middletown, CT 06457
(860) 347-8600
Fax: (860) 347-8434
www.connecticutcenterforhealth.
com

Dakota Medical Clinic
3408 Dakota Ave. South
St. Louis Park, MN 55416
(952) 924-1053
Fax: (952) 924-0254
www.dakotamc.com

Dallas Neurological Associates
403 West Campbell Rd., Suite 400
Richardson, TX 75080
(972) 783-8900
Fax: (972) 644-7926
www.dallasneurological.com

Dr. George J. Juetersonke
LifePulse Practice
3525 American Dr.
Colorado Springs, CO 80917
(719) 597-6075
Fax: (719) 573-6529
www.juetersonke.com


Dr. Teitelbaum's Clinic

Benmere Rd.
Glen Burnie, MD 21060
(410) 573-5389
Fax: 410-590-3047
office@endfatigue.com
www.endfatigue.com

Environmental Health and
Allergy Center
11585 W Florissant Ave.
Florissant, MO 63033
(314) 921-5600
Fax: (314) 921-8273
ehacstl@ehacstl.com
www.ehacstl.com

Fatigue Clinic of Michigan
G3494 Beecher Rd.
Flint, MI 48522
(810) 230-8677
www.cfids.com

Fatigue Consultation Clinic
1002 E South Temple St., Suite
408
Salt Lake City, UT 84102
(801) 359-7400
Fax: (801) 359-7404
FatigueConsultationClin-
ic@gmail.com
www.fcclinic.com

Fibromyalgia and Chronic
Fatigue Syndrome: Life Balance
PO Box 583
Stony Brook, NY 11790
(516) 702-4213
info@lifebalance7.com

www.lifebalance7.com

Fibromyalgia Treatment &
Learning Center
650 University Ave., Suite 200
Sacramento, CA 95825
(916) 922-8400
www.fmtlc.com

Four Rivers Naturopathic Clinic,
PC
1449 Lincoln Way
Auburn, CA 95603
(530) 823-1335
www.fourriversclinic.com

Gordon Medical Associates
3471 Regional Parkway
Santa Rosa, CA 95403
(707) 575- 5180
Fax: (707) 575- 5509
info@gordonmedical.com
www.gordonmedical.com

Greenhouse Naturopathic
Medicine
Spruce Park Professional Center
109 Ponemah Road, Suite 9
Amherst, NH 03031
(603) 249-5771
Fax: (603) 249-5924
www.greenhousemedicine.com

GW Medical Faculty Associates
2150 Pennsylvania Ave., NW
Washington, DC 20037
(202) 741-3000
www.gwdocs.com

Healing Arts Medical Center
Heights Medical Tower
427 W 20th St., Suite 602
Houston, TX 77008
(713) 802-1177
Fax: (713) 802-1277
info@awakenhealth.com
www.awakenhealth.com

Health Equations
PO Box 323
Newfane, VT 05345
(802) 365-9213
Fax: (802) 365-9218
service@healthequations.com
www.healthequations.com

Health for Life
2302 Amstel Lane
Vista, CA 92084
(760) 586-2627
info@alternativehealthandhealing.
com
www.alternativehealthandhealing.
com

Hillside Center for Behavioral
Services
8435 Holly Rd.
Grand Blanc, MI 48439
(810) 424-2400
www.genesys.org

Huber Natural Health, LLC
289 Main St.
Salem, NH 03079
(603) 890-9900

info@hubernaturalhealth.com
www.hubernaturalhealth.com

Hunter-Hopkins Center
7421 Carmel Executive Park Dr.
Charlotte, NC 28226
(704) 543-9692
drlapp@drlapp.net
www.drlapp.com

Infinity Wellness Center
205 Wild Basin Road S, Suite 2B
Austin, TX 78746
(512) 328-0505
info@austinholisticdr.com
www.austinholisticdr.com

Integrative Chiropractor Beverly
Hills
60 S Beverly Dr.
Beverly Hills, CA 90212
(310) 282-8882
www.wholebodycures.com

Integrative Healing Center
403 Main St., Suite 1
Port Washington, NY 11050
(516) 676-0200
Fax: (516) 676-2809
www.getintegrativehealth.com

Integrative Health Care of
Winona
356 E Sarnia St.
Winona, MN 55987
(507) 457-9000
Fax: (507) 457-9001
frontdesk@karenvrchota.com

www.karenvrchota.com

Jace Wellness Center
10843 Magnolia Blvd., Suite 1
North Hollywood, CA 91601
(818) 505-8610
www.jacemedical.com

Jeanne Hubbuch Family Practice
124 Watertown St., #2F
Watertown, MA 02472
(617) 744-0401
Fax: (617) 744-5346
drhubbuch@aol.com
www.drhubbuch.com

Johns Hopkins Medicine
1800 Orleans St.
Baltimore, MD 21287
(410) 955-5000
www.hopkinsmedicine.org

Lester Clinic
3700 Thomas Rd., #207
Santa Clara, CA 95054
(408) 844-0010
lesterclinic@gmail.com
www.lesterclinic.com

Manhattan Integrative Medicine
841 Broadway, 60th St., Suite
1012
New York, NY 10023
(917) 261-3771
Fax: (212) 262-2416
www.davidborensteinmd.com

Mary Claire Wise, MD

Holistic Medicine
4138 W Henrietta Rd.
Rochester, NY 14623
(585) 334-8020
marywisemd@yahoo.com
www.drmarywise.com

Mayo Clinic
13400 E Shea Blvd.
Scottsdale, AZ 85259
(480) 301-8000
Fax: (480) 301-9310
www.mayoclinic.org

Minneapolis Clinic of Neurology
4225 Golden Valley Rd.
Golden Valley, MN 55422
(763) 588-0661
www.minneapolisclinic.com

Nathanael Medical Center
1435 W Main St.
Dothan, AL 36301
(334) 702-8872
www.nathanaelmedicalcenter.com

Natural Health Medical Center,
Inc.
4469 Redondo Beach Blvd.
Lawndale, CA 90260
(310) 479-2266
Fax: (310) 479-2044
drhoang@naturalhealthmedical
center.com
www.naturalhealthmedicalcenter.
com

New Jersey's Family Holistic
Health & Acupuncture Center
206 Broad St.
Red Bank, NJ 07701
(732) 219-1900
info@NJHolistic.net
www.njholistic.net

New Seasons Natural Medicine
5 Oak Hill Rd.
Harvard, MA 01451
(978) 456-7789
Fax: (978) 456-7790
Janet@JanetBeaty.com
www.janetbeaty.com

New York ME/CFS Center
860 Fifth Ave., Suite 1C
New York, NY 10065
(212) 794-2000
Fax: (212) 327-2125
www.enlander.com

North Coast Family Health
500 Market St., Suite 1F
Portsmouth, NH 03801
(603) 427-6800
Fax: (603) 427-2801
info@naturopathic-doctors.com
www.naturopathic-doctors.com

Northampton Wellness Associates
395 Pleasant St.
Northampton, MA 01060
(413) 584-7787
Fax: (413) 584-7778
www.northamptonwellness.com

Perlmutter Health Center
800 Goodlette Rd. N, Suite 270
Naples, FL 34102
(239) 649-7400
Fax: (239) 649-6370
newpatient@perlhealth.com
www.perlhealth.com

Plymouth Integrative Medicine
Center
36650 Five Mile Rd., Suite 100
Livonia, MI 48154
(734) 432-1900
info@doctormetro.com
www.doctormetro.com

Rothfeld Center & Apothecary
411 Waverley Oaks Rd., Building
3, Suite 319
Waltham, MA 02452
(781) 736-1901
Fax: (781) 736-1911
info@rothfeldcenter.com
wholehealthne.com

Tahoma Clinic
6839 Fort Dent Way, #134
Tukwila, WA 98188
(206) 812-9988
Fax: (206) 812-9989
www.tahomaclinic.com

Tracy Darling, MD
Integrative Nutritional Medicine
31639 South Coast Hwy.
Laguna Beach, CA 92651
(949) 610-9950
Fax: (949) 612-6392

doc@darlingmd.com
www.darlingmd.com

Treatment Center for Chronic Fatigue Syndrome (CFS)
A. Martin Lerner, MD, MACP
32804 Pierce Rd.
Beverly Hills, MI 48025
(248) 540-9866
Fax: (248) 540-0139
drlerner@treatmentcenter
forcfs.com
www.treatmentcenterforcfs.com

UCSF Medical Center
500 Parnassus Ave.
San Francisco, CA 94143
(415) 476-1000
www.ucsfhealth.org

University of Maryland Medical
Center (UMMC)
22 S Greene St.
Baltimore, MD 21201
(410) 328-1500
webmaster@umms.org
www.umm.edu

University of Oklahoma College
of Medicine
Department of Neurology
1100 N Lindsay Ave.
Oklahoma City, OK 73104
(405) 271-4000
www.oumedicine.com

University of Pittsburgh Medical
Center (UPMC)

200 Lothrop St.
Pittsburgh, PA 15213
(412) 647-2345
www.upmc.edu

The Wellness Pros
471 Division St.
Campbell, CA 95008
(408) 871-8222
wellnesspros1@gmail.com
www.brainbasedcare.com

Whole Health Chicago
2522 North Lincoln Ave.
Chicago, IL 60614
(773) 296-6700
Fax: (773) 296-1131
www.wholehealthchicago.com

Winchester Natural Health Associates
10 Converse Place
Winchester, MA 01890
(781) 721-4585
Fax: (781) 569-0405
wnha@winchesternaturalhealth
.com
www.winchesternaturalhealth
.com

Woodlands Medical Center
5724 Clymer Rd.
Quakertown, PA 18951
( 215) 536-1890
Fax: (215) 529-9034
www.woodmed.com

# APPENDIX E

## For Further Reading

Bell, David S. *The Doctor's Guide to Chronic Fatigue Syndrome: Understanding, Treating, and Living with CFIDS.* Boston: Da Capo Press, 1995.

Bested, Alison, Russell Howe, and Alan Logan. *Hope and Help for Chronic Fatigue Syndrome and Fibromyalgia.* Nashville, TN: Cumberland House, 2008.

Campling, Frankie, and Michael Sharpe. *Chronic Fatigue Syndrome.* 2nd ed. New York: Oxford University Press, 2008.

Colbert, Don. *The New Bible Cure for Chronic Fatigue & Fibromyalgia: Ancient Truths, Natural Remedies, and the Latest Findings for Your Health Today.* Lake Mary, FL: Charisma House, 2011.

Cooper, Celeste, and Jeffrey Miller. *Integrative Therapies for Fibromyalgia, Chronic Fatigue Syndrome, and Myofascial Pain: The Mind-Body Connection.* Rochester, VT: Inner Traditions International, 2010.

Cox, Diane. *Occupational Therapy and Chronic Fatigue Syndrome.* Hoboken, NJ: John Wiley & Sons, 2000.

Craggs-Hinton, Christine. *How to Manage Chronic Fatigue.* New York: Perseus Book Group, 2012.

Dantini, Daniel C. *The New Fibromyalgia Remedy: Stop Your Pain Now with an Anti-Viral Regimen.* Omaha, NE: Addicus Books, 2008.

Engdahl, Sylvia. *Chronic Fatigue Syndrome.* Farmington Hills, MI: Greenhaven Press, 2012.

Englebienne, Patrick, and Kenny De Meirleir. *Chronic Fatigue Syndrome: A Biological Approach.* Boca Raton, FL: CRC Press, 2002.

Friedberg, Fred. *Coping with Chronic Fatigue Syndrome: Nine Things You Can Do.* Oakland, CA: New Harbinger Publications, 1995.

Jason, Leonard A., Patricia A. Fennell, and Renée R. Taylor. *Handbook of Chronic Fatigue Syndrome.* Hoboken, NJ: John Wiley & Sons, 2003.

Kenny, Timothy, and Paul R. Cheney. *Living with Chronic Fatigue Syndrome: A Personal Story of the Struggle for Recovery.* New York: Thunder's Mouth Press, 1994.

Montero, Roberto Patarca. *Chronic Fatigue Syndrome and the Body's Immune Defense System: What Does the Research Say?* Boca Raton, FL: CRC Press, 2002.

Montero, Roberto Patarca, and Kenny De Meirleir. *Chronic Fatigue Syndrome: Critical Reviews and Clinical Advances—What Does the Research Say?* Boca Raton, FL: CRC Press, 2000.

Murphree, Rodger H. *Treating and Beating Fibromyalgia and Chronic Fatigue Syndrome: A Step-by-Step Program Proven to Help You Get Well Again.* New York: Harrison & Hampton Publishing, 2008.

Pall, Martin. *Explaining Unexplained Illnesses: Disease Paradigm for Chronic Fatigue Syndrome, Multiple Chemical Sensitivity, Fibromyalgia, Post-Traumatic Stress Disorder, Gulf War Syndrome and Others.* Boca Raton, FL: CRC Press, 2007.

Perrin, Raymond. *The Perrin Technique: How to Beat Chronic Fatigue Syndrome/ME.* New York: Perseus Book Group, 2007.

Shlomo, Yehuda, and David I. Mostofsky. *Chronic Fatigue Syndrome.* New York: Plenum Press, 1997.

Shomon, Mary J. *Living Well with Chronic Fatigue Syndrome and Fibromyalgia: What Your Doctor Doesn't Tell You . . . That You Need to Know.* New York: Harper Collins Publishers, 2004.

Skloot, Floyd . *The Night-Side: Chronic Fatigue Syndrome & the Illness Experience.* Brownsville, OR: Story Line, 1996.

Stoff, Jesse A. *Chronic Fatigue Syndrome.* New York: Harper Perennial, 1992.

Taylor, Renee R. *Cognitive Behavioral Therapy for Chronic Illness and Disability.* New York: Springer, 2006.

Toenjes, Annette. *Musician, Heal Thyself! An Alternative Approach to Conquering Chronic Fatigue Syndrome.* Mustang, OK: Tate Publishing, 2014.

Wessely, Simon, Matthew Hotopf, and Michael Sharpe. *Chronic Fatigue and Its Syndromes.* New York: Oxford University Press, 1999.

# NOTES

## PREFACE

1. "Chronic Fatigue Syndrome," accessed May 17, 2014, www.nhs.uk/conditions/Chronic-fatigue-syndrome/Pages/Introduction.aspx; "Chronic Fatigue Syndrome," accessed May 17, 2014, www.cdc.gov/cfs.

2. "Chronic Fatigue Syndrome," accessed May 17, 2014, www.patient.co.uk/doctor/chronic-fatigue-syndrome.

3. "Chronic Fatigue Syndrome," accessed May 17, 2014, www.cdc.gov/cfs; "Chronic Fatigue Syndrome," accessed May 17, 2014, www.mayoclinic.org/diseases-conditions/chronic-fatigue-syndrome/basics/definition/con-20022009.

4. "Chronic Fatigue Syndrome," accessed May 17, 2014, www.mayoclinic.org/diseases-conditions/chronic-fatigue-syndrome/basics/definition/con-20022009.

5. "Chronic Fatigue Syndrome," accessed May 17, 2014, www.patient.co.uk/doctor/chronic-fatigue-syndrome.

6. "Chronic Fatigue Syndrome," accessed May 17, 2014, www.patient.co.uk/doctor/chronic-fatigue-syndrome.

7. "Chronic Fatigue Syndrome," accessed May 17, 2014, www.cdc.gov/cfs.

8. "Chronic Fatigue Syndrome," accessed May 17, 2014, www.patient.co.uk/doctor/chronic-fatigue-syndrome.

9. "Chronic Fatigue Syndrome," accessed May 17, 2014, www.patient.co.uk/doctor/chronic-fatigue-syndrome.

10. "Chronic Fatigue Syndrome," accessed May 17, 2014, www.cdc.gov/cfs.

11. "Chronic Fatigue Syndrome," accessed May 17, 2014, www.mayoclinic.org/diseases-conditions/chronic-fatigue-syndrome/basics/definition/con-20022009; "Chronic Fatigue Syndrome," accessed May 17, 2014,

www.nhs.uk/conditions/Chronic-fatigue-syndrome/Pages/Introduction.aspx; "Chronic Fatigue Syndrome," accessed May 17, 2014, www.cdc.gov/cfs.

12. "Chronic Fatigue Syndrome," accessed May 17, 2014, www.cdc.gov/cfs; "Chronic Fatigue Syndrome," accessed May 17, 2014, www.mayoclinic.org/diseases-conditions/chronic-fatigue-syndrome/basics/definition/con-20022009; "Chronic Fatigue Syndrome," accessed May 17, 2014, www.patient.co.uk/doctor/chronic-fatigue-syndrome.

13. "Chronic Fatigue Syndrome," accessed May 17, 2014, www.patient.co.uk/doctor/chronic-fatigue-syndrome.

14. "Chronic Fatigue Syndrome," accessed May 17, 2014, www.cdc.gov/cfs; "Chronic Fatigue Syndrome," accessed May 17, 2014, www.nlm.nih.gov/medlineplus/chronicfatiguesyndrome.html.

15. "Chronic Fatigue Syndrome," accessed May 17, 2014, www.cdc.gov/cfs.

16. "Chronic Fatigue Syndrome," accessed May 17, 2014, www.cdc.gov/cfs; "Chronic Fatigue Syndrome," accessed May 17, 2014, www.patient.co.uk/doctor/chronic-fatigue-syndrome.

17. "Chronic Fatigue Syndrome," accessed May 17, 2014, www.mayoclinic.org/diseases-conditions/chronic-fatigue-syndrome/basics/definition/con-20022009.

18. "Chronic Fatigue Syndrome," accessed May 17, 2014, www.mayoclinic.org/diseases-conditions/chronic-fatigue-syndrome/basics/definition/con-20022009.

19. "Chronic Fatigue Syndrome," accessed May 17, 2014, www.mayoclinic.org/diseases-conditions/chronic-fatigue-syndrome/basics/definition/con-20022009.

20. "Chronic Fatigue Syndrome," accessed May 17, 2014, www.nhs.uk/conditions/Chronic-fatigue-syndrome/Pages/Introduction.aspx.

21. D. Dorland, *Dorland's Illustrated Medical Dictionary*, 32nd ed. (New York: Elsevier Saunders), 167.

22. "Disease—Definition," accessed May 30, 2014, www.biology-online.org/dictionary/Disease.

23. "Chronic Fatigue Syndrome," accessed May 17, 2014, www.nhs.uk/conditions/Chronic-fatigue-syndrome/Pages/Introduction.aspx; "Chronic Fatigue Syndrome," accessed May 17, 2014, www.mayoclinic.org/diseases-conditions/chronic-fatigue-syndrome/basics/definition/con-20022009.

## I. ENERGY AND THE HUMAN BODY

1. J. Stedman, *Stedman's Medical Dictionary for the Health Professions and Nursing* (Baltimore: Lippincott Williams & Wilkins, 2005), 478.

2. National Sleep Foundation, "White Paper: Consequences of Drowsy Driving," accessed July 31, 2014, www.sleepfoundation.org.

3. H. Hildebrandt, M. Nübling, and V. Candia, "Increment of Fatigue, Depression, and Stage Fright during the First Year of High-level Education in Music Students," *Medical Problems of Performing Arts* 27, no. 1 (2012): 43–48.

4. G. Halvani, M. Zare, and S. Mirmohammadi, "The Relation between Shift Work, Sleepiness, Fatigue and Accidents in Iranian Industrial Mining Group Workers," *Industrial Health* 47, no. 2 (2009): 134–38.

5. B. Kozier, G. Erb, A. Berman, and S. Snyder, *Fundamentals of Nursing: Concepts, Process, and Practice* (Upper Saddle River, NJ: Pearson/Prentice Hall, 2004), 451; J. Stedman, *Stedman's Medical Dictionary for the Health Professions and Nursing* (Baltimore: Lippincott Williams & Wilkins, 2005), 1213.

6. K. Denniston, J. Topping, and R. Caret, *General, Organic, and Biochemistry* (New York: McGraw-Hill, 2007), 28.

7. B. Kozier, G. Erb, A. Berman, and S. Snyder, *Fundamentals of Nursing: Concepts, Process, and Practice* (Upper Saddle River, NJ: Pearson/Prentice Hall, 2004), 1077.

8. M. Cohen, B. Del Giorno, J. Harlan, A. McCormack, and J. Staver, *Science* (Glenview, IL: Scott Foresman & Co., 1984), 193.

9. M. Cohen, B. Del Giorno, J. Harlan, A. McCormack, and J. Staver, *Science* (Glenview, IL: Scott Foresman & Co., 1984), 6–7.

10. K. Denniston, J. Topping, and R. Caret, *General, Organic, and Biochemistry* (New York: McGraw-Hill, 2007), 28.

11. N. Campbell and J. Reece, *Essentials of Biology* (Singapore: Jurong, 2007), 1026; J. Stedman, *Stedman's Medical Dictionary for the Health Professions and Nursing* (Baltimore: Lippincott Williams & Wilkins, 2005), 155.

12. S. Smeltzer, B. Bare, J. Hinkle, and K. Cheever, *Brunner & Suddarth's Textbook of Medical-Surgical Nursing* (Baltimore: Lippincott Williams & Wilkins, 2008), 2129.

13. S. Smeltzer, B. Bare, J. Hinkle, and K. Cheever, *Brunner & Suddarth's Textbook of Medical-Surgical Nursing* (Baltimore: Lippincott Williams & Wilkins, 2008), 553.

14. L. Segers, R. Shannon, and B. Lindsey, "Interactions between Rostral Pontine and Ventral Medullary Respiratory Neurons," *Journal of Neurophysiology* 54, no. 2 (1985): 318–34.

15. N. Campbell and J. Reece, *Essentials of Biology* (Singapore: Jurong, 2007), 890.

16. S. Smeltzer, B. Bare, J. Hinkle, and K. Cheever, *Brunner & Suddarth's Textbook of Medical-Surgical Nursing* (Baltimore: Lippincott Williams & Wilkins, 2008), 2337–38.

## 2. HISTORY OF CHRONIC FATIGUE SYNDROME

1. L. Lorusso, S. Mikhaylova, E. Capelli, D. Ferrari, G. Ngonga, and G. Ricevuti, "Immunological Aspects of Chronic Fatigue Syndrome," *Autoimmunity Reviews* 8, no. 4 (2009): 287–91.

2. G. Holmes, J. Kaplan, N. Gantz, A. Komaroff, L. Schonberger, S. Straus, J. Jones, R. Dubois, C. Cunningham-Rundles, and S. Pahwa, "Chronic Fatigue Syndrome: A Working Case Definition," *Annals of Internal Medicine* 108, no. 3 (1988): 387– 89.

3. R. Manningham, *The Symptoms, Nature, Causes and Cure of the Februlica or Little Fever; Commonly Called the Nervous or Hysteric Fever; The Fever On The Spirits; Vapours, Hypo or Spleen* (London, 1750), 52– 53.

4. H. Deale and S. Adams, "Neurasthenia in Young Women," *American Journal of the Medical Sciences* 107, no. 4 (1894): 441.

5. G. Beard, "Neurasthenia, or Nervous Exhaustion," *The Boston Medical and Surgical Journal* (1869): 217–21.

6. H. Deale and S. Adams, "Neurasthenia in Young Women," *American Journal of the Medical Sciences* 107, no. 4 (1894): 441.

7. C. Neu, "Treatment and Management of the Neurasthenic Individual," in *Chronic Fatigue and Its Syndromes*, ed. S. Wessely, M. Hotopf, and M. Sharpe (Oxford: Oxford University Press, 1998), 106.

8. D. Young, "Florence Nightingale's Fever," *British Medical Journal* 311 (1995): 1697–1700.

9. S. Wessely, M. Hotopf, and M. Sharpe, eds., *Chronic Fatigue and Its Syndromes* (Oxford: Oxford University Press, 1998), 106.

10. D. Young, "Florence Nightingale's Fever," *British Medical Journal* 311 (1995): 1697–1700.

11. D. Young, "Florence Nightingale's Fever," *British Medical Journal* 311 (1995): 1697–1700.

12. D. Young, "Florence Nightingale's Fever," *British Medical Journal* 311 (1995): 1697–1700.

13. B. Evengard, R. Schacterle, and A. Komaroff, "Chronic Fatigue Syndrome: New Insights and Old Ignorance," *Journal of Internal Medicine* 246, no. 5 (1999): 455–69.

14. International Classification of Diseases, Tenth Revision (ICD-10) (Geneva: World Health Organization, 1992); J. Flaskerud, "Neurasthenia: Here and There, Now and Then," *Issues in Mental Health Nursing* 28, no. 6 (2007): 657–59.

15. A. MacIntyre, *M.E.: Chronic Fatigue Syndrome—A Practical Guide* (New York: Thorsons, 1998).

16. R. Patarca-Montero, *Medical Etiology, Assessment, and Treatment of Chronic Fatigue and Malaise* (Philadelphia: Haworth Press, 2004) 6–7.

17. A. Gilliam, "Epidemiological Study of an Epidemic Diagnosed as Poliomyelitis Occurring among the Personnel of the Los Angeles County General Hospital during the Summer of 1934," *Public Health Bulletin* 240 (1938).

18. R. Blattner, "Benign Myalgic Encephalomyelitis (Akureyri Disease, Iceland Disease)," *Journal of Pediatrics* 49, no. 4 (1956): 504–6.

19. A. MacIntyre, *M.E.: Chronic Fatigue Syndrome—A Practical Guide* (New York: Thorsons, 1998).

20. B. Sigurdsson, J. Sigursonsson, J. Sigurdsson, J. Thorkelsson, and K. Gudmondsson, "A Disease Epidemic in Iceland Simulating Poliomyelitis," *American Journal of Epidemiology* (1950): 222–38.

21. S. Wessely, *Chronic Fatigue and Its Syndromes* (Oxford: Oxford University Press, 1998), 105.

22. J. Parish, "Early Outbreaks of 'Epidemic Neuromyasthenia,'" *Postgraduate Medical Journal* 54, no. 637 (1978): 711– 17.

23. J. Parish, "Early Outbreaks of 'Epidemic Neuromyasthenia,'" *Postgraduate Medical Journal* 54, no. 637 (1978): 711– 17.

24. M. Ramsay, "Myalgic Encephalomyelitis: A Baffling Syndrome with a Tragic Aftermath," accessed June 24, 2014, www.meactionuk.org.uk/ramsey.html.

25. M. Ramsay, "Myalgic Encephalomyelitis: A Baffling Syndrome with a Tragic Aftermath," accessed June 24, 2014, www.meactionuk.org.uk/ramsey.html.

26. C. Shepherd, *Living with M.E.* (London: Vermillion, 1999), 21.

27. P. Levine, P. Snow, B. Ranum, C. Paul, and M. Holmes, "Epidemic Neuromyasthenia and Chronic Fatigue Syndrome in West Otago, New Zealand: A 10-year Follow-up," *Archives of Internal Medicine* 157, no. 7 (1997): 750–54.

28. N. Hashimoto, "History of Chronic Fatigue Syndrome [Article in Japanese]," *Nihon Rinsho* 65, no. 6 (2007): 975– 82.

29. N. Hashimoto, "History of Chronic Fatigue Syndrome [Article in Japanese]," *Nihon Rinsho* 65, no. 6 (2007): 975– 82.

30. N. Hashimoto, "History of Chronic Fatigue Syndrome [Article in Japanese]," *Nihon Rinsho* 65, no. 6 (2007): 975– 82.

31. W. Day, "Raggedy Ann Syndrome," *Hippocrates* July/August (1987).

32. C. Mulrow, G. Ramirez, J. Cornell, and K. Allsup, "Defining and Managing Chronic Fatigue Syndrome: Summary," in *AHRQ Evidence Report Summaries* (Rockville, MD: Agency for Healthcare Research and Quality, 1998–2005).

33.  P. Levine, J. Dale, E. Benson-Grigg, S. Fritz, S. Grufferman, and S. Straus, "A Cluster of Cases of Chronic Fatigue and Chronic Fatigue Syndrome: Clinical and Immunologic Studies," *Clinical Infectious Diseases* 23, no. 2 (1996): 408– 9.

34.  G. Holmes, J. Kaplan, N. Gantz, A. Komaroff, L. Schonberger, S. Straus, J. Jones, R. Dubois, C. Cunningham-Rundles, and S. Pahwa, "Chronic Fatigue Syndrome: A Working Case Definition," *Annals of Internal Medicine* 108, no. 3 (1988): 387 – 89.

35.  Tim Field Foundation, "Bullying, Stress and the Effects of Stress on Health: The Injury to Health Caused by Prolonged Negative Stress Including Fatigue, Anxiety, Depression, Immune System Suppression, IBS, Aches, Pains, Numbness and Panic Attacks," accessed August 21, 2014, www.bullyonline.org/stress/health.htm.

36.  J. Richman and L. Jason, "Gender Biases Underlying the Social Construction of Illness States: The Case of Chronic Fatigue Syndrome," *Current Sociology* 49, no. 3 (2001): 15– 29.

37.  G. Holmes, J. Kaplan, N. Gantz, A. Komaroff, L. Schonberger, S. Straus, J. Jones, R. Dubois, C. Cunningham-Rundles, and S. Pahwa, "Chronic Fatigue Syndrome: A Working Case Definition," *Annals of Internal Medicine* 108, no. 3 (1988): 387 – 89.

38.  R. Taylor, F. Friedberg, and L. Jason, *A Clinician's Guide to Controversial Illnesses: Chronic Fatigue Syndrome, Fibromyalgia, and Multiple Chemical Sensitivities* (Sarasota, FL: Professional Resource Press, 2001).

39.  L. Jason, R. Taylor, Z. Stepanek, and S. Plioplys, "Attitudes Regarding Chronic Fatigue Syndrome: The Importance of a Name," *Journal of Health Psychology* 6, no. 1 (2001): 61– 71; L. Jason, R. Taylor, S. Plioplys, Z. Stepanek, and J. Shlaes, "Evaluating Attributions for an Illness Based upon the Name: Chronic Fatigue Syndrome, Myalgic Encephalopathy and Florence Nightingale Disease," *American Journal of Community Psychology* 30, no. 1 (2002): 133– 48.

40.  J. Jason, R. Taylor, Z. Stepanek, and S. Plioplys, "Attitudes Regarding Chronic Fatigue Syndrome: The Importance of a Name," *Journal of Health Psychology* 6, no. 1 (2001): 61– 71; L. Jason, R. Taylor, S. Plioplys, Z. Stepanek, and J. Shlaes, "Evaluating Attributions for an Illness Based upon the Name: Chronic Fatigue Syndrome, Myalgic Encephalopathy and Florence Nightingale Disease," *American Journal of Community Psychology* 30, no. 1 (2002): 133– 48.

41.  L. Jason, C. Holbert, S. Torres-Harding, and R. Taylor, "Stigma and Chronic Fatigue Syndrome: Surveying a Name Change," *Journal of Disability Policy Studies* 14, no. 4 (2004): 222– 28.

42. L. Jason, C. Holbert, S. Torres-Harding, and R. Taylor, "Stigma and Chronic Fatigue Syndrome: Surveying a Name Change," *Journal of Disability Policy Studies* 14, no. 4 (2004): 222– 28.

43. L. Jason, C. Holbert, S. Torres-Harding, and R. Taylor, "Stigma and Chronic Fatigue Syndrome: Surveying a Name Change," *Journal of Disability Policy Studies* 14, no. 4 (2004): 222– 28.

44. L. Jason, C. Holbert, S. Torres-Harding, and R. Taylor, "Stigma and Chronic Fatigue Syndrome: Surveying a Name Change," *Journal of Disability Policy Studies* 14, no. 4 (2004): 222– 28.

45. L. Jason, C. Holbert, S. Torres-Harding, and R. Taylor, "Stigma and Chronic Fatigue Syndrome: Surveying a Name Change," *Journal of Disability Policy Studies* 14, no. 4 (2004): 222– 28.

46. L. Jason, J. Richman, F. Friedberg, L. Wagner, R. Taylor, and K. Jordan, "Politics, Science, and the Emergence of a New Disease: The Case of Chronic Fatigue Syndrome," *American Psychologist* 52, no. 9 (1997): 973– 83.

47. M. Akers, Standing Fast, Battles of a Champion (n.p.: JTC Sports, Inc. 1997).

48. S. Lisman and K. Dougherty, *Chronic Fatigue Syndrome for Dummies* (Indianapolis, IN: Wiley Publishing, 2007), 297– 302.

49. S. Lisman and K. Dougherty, *Chronic Fatigue Syndrome for Dummies* (Indianapolis, IN: Wiley Publishing, 2007), 297– 302.

50. S. Lisman and K. Dougherty, *Chronic Fatigue Syndrome for Dummies* (Indianapolis, IN: Wiley Publishing, 2007), 297– 302.

51. S. Lisman and K. Dougherty, *Chronic Fatigue Syndrome for Dummies* (Indianapolis, IN: Wiley Publishing, 2007), 297– 302.

52. S. Lisman and K. Dougherty, *Chronic Fatigue Syndrome for Dummies* (Indianapolis, IN: Wiley Publishing, 2007), 297– 302.

53. "Blake Edwards Biography," accessed July 29, 2014, www.thebiographychannel.co.uk.

54. "Blake Edwards Biography," accessed July 29, 2014, www.thebiographychannel.co.uk.

55. R. Shefchik, "World Short Track Speedskating Championships—Peterson Comes Home to Finish Skating Career," *St. Paul (MN) Pioneer Press* , March 31, 2006.

56. J. Weiner, "No Medals, but These Sports Have Own Gold—Short-track Speedskating Must Overcome Image Problem," *(MN) Star Tribune* , February 2, 1988.

57. B. Murphy, "On Track: Amy Peterson Has Something to Prove As She Bids for Her Fifth Olympic Games Berth," *St. Paul (MN) Pioneer Press* , December 14, 2001.

58. "100 Greatest Singers of All Time," *Rolling Stone*, accessed May 2, 2014, www.rollingstone.com./music/lists/100-greatest-singers-of-all-time-19691231/stevie-nicks-20101202.

59. M. Brown, "Stevie Nicks: A Survivor's Story," *The Daily Telegraph*, September 8, 2007, accessed June 3, 2014; M. Dennis, "Toronto Interview," CHUM Radio, May 6, 2001, accessed June 3, 2014.

60. M. Brown, "Stevie Nicks: A Survivor's Story," *The Daily Telegraph*, September 8, 2007, accessed June 3, 2014; M. Dennis, "Toronto Interview," CHUM Radio, May 6, 2001, accessed June 3, 2014.

61. D. Bell, *CFIDS: The Disease of a Thousand Names* (New York: Pollard Publications, 1991).

## 3. CAUSES AND RISK FACTORS

1. U.S. National Library of Medicine, "Chronic Fatigue Syndrome," accessed July 24, 2014, www.ncbi.nlm.nih.gov.

2. U.S. National Library of Medicine, "Chronic Fatigue Syndrome," accessed July 24, 2014, www.ncbi.nlm.nih.gov.

3. "Chronic Fatigue Syndrome (CFS)," CDC.gov, last updated May 14, 2012, accessed June 3, 2014, www.cdc.gov/cfs/causes.

4. H. Simon, "Chronic Fatigue Syndrome," University of Maryland Medical Center, last updated February 7, 2012, accessed June 3, 2014, www.umm.edu/health/medical/reports/articles/chronic-fatigue-syndrome.

5. H. Simon, "Chronic Fatigue Syndrome," University of Maryland Medical Center, last updated February 7, 2012, accessed June 3, 2014, www.umm.edu/health/medical/reports/articles/chronic-fatigue-syndrome.

6. H. Simon, "Chronic Fatigue Syndrome," University of Maryland Medical Center, last updated February 7, 2012, accessed June 3, 2014, www.umm.edu/health/medical/reports/articles/chronic-fatigue-syndrome.

7. "What are Cytokines?" Sino Biological Inc., accessed June 4, 2014, www.sinobiological.com/What-Is-Cytokine-Cytokine-Definition-a-5796.html.

8. R. Patarca, "Cytokines and Chronic Fatigue Syndrome," *Annals of the New York Academy of Sciences* 933 (2001): 185–200.

9. University of South Florida (USF Health), "Chronic Fatigue Syndrome: Inherited Virus Can Cause Cognitive Dysfunction and Fatigue," ScienceDaily, July 26, 2013, accessed June 5, 2014, www.sciencedaily.com/releases/2013/07/130726092427.htm.

10. University of South Florida (USF Health), "Chronic Fatigue Syndrome: Inherited Virus Can Cause Cognitive Dysfunction and Fatigue," ScienceDaily,

July 26, 2013, accessed June 5, 2014, www.sciencedaily.com/releases/2013/07/130726092427.htm.

11. L. Borish, K. Schmaling, J. DiClementi, J. Streib, J. Negri, and J. Jones, "Chronic Fatigue Syndrome: Identification of Distinct Subgroups on the Basis of Allergy and Psychologic Variables," *Journal of Allergy and Clinical Immunology* 102, no. 2 (1998): 222–30.

12. L. Borish, K. Schmaling, J. D. DiClementi, J. Streib, J. Negri, and J. F. Jones, "Chronic Fatigue Syndrome: Identification of Distinct Subgroups on the Basis of Allergy and Psychologic Variables," *Journal of Allergy and Clinical Immunology* 102, no. 2 (1998): 222–30.

13. "Causes of Chronic Fatigue Syndrome," NHS Choices, updated March 20, 2013, accessed June 6, 2014, www.nhs.uk/Conditions/Chronic-fatigue-syndrome/Pages/Causes.aspx.

14. M. Hanlon, "ME Is Possibly a Mental Illness—but That Does Not Mean That It Is Not Real," last updated on September 18, 2012, www.hanlonblog.dailymail.co.uk/2012/09/me-is-probably-a-mental-illness-after-all-but-that-does-not-mean-that-it-is-not-real.html.

15. "Chronic Fatigue Syndrome In-depth Report," accessed June 2, 2014, www.nytimes.com/health/guides/disease/chronic-fatigue-syndrome/print.html.

16. A. Cleare, J. Miell, E. Heap, S. Sookdeo, L. Young, G. Malhi, and V. O'Keane, "Hypothalamo-pituitary-adrenal Axis Dysfunction in Chronic Fatigue Syndrome, and the Effects of Low-dose Hydrocortisone Therapy," *The Journal of Clinical Endocrinology and Metabolism* 86, no. 8 (2001): 3545–54.

17. A. Cleare, J. Miell, E. Heap, S. Sookdeo, L. Young, G. Malhi, and V. O'Keane, "Hypothalamo-pituitary-adrenal Axis Dysfunction in Chronic Fatigue Syndrome, and the Effects of Low-dose Hydrocortisone Therapy," *The Journal of Clinical Endocrinology and Metabolism* 86, no. 8 (2001): 3545–54.

18. R. Rosmond, M. Dallman, and P. Björntorp, "Stress-related Cortisol Secretion in Men: Relationships with Abdominal Obesity and Endocrine, Metabolic and Hemodynamic Abnormalities," *The Journal of Clinical Endocrinology and Metabolism* 83, no. 6 (1998): 1853–59.

19. A. McGrady, P. Conran, D. Dickey, D. Garman, E. Farris, and C. Schumann-Brzezinski, "The Effects of Biofeedback-assisted Relaxation on Cell-mediated Immunity, Cortisol, and White Blood Cell Count in Healthy Adult Subjects," *Journal of Behavioral Medicine* 15, no. 4 (1992): 343–54.

20. H. Simon, "Chronic Fatigue Syndrome," University of Maryland Medical Center, last updated February 7, 2012, accessed June 3, 2014, www.umm.edu/health/medical/reports/articles/chronic-fatigue-syndrome.

21. "Chronic Fatigue Syndrome In-depth Report," accessed June 2, 2014, www.nytimes.com/health/guides/disease/chronic-fatigue-syndrome/print.html.

22. Mayo Clinic Staff, "Chronic Fatigue Syndrome Risk Factors," updated July 1, 2014, accessed July 5, 2014, www.mayoclinic.org/diseases-conditions/chronic-fatigue-syndrome/basics/risk-factors/con-20022009.

23. H. Simon, "Chronic Fatigue Syndrome," University of Maryland Medical Center, last updated February 7, 2012, accessed June 5, 2014, www.umm.edu/health/medical/reports/articles/chronic-fatigue-syndrome.

24. J. Issa, "The Personality of Chronic Fatigue," last updated October 22, 2010, accessed July 5, 2014, www.brainblogger.com/2010/10/22/the-personality-of-chronic-fatigue.

25. J. Issa, "The Personality of Chronic Fatigue," last updated October 22, 2010, accessed July 5, 2014, www.brainblogger.com/2010/10/22/the-personality-of-chronic-fatigue.

26. D. Ciccone, K. Busichio, M. Vickroy, and B. Natelson, "Psychiatric Morbidity in the Chronic Fatigue Syndrome: Are Patients with Personality Disorder More Physically Impaired?" *Journal of Psychosomatic Research* 54, no. 5 (2003): 445–52.

## 4. PATHOLOGY OF CHRONIC FATIGUE SYNDROME

1. K. Brurberg, M. Fonhus, L. Larun, S. Flottorp, and K. Malterud, "Case Definitions for Chronic Fatigue Syndrome/Myalgic Encephalomyelitis (CFS/ME): A Systematic Review," *BMJ Open* 4, no. 2 (2014): e003973.

2. E. Newsholme, E. Blomstrand, and B. Ekblom, "Physical and Mental Fatigue: Metabolic Mechanisms and Importance of Plasma Amino Acids," *British Medical Bulletin* 48, no. 3 (1992): 477–95.

3. Centers for Disease Control and Prevention, "Chronic Fatigue Syndrome: Diagnostic Tests to Exclude Other Causes," accessed May 13, 2014, www.cdc.gov/cfs/diagnosis/testing.html.

4. C. Ferri, *Chronic Fatigue Syndrome* (Quick Reference) (Chicago: Mosby, 2014), 10–12.

5. "Chronic Fatigue Syndrome/Myalgic Encephalomyelitis (or Encephalopathy) Diagnosis and Management," NICE Clinical Guideline (2007), accessed July 24, 2014, www.nice.org.uk.

6. A. Dellwo, "Chronic Fatigue Syndrome Basics Series #2," accessed May 3, 2014, www.about.com.

7. P. Plum, *Diagnosis of Stupor and Coma* (London: Oxford University Press, 2007), 5–6; Centers for Disease Control and Prevention, "Chronic Fatigue Syndrome (CFS): Symptoms," last updated May 5, 2012, accessed May 12, 2014, www.cdc.gov/cfs/symptoms/index.html.

8. L. Martínez-Martínez, T. Mora, A. Vargas, M. Fuentes-Iniestra, and M. Martínez-Lavín, "Sympathetic Nervous System Dysfunction in Fibromyalgia, Chronic Fatigue Syndrome, Irritable Bowel Syndrome, and Interstitial Cystitis: A Review of Case-control Studies," *Journal of Clinical Rheumatology* 20, no. 3 (2014): 146–50.

9. V. Giebels, H. Repping-Wuts, G. Bleijenberg, J. Kroese, N. Stikkelbroeck, and A. Hermus, "Severe Fatigue in Patients with Adrenal Insufficiency: Physical, Psychosocial and Endocrine Determinants," *Journal of Endocrinological Investigation* 37, no. 3 (2014): 293–301.

10. T. Hampton, "Researchers Find Genetic Clues to Chronic Fatigue Syndrome," *Journal of the American Medical Association* 295, no. 21 (2006): 2466–67.

11. T. Hampton, "Researchers Find Genetic Clues to Chronic Fatigue Syndrome," *Journal of the American Medical Association* 295, no. 21 (2006): 2466–67.

12. A. Pinching, "AIDS and CFS/ME: A Tale of Two Syndromes," *Clinical Medicine* 3, no. 1 (2003): 78–82.

13. E. Fuller-Thomson, R. Mehta, and J. Sulman, "Long-term Parental Unemployment in Childhood and Subsequent Chronic Fatigue Syndrome," *International Scholarly Research Notices: Family Medicine* (2013): 978250.

14. B. Natelson, M. Haghighi, and N. Ponzio, "Evidence for the Presence of Immune Dysfunction in Chronic Fatigue Syndrome," *Clinical and Diagnostic Laboratory Immunology* 9, no. 4 (2002): 747–52.

15. E. Acheson, "The Clinical Syndrome Variously Called Benign Myalgic Encephalomyelitis," *American Journal of Medicine* 26, no. 4 (1959): 569–95.

16. C. Davis, "Chronic Fatigue Syndrome: Symptoms," 2013, accessed June 23, 2014, www.medicinenet.com.

17. E. Acheson, "The Clinical Syndrome Variously Called Benign Myalgic Encephalomyelitis," *American Journal of Medicine* 26, no. 4 (1959): 569–95.

18. R. Moss-Morris V. Deary, and B. Castell, "Chronic Fatigue Syndrome," *Handbook of Clinical Neurology* 110 (2013): 303–14.

19. R. Moss-Morris, V. Deary, and B. Castell, "Chronic Fatigue Syndrome," *Handbook of Clinical Neurology* 110 (2013): 303–14.

20. R. Kilden, "Chronic Fatigue Syndrome: The Male Disorder That Became a Female Disorder," *Science Daily*, 2014, accessed August 2, 2014, www.Sciencedaily.com.

21. C. Davis, "Chronic Fatigue Syndrome: Symptoms," 2013, accessed June 23, 2014, www.medicinenet.com.

22. E. Gleichgerrcht and J. Decety, "The Relationship between Different Facets of Empathy, Pain Perception and Compassion Fatigue among Physicians," *Frontiers in Behavioral Neuroscience* 8 (2014): 243.

23. S. Love, *Menopause & Hormone Book: Making Informed Choices* (New York: Harmony, 2003), 103.

24. S. Love, *Menopause & Hormone Book: Making Informed Choices* (New York: Harmony, 2003), 103.

25. E. Crawley, "The Epidemiology of Chronic Fatigue Syndrome/Myalgic Encephalitis in Children," *Archives of Disease in Childhood* 99, no. 2 (2014): 171–74.

26. E. Crawley, "The Epidemiology of Chronic Fatigue Syndrome/Myalgic Encephalitis in Children," *Archives of Disease in Childhood* 99, no. 2 (2014): 171–74.

27. D. Barron, B. Cohen, M. Geraghty, R. Violand, and P. Rowe, "Joint Hypermobility Is More Common in Children with Chronic Fatigue Syndrome Than in Healthy Controls," *Journal of Pediatrics* 141, no. 3 (2002): 421.

28. D. Barron, B. Cohen, M. Geraghty, R. Violand, and P. Rowe, "Joint Hypermobility Is More Common in Children with Chronic Fatigue Syndrome Than in Healthy Controls," *Journal of Pediatrics* 141, no. 3 (2002): 421.

29. T. Chalder, J. Tong, and V. Deary, "Family Cognitive Behaviour Therapy for Chronic Fatigue Syndrome: An Uncontrolled Study," *Archives of Disease in Childhood* 86, no. 2 (2002): 95–97.

30. D. Cook, "Functional Neuroimaging Correlates of Mental Fatigue Induced by Cognition among Chronic Fatigue Syndrome Patients and Controls," *NeuroImage* 36, no. 1 (2007): 108–22.

31. D. Cook, "Functional Neuroimaging Correlates of Mental Fatigue Induced by Cognition among Chronic Fatigue Syndrome Patients and Controls," *NeuroImage* 36, no. 1 (2007): 108–22.

32. K. Miwa and M. Fujita, "Electrocardiographic QT Interval and Cardiovascular Reactivity in Fibromyalgia Differ from Chronic Fatigue Syndrome," *Clinical Cardiology* 19, no. 3 (2011): 782–86.

33. K. Rahman, A. Burton, S. Galbraith, A. Lloyd, and U. Vollmer-Conna, "Sleep-wake Behavior in Chronic Fatigue Syndrome," *Sleep* 34, no. 5 (2011): 671–78.

34. K. Rahman, A. Burton, S. Galbraith, A. Lloyd, and U. Vollmer-Conna, "Sleep-wake Behavior in Chronic Fatigue Syndrome," *Sleep* 34, no. 5 (2011): 671–78.

35. K. Rahman, A. Burton, S. Galbraith, A. Lloyd, and U. Vollmer-Conna, "Sleep-wake Behavior in Chronic Fatigue Syndrome," Sleep 34, no. 5 (2011): 671–78.

36. J. Naschitz, M. Fields, H. Isseroff, D. Sharif, E. Sabo, and I. Rosner, "Shortened QT Interval: A Distinctive Feature of the Dysautonomia of Chronic Fatigue Syndrome," *Journal of Electrocardiology* 39, no. 4 (2006): 389–94.

37.  J. Naschitz, M. Fields, H. Isseroff, D. Sharif, E. Sabo, and I. Rosner, "Shortened QT Interval: A Distinctive Feature of the Dysautonomia of Chronic Fatigue Syndrome," *Journal of Electrocardiology* 39, no. 4 (2006): 389–94.

38.  R. Antiel, J. Caudill, B. Burkhardt, C. Brands, and P. Fischer, "Iron, Insufficiency and Hypovitaminosis D in Adolescents with Chronic Fatigue and Orthostatic Intolerance," *Southern Medical Journal* 104, no.8 (2011): 609–11.

39.  A. Hoeck, *Vitamin D Deficiency Results in Chronic Fatigue and Multisystem Symptoms* (Cologne, Germany: International Association for Chronic Fatigue Syndrome/Myalgic Encaphalomyelitis, 2009), 1–6.

40.  A. Hoeck, *Vitamin D Deficiency Results in Chronic Fatigue and Multisystem Symptoms* (Cologne, Germany: International Association for Chronic Fatigue Syndrome/Myalgic Encaphalomyelitis, 2009), 1–6.

41.  B. Hurwitz, V. Coryell, M. Parker, P. Martin, A. Laperriere, N. Klimas, G. Sfakianakis, and M. Bilsker, "Chronic Fatigue Syndrome: Illness Severity, Sedentary Lifestyle, Blood Volume and Evidence of Diminished Cardiac Function," *Clinical Science* 118, no. 2 (2009): 125–35.

42.  B. Hurwitz, V. Coryell, M. Parker, P. Martin, A. Laperriere, N. Klimas, G. Sfakianakis, and M. Bilsker, "Chronic Fatigue Syndrome: Illness Severity, Sedentary Lifestyle, Blood Volume and Evidence of Diminished Cardiac Function," *Clinical Science* 118, no. 2 (2009): 125–35.

43.  A. Lerner, "Prevalence of Abnormal Cardiac Wall Motion in the Cardiomyopathy Associated with Incomplete Multiplication of Epstein-Barr Virus and/or Cytomegalovirus in Patients with Chronic Fatigue Syndrome," *In Vivo* 18, no. 4 (2004): 417–24.

44.  Centers for Disease Control and Prevention, "Chronic Fatigue Syndrome (CFS), Symptoms," last updated May 5, 2012, accessed June 2, 2014, www.cdc.gov/cfs/symptoms/index.html.

45.  T. Muayqil, G. Gronseth, and R. Camicioli, "Evidence-based Guideline: Diagnostic Accuracy of CSF 14-3-3 Protein in Sporadic Creutzfeldt-Jakob Disease: Report of the Guideline Development Subcommittee of the American Academy of Neurology," *Neurology* 79, no. 14 (2012): 1499–506.

46.  E. Verrillo, *Chronic Fatigue Syndrome: A Treatment Guide*, 2nd ed. (Seattle, WA: Erica Verrillo, 2012).


## 5. DIAGNOSING CHRONIC FATIGUE SYNDROME


1.  M. Sharpe, L. Archard, J. Banatvala, L. Borysiewicz, A. Clare, A. David, R. Edwards, K. Hawton, H. Lambert, R. Lane, E. McDonald, J. Mowbray, D. Pearson, T. Peto, V. Preedy, A. Smith, D. Smith, D. Taylor, D. Tyrrell, S.

Wessely, and P. White, "A Report: Chronic Fatigue Syndrome: Guidelines for Research," *Journal of the Royal Society of Medicine* 84, no. 2 (1991): 118–21.

2. M. Sharpe, L. Archard, J. Banatvala, L. Borysiewicz, A. Clare, A. David, R. Edwards, K. Hawton, H. Lambert, R. Lane, E. McDonald, J. Mowbray, D. Pearson, T. Peto, V. Preedy, A. Smith, D. Smith, D. Taylor, D. Tyrrell, S. Wessely, and P. White, "A Report: Chronic Fatigue Syndrome: Guidelines for Research," *Journal of the Royal Society of Medicine* 84, no. 2 (1991): 118–21.

3. E. Lattie, M. Antoni, M. Fletcher, S. Czaja, D. Perdomo, A. Sala, S. Nair, S. Hua Fu, F. Penedo, and N. Klimas, "Beyond Myalgic Encephalomyelitis/Chronic Fatigue Syndrome (ME/CFS) Symptom Severity: Stress Management Skills Are Related to Lower Illness Burden," *Fatigue* 1, no. 4 (2013): 210–22.

4. D. Bates, D. Buchwald, J. Lee, P. Kith, T. Doolittle, C. Rutherford, W. Churchill, P. Schur, M. Wener, and D. Wybenga, "Clinical Laboratory Test Findings in Patients with Chronic Fatigue Syndrome," *Archives of Internal Medicine* 155, no. 1 (1995): 97–103.

5. C. Shepherd, *Diagnosis: Delay Harms Health—Early Diagnosis: Why Is It So Important?* (London: ME Alliance, 2005), 11.

6. M. Sharpe, L. Archard, J. Banatvala, L. Borysiewicz, A. Clare, A. David, R. Edwards, K. Hawton, H. Lambert, R. Lane, E. McDonald, J. Mowbray, D. Pearson, T. Peto, V. Preedy, A. Smith, D. Smith, D. Taylor, D. Tyrrell, S. Wessely, and P. White, "A Report: Chronic Fatigue Syndrome: Guidelines for Research," *Journal of the Royal Society of Medicine* 84, no. 2 (1991): 118–21.

7. C. Shepherd, *Living with M.E.: The Chronic/Post-viral Fatigue Syndrome*, 3rd ed. (London: Random House UK, 1999).

8. G. Norman and K. Eva, "Diagnostic Error and Clinical Reasoning," *Medical Education* 44, no. 1 (2010): 94–100.

9. J. Valdizán Usón and I. Alecha, "Diagnostic and Treatment Challenges of Chronic Fatigue Syndrome: Role of Immediate-release Methylphenidate," *Expert Review of Neurotherapeutics* 8, no. 6 (2008): 917–27.

10. C. Shepherd, *Living with M.E.: The Chronic/Post-viral Fatigue Syndrome*, 3rd ed. (London: Random House UK, 1999).

11. S. Shor, "Lyme Disease Presenting As Chronic Fatigue Syndrome," *Journal of Chronic Fatigue Syndrome*, 13, no. 4 (2006).

12. S. Shor, "Lyme Disease Presenting As Chronic Fatigue Syndrome," *Journal of Chronic Fatigue Syndrome*, 13, no. 4 (2006).

13. C. Shepherd, *Living with M.E.: The Chronic/Post-viral Fatigue Syndrome*, 3rd ed. (London: Random House UK, 1999).

14. C. Ray, S. Jefferies, and W. Weir, "Life Events and the Course of Chronic Fatigue Syndrome," *British Journal of Medical Psychology*, 68, no. 4 (1995): 323–31.

15. P. White, J. Thomas, H. Kangro, W. Bruce-Jones, J. Amess, D. Crawford, S. Grover, and A. Clare, "Predictions and Associations of Fatigue Syndromes and Mood Disorders That Occur after Infectious Mononucleosis," *Lancet* 358, no. 9297 (2001): 1946–54.

16. A. House and H. Andrews, "Life Events and Difficulties Preceding the Onset of Functional Dysphonia," *Journal of Psychosomatic Research* 32, no. 3 (1988): 311–19; H. Andrews and A House, "Functional Dysphonia: Establishing a New Dimension of Life Events and Difficulties," in *Life Events and Illness*, ed. G. Brown and T. Harris (London: Guilford Press, 1989), 343–53.

17. C. Werker, S. Nijhof, and E. Van de Putte, "Clinical Practice: Chronic Fatigue Syndrome," *European Journal of Pediatrics* 172, no. 10 (2013): 1293–98.

18. M. Huibers, I. Kant, J. Knottnerus, G. Bleijenberg, G. Swaen, and S. Kasl, "Development of the Chronic Fatigue Syndrome in Severely Fatigued Employees: Predictors of Outcome in the Maastricht Cohort Study," *Journal of Epidemiology & Community Health* 58, no. 10 (2004): 877–82.

19. D. Buchwald and D. Garrity, "Comparison of Patients with Chronic Fatigue Syndrome, Fibromyalgia, and Multiple Chemical Sensitivities," *Archives of Internal Medicine* 154, no. 18 (1994): 2049–53.

20. D. Buchwald and D. Garrity, "Comparison of Patients with Chronic Fatigue Syndrome, Fibromyalgia, and Multiple Chemical Sensitivities," *Archives of Internal Medicine* 154, no. 18 (1994): 2049–53.

21. R. Dietert and J. Dietert, "Possible Role for Early-life Immune Insult Including Developmental Immunotoxicity in Chronic Fatigue Syndrome (CFS) or Myalgic Encephalomyelitis (ME)," *Toxicology* 247, no. 1 (2008).

22. J. Fenaux, R. Gogal Jr, and S. Ahmed, "Diethylstilbesterol Exposure during Fetal Development Affects Thymus: Studies in Fourteen-month-old Mice," *Journal of Reproductive Immunology* 64 nos. 1–2 (2004): 75–90.

23. R. Dietert and J. Dietert, "Possible Role for Early-life Immune Insult Including Developmental Immunotoxicity in Chronic Fatigue Syndrome (CFS) or Myalgic Encephalomyelitis (ME)," *Toxicology* 247, no. 1 (2008).

24. M. Espey, D. Thomas, K. Miranda, and D. Wink, "Focusing of Nitric Oxide Mediated Nitrosation and Oxidative Nitrosylation As a Consequence of Reaction with Superoxide," *Proceedings of the National Academy of Sciences* 99, no. 17 (2002): 11127–32.

25. M. Espey, D. Thomas, K. Miranda, and D. Wink, "Focusing of Nitric Oxide Mediated Nitrosation and Oxidative Nitrosylation As a Consequence of Reaction with Superoxide," *Proceedings of the National Academy of Sciences* 99, no. 17 (2002): 11127–32.

26. M. Caliguri, C. Murray, D. Buchwald, H. Levine, P. Cheney, D. Peterson, A. Komaroff, and J. Ritz, "Phenotypic and Functional Deficiency of Natu-

ral Killer Cells in Patients with Chronic Fatigue Syndrome," *Journal of Immunology* 130 (1987): 3306–13.

27.  "Chronic Fatigue Syndrome," University of Maryland Medical Center (UMMC), accessed May 3, 2014, www.umm.edu/health/medical/altmed/condition/chronic-fatigue-syndrome.

28.  C. Shepherd, *Living with M.E.: The Chronic/Post-viral Fatigue Syndrome*, 3rd ed. (London: Random House UK, 1999).

29.  D. Goldenberg, R. Simms, A. Geiger, and A. Komaroff, "High Frequency of Fibromyalgia in Patients with Chronic Fatigue Seen in Primary Care Practice," *Arthritis & Rheumatology* 33, no. 3 (1990): 381–87.

30.  C. Shepherd, *Living with M.E.: The Chronic/Post-viral Fatigue Syndrome*, 3rd ed. (London: Random House UK, 1999).

31.  I. Hickie, B. Bennett, A. Lloyd, A. Heath, and N. Martin, "Complex Genetic and Environmental Relationships between Psychological Distress, Fatigue and Immune Functioning: A Twin Study," *Psychological Medicine* 29, no. 2 (1999): 269–77.

32.  A. Farmer, J. Scourfield, N. Martin, A. Cardeno, and P. McGuffin, "Is Disabling Fatigue in Childhood Influenced by Genes?" *Psychological Medicine* 29, no. 2 (1999): 279–82.

33.  A. Farmer, J. Scourfield, N. Martin, A. Cardeno, and P. McGuffin, "Is Disabling Fatigue in Childhood Influenced by Genes?" *Psychological Medicine* 29, no. 2 (1999): 279–82.

34.  N. Afari and D. Buchwald, "Chronic Fatigue Syndrome: A Review," *American Journal of Psychiatry* 160 (2003): 221–36.

35.  B. Natelson, J. Cohen, I. Brassloff, and H. Lee, "A Controlled Study of Brain Magnetic Resonance Imaging in Patients with Fatiguing Illnesses," *Journal of Neurological Science* 120, no. 2 (1993): 213–17.

36.  R. Schwartz, B. Garada, A. Komaroff, H. Tice, M. Gleit, F. Jolesz, and B. Holman, "Detection of Intracranial Abnormalities in Patients with Chronic Fatigue Syndrome: Comparison of MR Imaging and SPECT," *American Journal of Roentgenology* 162, no. 4 (1994): 935–41.

37.  D. Lewis, H. Mayberg, M. Fischer, J. Goldberg, S. Ashton, M. Graham, and D. Buchwald, "Monozygotic Twins Discordant for Chronic Fatigue Syndrome: Regional Cerebral Blood Flow SPECT," *Radiology* 219, no. 3 (2001): 766–73.

38.  D. Torpy, A. Bachmann, J. Grice, S. Fitzgerald, P. Phillips, J. Whitworth, and R. Jackson, "Familial Corticosteroid-binding Globulin Deficiency Due to a Novel Null Mutation: Association with Fatigue and Relative Hypotension," *Journal of Clinical Endocrinology and Metabolism* 86, no. 8 (2001): 3692–700.

39. D. Torpy, A. Bachmann, J. Grice, S. Fitzgerald, P. Phillips, J. Whitworth, and R. Jackson, "Familial Corticosteroid-binding Globulin Deficiency Due to a Novel Null Mutation: Association with Fatigue and Relative Hypotension," *Journal of Clinical Endocrinology and Metabolism* 86, no. 8 (2001): 3692–700.

40. N. Afari and D. Buchwald, "Chronic Fatigue Syndrome: A Review," *American Journal of Psychiatry* 160, no. 2 (2003): 221–36.

41. S. Wessely, T. Chalder, S. Hirsch, P. Wallace, and D. Wright, "Psychological Symptoms, Somatic Symptoms, and Psychiatric Disorder in Chronic Fatigue and Chronic Fatigue Syndrome: A Prospective Study in the Primary Care Setting," *American Journal of Psychiatry* 153, no. 8 (1996): 1050–59.

42. I. Hickie, A. Lloyd, D. Wakefield, and G. Parker, "The Psychiatric Status of Patients with Chronic Fatigue Syndrome," *British Journal of Psychiatry* 156 (1990): 534–40.

43. N. Afari and D. Buchwald, "Chronic Fatigue Syndrome: A Review," *American Journal of Psychiatry* 160, no. 2 (2003): 221–36.

44. C. Surawy, A. Hackman, K. Hawton, and M. Sharpe, "Chronic Fatigue Syndrome: A Cognitive Approach," *Behaviour Research and Therapy* 33, no. 5 (1995): 534–44.

45. C. Whelton, I. Salit, and H. Moldofsky, "Sleep, Epstein-Barr Virus Infection, Musculoskeletal Pain, and Depressive Symptoms in Chronic Fatigue Syndrome," *Journal of Rheumatology* 19, no. 6 (1992): 939–43; R. Morris, M. Sharpe, A. Sharpley, P. Cowen, K. Hawton, and J. Morris, "Abnormalities of Sleep in Patients with Chronic Fatigue Syndrome," *British Medical Journal* 306 (1993): 1161–64.

46. O. Ortega-Hernandez and Y. Shoenfeld, "Infection, Vaccination, and Autoantibodies in Chronic Fatigue Syndrome, Cause or Coincidence?" *Annals of the New York Academy of Sciences* 1173 (2009): 600–609.

47. M. Hotopf and S. Wessely, "Viruses, Neurosis and Fatigue," *Journal of Psychosomatic Research* 38, no. 6 (1994): 499–514.

## 6. ROLES OF THE FAMILY PHYSICIAN, INTERNIST, AND NEUROLOGIST IN CHRONIC FATIGUE SYNDROME

1. J. Bowen, D. Pheby, A. Charlett, and C. McNulty, "Chronic Fatigue Syndrome: A Survey of GPs' Attitudes and Knowledge," *Family Practice* 22, no. 4 (2005): 389–93.

2. D. Stevens, "Chronic Fatigue," *Western Journal of Medicine* 175, no. 5 (2001): 315–19.

3. A. Mcgaha, E. Garrett, A. Jobe, P. Nalin, W. Newton, P. Pugno, and N. Kahn, "Responses to Medical Students' Frequently Asked Questions about Family Medicine," *American Family Physician* 76, no. 1 (2007): 99–106.

4. "What Does a Family Physician Do?" Virginia Commonwealth University Medical Center Department of Family Medicine and Population Health, last modified February 8, 2013, accessed May 23, 2014, www.familymedicine.vcu.edu/patient/physician.

5. "What Does a Family Physician Do?" Virginia Commonwealth University Medical Center Department of Family Medicine and Population Health, last modified February 8, 2013, accessed May 23, 2014, www.familymedicine.vcu.edu/patient/physician.

6. L. McNaughton-Filion, "The Role of a Community Family Physician from a Resident's Viewpoint," *Canadian Family Physician* 37 (1991): 1843–45.

7. A. Mcgaha, E. Garrett, A. Jobe, P. Nalin, W. Newton, P. Pugno, and N. Kahn, "Responses to Medical Students' Frequently Asked Questions about Family Medicine," *American Family Physician* 76, no. 1 (2007): 99–106.

8. D. Mueller, "Medical Student Perspectives: What Are the Differences between Internal Medicine and Family Medicine," American College of Physicians, last modified 2011, accessed June 2, 2014, www.acponline.org/medical_students/impact/archives/2010/12/perspect/.

9. D. Mueller, "Medical Student Perspectives: What Are the Differences between Internal Medicine and Family Medicine," American College of Physicians, last modified 2011, accessed June 2, 2014, www.acponline.org/medical_students/impact/archives/2010/12/perspect/.

10. D. Mueller, "Medical Student Perspectives: What Are the Differences between Internal Medicine and Family Medicine," American College of Physicians, last modified 2011, accessed June 2, 2014, www.acponline.org/medical_students/impact/archives/2010/12/perspect/.

11. D. Robinson, "The Internist's Role in Treating Fibromyalgia & Chronic Fatigue Syndrome," ProHealth, October 20, 2003, accessed June 4, 2014, www.prohealth.com/library/showarticle.cfm?libid=9927.

12. Y. Cheng-Chee, "1st College of Physicians Lecture: The Role of Internal Medicine As a Specialty in the Era of Subspecialisation," *Annals of the Academy of Medicine* 33, no. 6 (2004): 725–32.

13. D. Robinson, "The Internist's Role in Treating Fibromyalgia & Chronic Fatigue Syndrome," ProHealth, October 20, 2003, accessed June 4, 2014, www.prohealth.com/library/showarticle.cfm?libid=9927.

14. D. Mueller, "Medical Student Perspectives: What Are the Differences between Internal Medicine and Family Medicine," American College of Physicians, last modified 2011, accessed June 2, 2014, www.acponline.org/medical_students/impact/archives/2010/12/perspect/.

15. Y. Cheng-Chee, "1st College of Physicians Lecture: The Role of Internal Medicine As a Specialty in the Era of Subspecialisation," *Annals of the Academy of Medicine* 33, no. 6 (2004): 725–32.

16. S. Cohn and D. Macpherson, "Overview of the Principles of Medical Consultation and Perioperative Medicine," UpToDate, last modified June 28, 2013, accessed June 5, 2014, www.uptodate.com/contents/overview-of-the-principles-of-medical-consultation-and-perioperative-medicine.

17. S. Cohn and D. Macpherson, "Overview of the Principles of Medical Consultation and Perioperative Medicine," UpToDate, last modified June 28, 2013, accessed June 5, 2014, www.uptodate.com/contents/overview-of-the-principles-of-medical-consultation-and-perioperative-medicine.

18. W. Levinson, "Preoperative Evaluations by an Internist—Are They Worthwhile?" *Western Journal of Medicine* 141, no. 3 (1984): 395–98.

19. American Academy of Neurology and American Academy of Neurology Education & Research Foundation, "What Is Neurology," Montana Neurological Associates, accessed July 9, 2014, www.montananeurosurgery.com/What_is_Neurology.

20. American Academy of Neurology and American Academy of Neurology Education & Research Foundation, "What Is Neurology," Montana Neurological Associates, accessed July 9, 2014, www.montananeurosurgery.com/What_is_Neurology.

21. T. Sabin, "An Approach to Chronic Fatigue Syndrome in Adults," *Neurologist* 9, no. 1 (2003): 28–34.

22. American Academy of Neurology and American Academy of Neurology Education & Research Foundation, "What Is Neurology," Montana Neurological Associates, accessed July 9, 2014, http://www.montananeurosurgery.com/What_is_Neurology.

23. L. Kelchner, "The Duties of a Neurologist," accessed July 9, 2014, www.work.chron.com/duties-neurologist-12344.html.

24. L. Kelchner, "The Duties of a Neurologist," accessed July 9, 2014, www.work.chron.com/duties-neurologist-12344.html.

25. T. Sabin, "An Approach to Chronic Fatigue Syndrome in Adults," *Neurologist* 9, no. 1 (2003): 28–34.

26. L. Kelchner, "The Duties of a Neurologist," accessed July 9, 2014, www.work.chron.com/duties-neurologist-12344.html.

27. L. Kelchner, "The Duties of a Neurologist," accessed July 9, 2014, www.work.chron.com/duties-neurologist-12344.html.

28. L. Kelchner, "The Duties of a Neurologist," accessed July 9, 2014, www.work.chron.com/duties-neurologist-12344.html.

29. S. Gluckman, "Clinical Features and Diagnosis of Chronic Fatigue Syndrome," UpToDate, last modified November 26, 2013, accessed May 23, 2014,

www.uptodate.com/contents/clinical-features-and-diagnosis-of-chronic-fa-tigue-syndrome.

30. J. McSherry, "Chronic Fatigue Syndrome: A Fresh Look at an Old Problem, *Canadian Family Physician* 39 (1993): 336–40.

31. C. DiMaria, "CFS (Chronic Fatigue Syndrome)," Healthline, July 18, 2012, accessed May 23, 2014, www.healthline.com/health/chronic-fatigue-syndrome#Overview1.

32. F. Albright, K. Light, A. Light, L. Bateman, and L. Cannon-Albright, "Evidence for a Heritable Predisposition to Chronic Fatigue Syndrome," *BMC Neurology* 11 (2011): 62.

33. C. DiMaria, "CFS (Chronic Fatigue Syndrome)," Healthline, July 18, 2012, accessed May 23, 2014, www.healthline.com/health/chronic-fatigue-syndrome#Overview1.

34. S. Gluckman, "Patient Information: Chronic Fatigue Syndrome (Beyond the Basics)," UpToDate, last modified March 3, 2014, accessed May 23, 2014, www.uptodate.com/contents/chronic-fatigue-syndrome-beyond-the-basics.

35. S. Gluckman, "Patient Information: Chronic Fatigue Syndrome (Beyond the Basics)," UpToDate, last modified March 3, 2014, accessed May 23, 2014, www.uptodate.com/contents/chronic-fatigue-syndrome-beyond-the-basics.

36. S. Gluckman, "Patient Information: Chronic Fatigue Syndrome (Beyond the Basics)," UpToDate, last modified March 3, 2014, accessed May 23, 2014, www.uptodate.com/contents/chronic-fatigue-syndrome-beyond-the-basics.

37. A. Bested, P. Saunders, and A. Logan, "Chronic Fatigue Syndrome: Neurological Findings May Be Related to Blood-Brain Barrier Permeability," *Medical Hypotheses* 57, no. 2 (2001): 231–37.

38. Georgetown University Medical Center, "Research Provides More Evidence That Chronic Fatigue Syndrome Is a Legitimate Medical Condition," Science Daily, accessed July 9, 2014, www.sciencedaily.com/releases/2006/01/060110013424.htm.

39. Georgetown University Medical Center, "Research Provides More Evidence That Chronic Fatigue Syndrome Is a Legitimate Medical Condition," Science Daily, accessed July 9, 2014, www.sciencedaily.com/releases/2006/01/060110013424.htm.

40. A. Fernandez, A. Martin, M. Martinez, M. Bustillo, F. Hernandez, J. Labrado, R. Peñas, E. Rivas, C. Delgado, J. Redondo, and J. Gimenez, "Chronic Fatigue Syndrome: Aetiology, Diagnosis, and Treatment," *BioMed Central Psychiatry* 9, Suppl. 1 (2009): S1.

41. J. McSherry, "Chronic Fatigue Syndrome: A Fresh Look at an Old Problem," *Canadian Family Physician* 39 (1993): 336–40.

42. S. Kreijkamp-Kaspers, E. Brenu, S. Marshall, D. Staines, and M. Van Driel, "Treating Chronic Fatigue Syndrome—A Study into the Scientific Evidence for Pharmacological Treatments," *Australian Family Physician* 40, no. 11 (2011): 907–12.

43. Georgetown University Medical Center, "Research Provides More Evidence That Chronic Fatigue Syndrome Is a Legitimate Medical Condition," Science Daily, accessed July 9, 2014, www.sciencedaily.com/releases/2006/01/060110013424.htm.

44. A. Fernandez, A. Martin, M. Martinez, M. Bustillo, F. Hernandez, J. Labrado, R. Peñas, E. Rivas, C. Delgado, J. Redondo, and J. Gimenez, "Chronic Fatigue Syndrome: Aetiology, Diagnosis, and Treatment," *BioMed Central Psychiatry* 9, Suppl. 1 (2009): S1.

45. J. McSherry, "Chronic Fatigue Syndrome: A Fresh Look at an Old Problem," *Canadian Family Physician* 39 (1993): 336–40.

46. A. Fernandez, A. Martin, M. Martinez, M. Bustillo, F. Hernandez, J. Labrado, R. Peñas, E. Rivas, C. Delgado, J. Redondo, and J. Gimenez, "Chronic Fatigue Syndrome: Aetiology, Diagnosis, and Treatment," *BioMed Central Psychiatry* 9, Suppl. 1 (2009): S1.

47. A. Fernandez, A. Martin, M. Martinez, M. Bustillo, F. Hernandez, J. Labrado, R. Peñas, E. Rivas, C. Delgado, J. Redondo, and J. Gimenez, "Chronic Fatigue Syndrome: Aetiology, Diagnosis, and Treatment," *BioMed Central Psychiatry* 9, Suppl. 1 (2009): S1.

48. A. Fernandez, A. Martin, M. Martinez, M. Bustillo, F. Hernandez, J. Labrado, R. Peñas, E. Rivas, C. Delgado, J. Redondo, and J. Gimenez, "Chronic Fatigue Syndrome: Aetiology, Diagnosis, and Treatment," *BioMed Central Psychiatry* 9, Suppl. 1 (2009): S1.

49. S. Attfield, A. Adams, and A. Blandford, "Patient Information Needs: Pre- and Post-consultation," *Health Informatics Journal* 12, no. 2 (2006): 165–77.

50. C. King and L. Jason, "Improving the Diagnostic Criteria and Procedures for Chronic Fatigue Syndrome," *Biological Psychology* 68, no. 2 (2005): 87–106.

51. A. Fernandez, A. Martin, M. Martinez, M. Bustillo, F. Hernandez, J. Labrado, R. Peñas, E. Rivas, C. Delgado, J. Redondo, and J. Gimenez, "Chronic Fatigue Syndrome: Aetiology, Diagnosis, and Treatment," *BioMed Central Psychiatry* 9, Suppl. 1 (2009): S1.

52. M. Brown, A. Brown, and L. Jason, "Illness Duration and Coping Style in Chronic Fatigue Syndrome," *Psychological Reports* 106, no. 2 (2010): 383–93.

53. M. Brown, A. Brown, and L. Jason, "Illness Duration and Coping Style in Chronic Fatigue Syndrome," *Psychological Reports* 106, no. 2 (2010): 383–93.

54. L. Cordingley, A. Wearden, L. Appleby, and L. Fisher, "The Family Response Questionnaire: A New Scale to Assess the Responses of Family Members to People with Chronic Fatigue Syndrome," *Journal of Psychosomatic Research* 51, no. 2 (2001): 417–24.

55. L. Cordingley, A. Wearden, L. Appleby, and L. Fisher, "The Family Response Questionnaire: A New Scale to Assess the Responses of Family Members to People with Chronic Fatigue Syndrome," *Journal of Psychosomatic Research* 51, no. 2 (2001): 417–24.

56. "Causes of Chronic Fatigue Syndrome," NHS Choices, last modified March 20, 2013, accessed May 24, 2014, www.nhs.uk/Conditions/Chronic-fatigue-syndrome/Pages/Causes.aspx.

57. "Causes of Chronic Fatigue Syndrome," NHS Choices, last modified March 20, 2013, accessed May 24, 2014, www.nhs.uk/Conditions/Chronic-fatigue-syndrome/Pages/Causes.aspx.

58. "Causes of Chronic Fatigue Syndrome," NHS Choices, last modified March 20, 2013, accessed May 24, 2014, www.nhs.uk/Conditions/Chronic-fatigue-syndrome/Pages/Causes.aspx.

59. D. Saltman, N. O'Dea, and M. Kidd, "Conflict Management: A Primer for Doctors in Training," *Postgraduate Medical Journal* 82, no. 963 (2006): 9–12.

60. S. Gluckman, "Treatment of Chronic Fatigue Syndrome," UpToDate, last modified June 25, 2013, accessed May 24, 2014, www.uptodate.com/contents/treatment-of-chronic-fatigue-syndrome.

61. A. Helfer, A. Camargo, N. Tavares, P. Kanavos, and A. Bertoldi, "Affordability and Availability of Drugs for Treatment of Chronic Diseases in the Public Health Care System [Article in Portuguese]," *Revista Panamericana de Salud Pública* 31, no. 3 (2012): 225–32.

# 7. ROLE OF THE HOSPITAL IN CHRONIC FATIGUE SYNDROME

1. "Chronic Fatigue Syndrome (CFS)/Diagnosis," Centers for Disease Control and Prevention, last modified May 14, 2012, accessed July 4, 2014. www.cdc.gov/cfs/diagnosis.

2. "Chronic Fatigue Syndrome (CFS)/Diagnosis," Centers for Disease Control and Prevention, last modified May 14, 2012, accessed July 4, 2014. www.cdc.gov/cfs/diagnosis.

3. S. Gluckman, "Patient Information: Chronic Fatigue Syndrome (Beyond the Basics)," last updated March 3, 2014, accessed July 5, 2014, www.uptodate.com.

4. S. Gluckman, "Patient Information: Chronic Fatigue Syndrome (Beyond the Basics)," last updated March 3, 2014, accessed July 5, 2014, www.uptodate.com.

5. H. Aiken, P. Clarke, M. Sloane, T. Lake, and T. Cheney, "Effects of Hospital Environment on Patient Mortality and Nurse Outcome," *The Journal of Nursing Administration* 38, no. 5 (2008): 223–29.

6. H. Aiken, P. Clarke, M. Sloane, T. Lake, and T. Cheney, "Effects of Hospital Environment on Patient Mortality and Nurse Outcome," *The Journal of Nursing Administration* 38, no. 5 (2008): 223–29.

7. H. Aiken, P. Clarke, M. Sloane, T. Lake, and T. Cheney, "Effects of Hospital Environment on Patient Mortality and Nurse Outcome," *The Journal of Nursing Administration* 38, no. 5 (2008): 223–29.

8. J. Pols, "Politics of Mental Illness: Myth and Power in the Work of Thomas S. Szasz," 2005, accessed July 4, 2014, www.janpols.net/Chapter-6/5.html.

9. J. Pols, "Politics of Mental Illness: Myth and Power in the Work of Thomas S. Szasz," 2005, accessed July 4, 2014, www.janpols.net/Chapter-6/5.html.

10. A. Coulter and P. Cleary, "Patients' Experiences with Hospital Care in Five Countries," *Health Affairs* 20, no. 3 (2001): 244–52.

11. E. Jacobson, W. Keough, B. Dalton, and D. Giansiracusa, "A Comparison of Inpatient and Outpatient Experiences during an Internal Medicine Clerkship," *American Journal of Medicine* 104, no. 2 (1998): 159–62.

12. E. Jacobson, W. Keough, B. Dalton, and D. Giansiracusa, "A Comparison of Inpatient and Outpatient Experiences during an Internal Medicine Clerkship," *American Journal of Medicine* 104, no. 2 (1998): 159–62.

13. D. Cox and L. Findley, "The Management of Chronic Fatigue Syndrome in an Inpatient Setting: Presentation of an Approach and Perceived Outcome," *British Journal of Occupational Therapy* 61, no. 9 (1998): 405–9.

14. E. Jacobson, W. Keough, B. Dalton, and D. Giansiracusa, "A Comparison of Inpatient and Outpatient Experiences during an Internal Medicine Clerkship," *American Journal of Medicine* 104, no. 2 (1998): 159–62.

15. B. Kozier, G. Erb, A. Berman, and S. Snyder, *Fundamentals of Nursing: Concepts, Process, and Practice*, 7th ed. (Singapore: Pearson Education South East Asia, 2004), 91.

16. S. Gluckman, "Patient Information: Chronic Fatigue Syndrome (Beyond the Basics)," last updated March 3, 2014, accessed July 5, 2014, www.uptodate.com.

17.  E. Jacobson, W. Keough, B. Dalton, and D. Giansiracusa, "A Comparison of Inpatient and Outpatient Experiences during an Internal Medicine Clerkship," *American Journal of Medicine* 104, no. 2 (1998): 159–62.

18.  R. Viner, A. Gregorowski, C. Wine, M. Bladen, D. Fisher, M. Miller, and S. El Neil, "Outpatient Rehabilitative Treatment of Chronic Fatigue Syndrome (CFS/ME)," *Archives of Disease in Childhood* 89, no. 7 (2004): 615–19.

19.  B. Kozier, G. Erb, A. Berman, and S. J. Snyder, *Fundamentals of Nursing: Concepts, Process, and Practice*, 7th ed. (Singapore: Pearson Education South East Asia, 2004), 91.

20.  R. Viner, A. Gregorowski, C. Wine, M. Bladen, D. Fisher, M. Miller, and S. El Neil, "Outpatient Rehabilitative Treatment of Chronic Fatigue Syndrome (CFS/ME)," *Archives of Disease in Childhood* 89, no. 7 (2004): 615–19.

21.  R. Viner, A. Gregorowski, C. Wine, M. Bladen, D. Fisher, M. Miller, and S. El Neil, "Outpatient Rehabilitative Treatment of Chronic Fatigue Syndrome (CFS/ME)," *Archives of Disease in Childhood* 89, no. 7 (2004): 615–19.

22.  R. Viner R, A. Gregorowski, C. Wine, M. Bladen, D. Fisher, M. Miller, and S. El Neil, "Outpatient Rehabilitative Treatment of Chronic Fatigue Syndrome (CFS/ME)," *Archives of Disease in Childhood* 89, no. 7 (2004): 615–19.

23.  Y. Gist and L. Hetzal, "We the People: Aging in the United States," U.S. Census Bureau, 2004, accessed July 4, 2014, www.census.gov/prod/2004pubs/censr-19.pdf.

24.  B. Kozier, G. Erb, A. Berman, and S. Snyder, *Fundamentals of Nursing: Concepts, Process, and Practice*, 7th ed. (Singapore: Pearson Education South East Asia, 2004), 95.

25.  B. Kozier, G. Erb, A. Berman, and S. Snyder, *Fundamentals of Nursing: Concepts, Process, and Practice*, 7th ed. (Singapore: Pearson Education South East Asia, 2004), 96.

26.  H. Cho, P. Menezes, D. Bhugra, and S. Wessely, "The Awareness of Chronic Fatigue Syndrome: A Comparative Study in Brazil and the United Kingdom," *Journal of Psychosomatic Research* 64, no. 4 (2008): 351–55.

27.  P. McCrone, L. Darbishire, L. Ridsdale, and P. Seed, "The Economic Cost of Chronic Fatigue and Chronic Fatigue Syndrome in UK Primary Care," *Psychological Medicine* 33, no. 2 (2003): 253–61.

28.  B. Kozier, G. Erb, A. Berman, and S. Snyder, *Fundamentals of Nursing: Concepts, Process, and Practice*, 7th ed. (Singapore: Pearson Education South East Asia, 2004), 96.

29.  B. Kozier, G. Erb, A. Berman, and S. Snyder, *Fundamentals of Nursing: Concepts, Process, and Practice*, 7th ed. (Singapore: Pearson Education South East Asia, 2004), 95.

30. J. Weissman, J. Ayanian, S. Chasan-Taber, M. Sherwood, C. Roth, and A. Epstein, "Hospital Readmissions and Quality of Care," *Medical Care* 37, no. 5 (1999): 490–501.

31. A. Deale and S. Wessely, "Patients' Perceptions of Medical Care in Chronic Fatigue Syndrome," *Social Science and Medicine* 52, no. 12 (2001): 1859–64.

32. A. Deale and S. Wessely, "Patients' Perceptions of Medical Care in Chronic Fatigue Syndrome," *Social Science and Medicine* 52, no. 12 (2001): 1859–64.

33. A. Deale and S. Wessely, "Patients' Perceptions of Medical Care in Chronic Fatigue Syndrome," *Social Science and Medicine* 52, no. 12 (2001): 1859–64.

34. A. Deale and S. Wessely, "Patients' Perceptions of Medical Care in Chronic Fatigue Syndrome," *Social Science and Medicine* 52, no. 12 (2001): 1859–64.

35. R. Webb, "Addressing the Global Health Work Force Crisis: Challenges for France, Germany, Italy, Spain and the UK," Action for Global Health 2011, accessed July 6, 2014, www.actionforglobalhealth.eu.

36. B. Kozier, G. Erb, A. Berman, and S. J. Snyder, *Fundamentals of Nursing: Concepts, Process, and Practice*, 7th ed. (Singapore: Pearson Education South East Asia, 2004), 94.

37. J. Penrod, P. Deb, C. Luhrs, C. Dellenbaugh, C. Zhu, T. Hochman, M. Maciejewski, E. Granieri, and R. Morrison, "Cost and Utilization Outcomes of Patients Receiving Hospital-based Palliative Care Consultation," *Journal of Palliative Medicine* 9, no. 4 (2006): 855–60.

38. B. Lucas, W. Trick, A. Evans, B. Mba, J. Smith, K. Das, P. Clarke, A. Varkey, S. Mathew, and R. Weinstein, "Effects of 2- vs. 4-week Attending Physician Inpatient Rotations on Unplanned Patient Revisits, Evaluations by Trainees, and Attending Physician Burnout: A Randomized Trial," *Journal of the American Medical Association* 308, no. 21 (2012): 2199–207.

39. C. Hawk, L. Jason, and S. Torres-Harding, "Differential Diagnosis of Chronic Fatigue Syndrome and Major Depressive Disorder," *International Journal of Behavioral Medicine* 13, no. 3 (2006): 244–51.

40. C. Blatch and T. Blatt, "Chronic Fatigue Syndrome: Role of Psychological Factors Overemphasised," *British Medical Journal* 308, no. 6939 (1994): 1297.

## 8. FATIGUE AND THE HUMAN BODY

1. H. Dong, I. Ugalde, N. Figueroa, and A. El-Saddik, "Towards Whole Body Fatigue Assessment of Human Movement: A Fatigue-tracking System Based on Combined sEMG and Accelerometer Signals," *Sensors* 14, no. 2 (2014): 2052–70.

2. C. Luca, "Myoelectrical Manifestations of Localized Muscular Fatigue in Humans," *CRC Critical Reviews in Biomedical Engineering* 11, no. 4 (1984): 251–79.

3. C. Luca, "Myoelectrical Manifestations of Localized Muscular Fatigue in Humans," *CRC Critical Reviews in Biomedical Engineering* 11, no. 4 (1984): 251–79.

4. National Collaborating Centre for Primary Care (UK), *Chronic Fatigue Syndrome/Myalgic Encephalomyelitis (or Encephalopathy): Diagnosis and Management of Chronic Fatigue Syndrome/Myalgic Encephalomyelitis (or Encephalopathy) in Adults and Children* (London: Royal College of General Practitioners, 2007).

5. H. Dong, I. Ugalde, N. Figueroa, and A. El-Saddik, "Towards Whole Body Fatigue Assessment of Human Movement: A Fatigue-tracking System Based on Combined sEMG and Accelerometer Signals," *Sensors* 14, no. 2 (2014): 2052–70.

6. H. Dong, I. Ugalde, N. Figueroa, and A. El-Saddik, "Towards Whole Body Fatigue Assessment of Human Movement: A Fatigue-tracking System Based on Combined sEMG and Accelerometer Signals," *Sensors* 14, no. 2 (2014): 2052–70.

7. R. Nardone, Y. Höller, F. Brigo, P. Höller, M. Christova, F. Tezzon, S. Golaszewski, and E. Trinka, "Fatigue-induced Motor Cortex Excitability Changes in Subjects with Spinal Cord Injury," *Brain Research Bulletin* 99 (2013): 9–12.

8. J. Davis, N. Anderson, and R. Welch, "Serotonin and Central Nervous System Fatigue: Nutritional Considerations," *American Journal for Clinical Nutrition* 72, Suppl. 2 (2000): 573S–578S.

9. A. Gualano, T. Bozza, P. Lopes De Campos, H. Roschel, A. Dos Santos Costa, M. Luiz Marquezi, F. Benatti, and A. Lancha Jr., "Branched-chain Amino Acids Supplementation Enhances Exercise Capacity and Lipid Oxidation during Endurance Exercise after Muscle Glycogen Depletion," *The Journal of Sports Medicine and Physical Fitness* 51, no. 1 (2011): 82–88.

10. A. Strachan and R. Maughan, "Platelet Serotonin Transporter Density and Related Parameters in Endurance-trained and Sedentary Male Subjects," *Acta Physiologica* 163, no. 2 (1998): 165–71.

11. E. Newsholme and E. Blomstrand, "Branched-chain Amino Acids and Central Fatigue," *Journal of Nutrition* 136, Suppl. 1 (2006): 274S–6S.

12. T. Friedman and C. Kimbal, "Endocrine Causes of Chronic Fatigue Syndrome (CFS)/Chronic Fatigue Immune: A Brief Guide for Primary Care Physicians," accessed May 23, 2014, www.goodhormonehealth.com/endo-causes.pdf.

13. K. Evans, D. Flanagan, and T. Wilkin, "Chronic Fatigue: Is It Endocrinology? *Clinical Medicine* 9, no. 1 (2009): 34–38.

14. K. Evans, D. Flanagan, and T. Wilkin, "Chronic Fatigue: Is It Endocrinology? *Clinical Medicine* 9, no. 1 (2009): 34–38.

15. J. Dempsey, M. Amann, L. Romer, and J. Miller, "Respiratory System Determinants of Peripheral Fatigue and Endurance Performance," *Medicine & Science in Sports & Exercise* 40, no. 3 (2008): 457–61.

16. J. Dempsey, M. Amann, L. Romer, and J. Miller, "Respiratory System Determinants of Peripheral Fatigue and Endurance Performance," *Medicine & Science in Sports & Exercise* 40, no. 3 (2008): 457–61.

17. J. Dempsey, M. Amann, L. Romer, and J. Miller, "Respiratory System Determinants of Peripheral Fatigue and Endurance Performance," *Medicine & Science in Sports & Exercise* 40, no. 3 (2008): 457–61.

18. J. Dempsey, M. Amann, L. Romer, and J. Miller, "Respiratory System Determinants of Peripheral Fatigue and Endurance Performance," *Medicine & Science in Sports & Exercise* 40, no. 3 (2008): 457–61.

19. B. Carruthers, A. Jain, K. De Meirleir, D. Peterson, N. Klimas, and A. Lerner, "Myalgic Encephalomyelitis/Chronic Fatigue Syndrome: Clinical Working Case Definition, Diagnostics, and Treatment Protocols," *Journal of Chronic Fatigue Syndrome* 11, no. 1 (2003): 7–36.

20. B. Carruthers, A. Jain, K. De Meirleir, D. Peterson, N. Klimas, and A. Lerner, "Myalgic Encephalomyelitis/Chronic Fatigue Syndrome: Clinical Working Case Definition, Diagnostics, and Treatment Protocols," *Journal of Chronic Fatigue Syndrome* 11, no. 1 (2003): 7–36.

21. B. Carruthers, A. Jain, K. De Meirleir, D. Peterson, N. Klimas, and A. Lerner, "Myalgic Encephalomyelitis/Chronic Fatigue Syndrome: Clinical Working Case Definition, Diagnostics, and Treatment Protocols," *Journal of Chronic Fatigue Syndrome* 11, no. 1 (2003): 7–36.

22. B. Carruthers, A. Jain, K. De Meirleir, D. Peterson, N. Klimas, and A. Lerner, "Myalgic Encephalomyelitis/Chronic Fatigue Syndrome: Clinical Working Case Definition, Diagnostics, and Treatment Protocols," *Journal of Chronic Fatigue Syndrome* 11, no. 1 (2003): 7–36.

23. S. Zakynthinos and C. Roussos, "Respiratory Muscle Fatigue," in *Physiologic Basis of Respiratory Disease*, ed. Q. Hamid, J. Shannon and J. Martin (Ontario, Canada: BC Decker Inc., 2005).

24. S. Zakynthinos and C. Roussos, "Respiratory Muscle Fatigue," in *Physiologic Basis of Respiratory Disease*, ed. Q. Hamid, J. Shannon, and J. Martin (Ontario, Canada: BC Decker Inc., 2005); J. Davis, N. Andeson, and R. Welch, "Serotonin and Central Nervous System Fatigue: Nutritional Considerations," *Americal Journal for Clincal Nutrition* 72, Suppl. 2 (2000): 573S–578S.

25. S. Zakynthinos and C. Roussos, "Respiratory Muscle Fatigue," in *Physiologic Basis of Respiratory Disease*, ed. Q. Hamid, J. Shannon, and J. Martin, (Ontario, Canada: BC Decker Inc., 2005); J. Davis, N. Andeson, and R. Welch, "Serotonin and Central Nervous System Fatigue: Nutritional Considerations," *Americal Journal for Clincal Nutrition* 72, Suppl. 2 (2000): 573S–578S.

26. M.-R. Huerta-Franco, M. Vargas-Luna, P. Tienda, I. Delgadillo-Holt-fort, M. Balleza-Ordaz, and C. Flores-Hernandez, "Effects of Occupational Stress on the Gastrointestinal Tract," *World Journal of Gastrointestinal Pathophysiology* 4, no. 4 (2013): 108–18.

27. B. Carruthers, A. Jain, K. De Meirleir, D. Peterson, N. Klimas, and A. Lerner, "Myalgic Encephalomyelitis/Chronic Fatigue Syndrome: Clinical Working Case Definition, Diagnostics, and Treatment Protocols," *Journal of Chronic Fatigue Syndrome* 11, no. 1 (2003): 7–36.

28. K. Kahol, M. Smith, S. Mayes, M. Deka, V. Deka, J. Ferrara, and S. Panchanatan, "The Effects of Fatigue on Cognitive and Psychomotor Skills of Surgical Residents," 3rd International Conference on Foundation of Augmented Cognition (Heidelberg: Springer-Verlag Hesling, 2007), 304–13.

## 9. VIRAL, NEUROPSYCHIATRIC, AND NEUROENDOCRINE HYPOTHESES

1. P. Forterre, "The Origin of Viruses and their Possible Roles in Major Evolutionary Transitions," *Virus Research* 117, no. 1 (2006): 5–16.

2. E. Holmes, "What Does Virus Evolution Tell Us about Virus Origins?" *Journal of Virology* 85, no. 11 (2011): 5247–51.

3. E. Holmes, "What Does Virus Evolution Tell Us about Virus Origins?" *Journal of Virology* 85, no. 11 (2011): 5247–51.

4. C. Johnson, "One Theory to Explain Them All? The Vagus Nerve Infection Hypothesis for Chronic Fatigue Syndrome," Simmaron Research, accessed December 28, 2013, www.simmaronresearch.com/2013/12/one-theory-explain-vagus-nerve-infection-chronic-fatigue-syndrome/ #sthash.hipkT6P6.dpuf.

5. M. Van Elzakker, "Chronic Fatigue Syndrome from Vagus Nerve Infection: A Psychoneuroimmunological Hypothesis," *Medical Hypotheses* 81, no. 3 (2013): 414–23.

6. M. Van Elzakker, "Chronic Fatigue Syndrome from Vagus Nerve Infection: A Psychoneuroimmunological Hypothesis," Medical Hypotheses 81, no. 3 (2013): 414–23.

7. C. Johnson, "One Theory to Explain Them All? The Vagus Nerve Infection Hypothesis for Chronic Fatigue Syndrome," Simmaron Research, accessed December 28, 2013, www.simmaronresearch.com/2013/12/one-theory-explain-vagus-nerve-infection-chronic-fatigue-syndrome/ #sthash.hipkT6P6.dpuf.

8. C. Johnson, "One Theory to Explain Them All? The Vagus Nerve Infection Hypothesis for Chronic Fatigue Syndrome," Simmaron Research, accessed December 28, 2013, www.simmaronresearch.com/2013/12/one-theory-explain-vagus-nerve-infection-chronic-fatigue-syndrome/ #sthash.hipkT6P6.dpuf.

9. C. Johnson, "One Theory to Explain Them All? The Vagus Nerve Infection Hypothesis for Chronic Fatigue Syndrome," Simmaron Research, accessed December 28, 2013, www.simmaronresearch.com/2013/12/one-theory-explain-vagus-nerve-infection-chronic-fatigue-syndrome/ #sthash.hipkT6P6.dpuf.

10. C. Johnson, "One Theory to Explain Them All? The Vagus Nerve Infection Hypothesis for Chronic Fatigue Syndrome," Simmaron Research, accessed December 28, 2013, www.simmaronresearch.com/2013/12/one-theory-explain-vagus-nerve-infection-chronic-fatigue-syndrome/ #sthash.hipkT6P6.dpuf.

11. G. Morris and M. Maes, "A Neuro-immune Model of Myalgic Encephalomyelitis/Chronic Fatigue Syndrome," *Metabolic Brain Disease* 28, no. 4 (2013): 523–40.

12. G. Morris and M. Maes, "Myalgic Encephalomyelitis/Chronic Fatigue Syndrome and Encephalomyelitis Disseminata/Multiple Sclerosis Show Remarkable Levels of Similarity in Phenomenology and Neuroimmune Characteristics," *BMC Medicine* 11 (2013): 205.

13. D. Schrijvers, F. Van Den Eede, Y. Maas, P. Cosyns, W. Hulstijn, and B. Sabbe, "Psychomotor Functioning in Chronic Fatigue Syndrome and Major Depressive Disorder: A Comparative Study," *Journal of Affective Disorders* 115, nos. 1–2 (2009): 46–53.

14. M. Maes, "Inflammatory and Oxidative and Nitrosative Stress Pathways Underpinning Chronic Fatigue, Somatization and Psychosomatic Symptoms," *Current Opinion in Psychiatry* 22, no. 1 (2009): 75–83.

15. E. Fuller-Thomson and J. Nimigon, "Factors Associated with Depression among Individuals with Chronic Fatigue Syndrome: Findings from a Nationally Representative Survey," *Family Practice* 25, no. 6 (2008): 414–22; M. Offenbaecher, K. Glatzeder, and M. Ackenheil, "Self-reported Depression, Familial History of Depression and Fibromyalgia (FM), and Psychological Distress in Patients with FM," *Zeitschrift für Rheumatologie* 57, Suppl. 2 (1998): 94–96; D. Buchwald, T. Pearlman, P. Kith, W. Katon, and K. Schmaling, "Screening for Psychiatric Disorders in Chronic Fatigue and Chronic Fatigue Syndrome," *Journal of Psychosomatic Research* 42, no. 1 (1997): 87–94; Y. Christley, T. Duffy, I. Everall, and C. Martin, "The Neuropsychiatric and Neuropsychological Features of Chronic Fatigue Syndrome: Revisiting the Enigma," *Current Psychiatry Reports* 15, no. 4 (2013): 353.

16. E. Fuller-Thomson and J. Nimigon, "Factors Associated with Depression among Individuals with Chronic Fatigue Syndrome: Findings from a Nationally Representative Survey," *Family Practice* 25, no. 6 (2008): 414–22; M. Offenbaecher, K. Glatzeder, and M. Ackenheil, "Self-reported Depression, Familial History of Depression and Fibromyalgia (FM), and Psychological Distress in Patients with FM," *Zeitschrift für Rheumatologie* 57, Suppl 2 (1998): 94–96; D. Buchwald, T. Pearlman, P. Kith, W. Katon, and K Schmaling, "Screening for Psychiatric Disorders in Chronic Fatigue and Chronic Fatigue Syndrome," *Journal of Psychosomatic Research* 42, no. 1 (1997): 87–94; Y. Christley, T. Duffy, I. Everall, and C. Martin, "The Neuropsychiatric and Neuropsychological Features of Chronic Fatigue Syndrome: Revisiting the Enigma," *Current Psychiatry Reports* 15, no. 4 (2013): 353.

17. L. Aaron, M. Burke, and D. Buchwald, "Overlapping Conditions among Patients with Chronic Fatigue Syndrome, Fibromyalgia, and Temporomandibular Disorder," *Archives of Internal Medicine* 160, no. 2 (2000): 221–27.

18. P. Sanders and J. Korf, "Neuroaetiology of Chronic Fatigue Syndrome: An Overview," *The World Journal of Biological Psychiatry* 9, no. 3 (2008): 165–71.

19. S. Johnson, J. DeLuca, and B. Natelson, "Depression in Fatiguing Illness: Comparing Patients with Chronic Fatigue Syndrome, Multiple Sclerosis and Depression," *Journal of Affective Disorders* 39, no. 1 (1996): 21–30.

20. S. Johnson, J. DeLuca, and B. Natelson, "Depression in Fatiguing Illness: Comparing Patients with Chronic Fatigue Syndrome, Multiple Sclerosis and Depression," *Journal of Affective Disorders* 39, no. 1 (1996): 21–30.

21. C. Hawk, L. Jason, and S. Torres-Harding, "Differential Diagnosis of Chronic Fatigue Syndrome and Major Depressive Disorder," *International Journal of Behavioral Medicine* 13, no. 3 (2006): 244–51.

22. E. Axe, P. Satz, N. Rasgon, and F. Fawzy, "Major Depressive Disorder in Chronic Fatigue Syndrome: A CDC Surveillance Study," *Journal of Chronic*

*Fatigue Syndrome* 12, no. 3 (2004): 7–23; L. Jason, J. Richman, F. Friedberg, L. Wagner, R. Taylor, and K. Jordan, "Politics, Science, and the Emergence of a New Disease, The Case of Chronic Fatigue Syndrome," *American Psychologist* 52, no. 9 (1997): 973–83.

23. A. Silver, M. Haeney, P. Vijayadurai, D. Wilks, M. Pattrick, and C. Main, "The Role of Fear of Physical Movement and Activity in Chronic Fatigue Syndrome," *Journal of Psychosomatic Research* 52, no. 6 (2002): 485–93.

24. E. Axe, P. Satz, N. Rasgon, and F. Fawzy, "Major Depressive Disorder in Chronic Fatigue Syndrome: A CDC Surveillance Study," *Journal of Chronic Fatigue Syndrome* 12, no. 3 (2004): 7–23.

25. B. Leonard and M. Maes, "Mechanistic Explanations How Cell-mediated Immune Activation, Inflammation and Oxidative and Nitrosative Stress Pathways and Their Sequels and Concomitants Play a Role in the Pathophysiology of Unipolar Depression," *Neuroscience and Biobehavioral Reviews* 36, no. 2 (2012): 764–85.

26. M. Maes, I. Mihaylova, and J. Leunis, "Increased Serum IgM Antibodies Directed against Phosphatidyl Inositol (Pi) in Chronic Fatigue Syndrome (CFS) and Major Depression: Evidence that an IgMmediated Immune Response against Pi Is One Factor Underpinning the Comorbidity between Both CFS and Depression," *Neuroendocrinology Letters* 28, no. 6 (2007): 861–67.

27. A. Roberts, A. Papadopoulos, S. Wessely, T. Chalder, and A. Cleare, "Salivary Cortisol Output before and after Cognitive Behavioural Therapy for Chronic Fatigue Syndrome," *Journal of Affective Disorders* 115, nos. 1–2 (2009): 280–86; A. Cleare, "The Neuroendocrinology of Chronic Fatigue Syndrome," *Endocrine Reviews* 24, no. 2 (2003): 236–52.

28. M. Maes and F. Twisk, "Chronic Fatigue Syndrome: Harvey and Wessely's (Bio)Psychosocial Model versus a Bio(Psychosocial) Model Based on Inflammatory and Oxidative and Nitrosative Stress Pathways," *Biomed Central Medicine* 8 (2010): 35.

29. K. Hinkelmann, S. Moritz, J. Botzenhardt, C. Muhtz, K. Wiedemann, M. Kellner, and C. Otte, "Changes in Cortisol Secretion during Antidepressive Treatment and Cognitive Improvement in Patients with Major Depression: A Longitudinal Study," *Psychoneuroendocrinology* 37, no. 5 (2011): 685–92.

30. K. Hinkelmann, S. Moritz, J. Botzenhardt, K. Riedesel, K. Wiedemann, and M. Kellner, "Cognitive Impairment in Major Depression: Association with Salivary Cortisol," *Biological Psychiatry* 66, no. 9 (2009): 879–85; R. Gomez, J. Posener, J. Keller, C. DeBattista, B. Solvason, and A. Schatzberg, "Effects of Major Depression Diagnosis and Cortisol Levels on Indices of Neurocognitive Function," *Psychoneuroendocrinology* 34, no. 7 (2009): 1012–18; A. Roberts, A. Papadopoulos, S. Wessely, T. Chalder, and A. Cleare, "Salivary Cortisol

Output before and after Cognitive Behavioral Therapy for Chronic Fatigue Syndrome," *Journal of Affective Disorders* 115, nos. 1–2 (2009): 280–86.

31. T. Turan, H. Izgi, S. Ozsoy, F. Tanriverdi, M. Basturk, and A. Asdemir, "The Effects of Galantamine Hydrobromide Treatment on Dehydroepiandrosterone Sulfate and Cortisol Levels in Patients with Chronic Fatigue Syndrome," *Psychiatry Investigation* 6, no. 3 (2009): 204–10.

32. L. Parker, E. Levin, and E. Lifrak, "Evidence for Adrenocortical Adaptation to Severe Illness," *The Journal of Clinical Endocrinology and Metabolism* 60, no. 5 (1985): 947–52.

33. L. Scott, F. Svec, and T. Dinan, "A Preliminary Study of Dehydroepiandrosterone Response to Low-dose ACTH in Chronic Fatigue Syndrome and in Healthy Subjects," *Psychiatric Research* 97, no. 1 (2000): 21–28.

34. P. Himmel and T. Seligman, "A Pilot Study Employing Dehydroepiandrosterone (DHEA) in the Treatment of Chronic Fatigue Syndrome," *Journal of Clinical Rheumatology* 5, no. 2 (1999): 56–59.

35. P. Manu, G. Affleck, H. Tennen, P. Morse, and J. Escobar, "Hypochondriasis Influences Quality-of-life Outcomes in Patients with Chronic Fatigue," *Psychotherapy and Psychosomatics* 65, no. 2 (1996): 76–81.

36. C. Pepper, L. Krupp, F. Friedberg, C. Doscher, and P. Coyle, "A Comparison of Neuropsychiatric Characteristics in Chronic Fatigue Syndrome, Multiple Sclerosis, and Major Depression," *The Journal of Neuropsychiatry and Clinical Neurosciences* 5, no. 2 (1993): 200–205.

37. B. Fischler, P. Dendale, V. Michiels, R. Cluydts, L. Kaufman, and K. De Meirleir, "Physical Fatigability and Exercise Capacity in Chronic Fatigue Syndrome: Association with Disability, Somatization and Psychopathology," *Journal of Psychosomatic Research* 42, no. 4 (1997): 369–78.

38. B. Fischler, P. Dendale, V. Michiels, R. Cluydts, L. Kaufman, and K. De Meirleir, "Physical Fatigability and Exercise Capacity in Chronic Fatigue Syndrome: Association with Disability, Somatization and Psychopathology," *Journal of Psychosomatic Research* 42, no. 4 (1997): 369–78.

39. Z. Lipowski, "Somatization: The Concept and Its Clinical Application," *American Journal of Psychiatry* 145 (1988): 1358–68.

40. L. Kirmayer, J. Robbins, and J. Paris, "Somatoform Disorders: Personality and the Social Matrix of Somatic Distress," *Journal of Abnormal Psychology* 103, no. 1 (1994): 125–36.

41. S. Abbey, "Somatization, Illness Attribution and the Sociocultural Psychiatry of Chronic Fatigue Syndrome," *Ciba Foundation Symposium* 173 (1993): 238–52.

42. C. Pepper, B. Krupp, F. Friedberg, C. Doscher, and P. Coyle, "A Comparison of Neuropsychiatric Characteristics in Chronic Fatigue Syndrome, Multiple Sclerosis, and Major Depression," *The Journal of Neuropsychiatry*

*and Clinical Neurosciences* 5, no. 2 (1993): 200–205; S. Johnson, J. DeLuca, and B. Natelson, "Assessing Somatization Disorder in the Chronic Fatigue Syndrome," *Psychosomatic Medicine* 58, no. 1 (1996): 50–57; P. Manu, T. Lane, D. Matthews, and J. Escobar, "Screening for Somatization Disorder in Patients with Chronic Fatigue," *General Hospital Psychiatry* 11 (1989): 294–97; S. Johnson, J. DeLuca, and B. Natelson, "Assessing Somatization Disorder in the Chronic Fatigue Syndrome," *Psychosomatic Medicine* 58, no. 1 (1996): 50–57.

43. J. Johnson, J. DeLuca, and B. Natelson, "Assessing Somatization Disorder in the Chronic Fatigue Syndrome," *Psychosomatic Medicine* 58, no. 1 (1996): 50–57.

44. M. Demitrack, "Neuroendocrine Research Strategies in Chronic Fatigue Syndrome," in *Chronic Fatigue and Related Immune Deficiency Syndromes*, ed. P. Goodnick and N. Klimas (Washington: American Psychiatric Press, 1993), 45–66.

45. W. Katon and E. Walker, "The Relationship of Chronic Fatigue to Psychiatric Illness in Community, Primary Care and Tertiary Care Samples," *Ciba Foundation Symposium* 173, no. (1993): 193–204.

46. W. Katon and J. Russo, "Chronic Fatigue Syndrome Criteria: A Critique of the Requirement for Multiple Physical Complaints," *Archives of Internal Medicine* 152, no. 8 (1992): 1604–9.

47. S. Johnson, J. DeLuca, and B. Natelson, "Personality Dimensions in the Chronic Fatigue Syndrome: A Comparison with Multiple Sclerosis and Depression," *Journal of Psychiatric Research* 30, no. 1 (1996): 9–20.

48. S. Johnson, J. DeLuca, and B. Natelson, "Personality Dimensions in the Chronic Fatigue Syndrome: A Comparison with Multiple Sclerosis and Depression," *Journal of Psychiatric Research* 30, no. 1 (1996): 9–20.

49. S. Johnson, J. DeLuca, and B. Natelson, "Personality Dimensions in the Chronic Fatigue Syndrome: A Comparison with Multiple Sclerosis and Depression," *Journal of Psychiatric Research* 30, no. 1 (1996): 9–20.

50. J. Deluca, C. Christodoulou, B. Diamond, E. Rosenstein, N. Kramer, and B. Natelson, "Working Memory Deficits in Chronic Fatigue Syndrome: Differentiating between Speed and Accuracy of Information Processing," *Journal of the International Neuropsychological Society* 10, no. 1 (2004): 101–9.

51. M. Majer, L. Welberg, L. Capuron, A. Miller, G. Pagnoni, and W. Reeves, "Neuropsychological Performance in Persons with Chronic Fatigue Syndrome: Results from a Population-based Study," *Psychosomatic Medicine* 70, no. 7 (2008): 829–36; A. Wearden and L. Appleby, "Cognitive Performance and Complaints of Cognitive Impairment in Chronic Fatigue Syndrome (CFS)," *Psychological Medicine* 27, no. 1 (1997): 81–90.

52. M. Majer, L. Welberg, L. Capuron, A. Miller, G. Pagnoni, and W. Reeves, "Neuropsychological Performance in Persons with Chronic Fatigue Syndrome: Results from a Population-based Study," *Psychosomatic Medicine* 70, no. 7 (2008): 829–36.

53. S. Lutgendorf, M. Antoni, G. Ironson, M. Fletcher, F. Penedo, A. Baum, N. Schniederman, and N. Klimas, "Physical Symptoms of Chronic Fatigue Syndrome Are Exacerbated by the Stress of Hurricane Andrew," *Psychosomatic Medicine* 57, no. 4 (1995): 310–23.

54. V. Michiels and R. Cluydts, "Neuropsychological Functioning in Chronic Fatigue Syndrome: A Review," *Acta Psychiatrica Scandinavica* 103, no. 2 (2001): 84–93.

55. V. Michiels and R. Cluydts, "Neuropsychological Functioning in Chronic Fatigue Syndrome: A Review," *Acta Psychiatrica Scandinavica* 103, no. 2 (2001): 84–93; L. Tiersky, S. Johnson, G. Lange, B. Natelson, and J. DeLuca, "Neuropsychology of Chronic Fatigue Syndrome: A Critical Review," *Journal of Clinical and Experimental Neuropsychology* 19, no. 4 (1997): 560–86.

56. R. Mahurin, K. Claypoole, J. Goldberg, L. Arguelles, S. Ashton, and D. Buchwald, "Cognitive Processing in Monozygotic Twins Discordant for Chronic Fatigue Syndrome," Neuropsychology 18, no. 2 (2004): 232–39; J. Deluca, C. Christodoulou, B. Diamond, E. Rosenstein, N. Kramer, and B. Natelson, "Working Memory Deficits in Chronic Fatigue Syndrome: Differentiating between Speed and Accuracy of Information Processing," *Journal of the International Neuropsychological Society* 10, no. 1 (2004): 101–9; M. Majer, L. Welberg, L. Capuron, A. Miller, G. Pagnoni, and W. Reeves, "Neuropsychological Performance in Persons with Chronic Fatigue Syndrome: Results from a Population-based Study," *Psychosomatic Medicine* 70, no. 7 (2008): 829–36; L. Capuron, L. Welberg, C. Heim, D. Wagner, L. Solomon, D. Papanicolaou, R. Craddock, A. Miller, and W. Reeves, "Cognitive Dysfunction Relates to Subjective Report of Mental Fatigue in Patients with Chronic Fatigue Syndrome," *Neuropsychopharmacology* 31, no. 8 (2006): 1777–84.

57. S. Crowe and A. Casey, "A Neuropsychological Study of the Chronic Fatigue Syndrome: Support for a Deficit in Memory Function Independent of Depression," *Australian Psychological Society* 34, no. 1 (1999): 70–75; N. Fiedler, H. Kipen, J. DeLuca, K. Kelly-McNeil, and B. Natelson, "Controlled Comparison of Multiple Chemical Sensitivities and Chronic Fatigue Syndrome," *Psychosomatic Medicine* 58, no. 1 (1996): 38–49.

58. V. Michiels and R. Cluydts, "Neuropsychological Functioning in Chronic Fatigue Syndrome: A Review," *Acta Psychiatrica Scandinavica* 103, no. 2 (2001): 84–93; L. Tiersky, S. Johnson, G. Lange, B. Natelson, and J. DeLuca, "Neuropsychology of Chronic Fatigue Syndrome: A Critical Review," *Journal of Clinical and Experimental Neuropsychology* 19, no. 4 (1997): 560–86.

59. S. Cockshell and J. Mathias, "Cognitive Functioning in Chronic Fatigue Syndrome: A Meta-Analysis," *Psychological Medicine* 40, no. 8 (2010): 1253–67; J. Deluca, C. Christodoulou, B. Diamond, E. Rosenstein, N. Kramer, and B. Natelson, "Working Memory Deficits in Chronic Fatigue Syndrome: Differentiating between Speed and Accuracy of Information Processing," *Journal of the International Neuropsychological Society* 10, no. 1 (2004): 101–9; M. Majer, L. Welberg, L. Capuron, A. Miller, G. Pagnoni, and W. Reeves, "Neuropsychological Performance in Persons with Chronic Fatigue Syndrome: Results from a Population-based Study," *Psychosomatic Medicine* 70, no. 7 (2008): 829–36; L. Tiersky, R. Matheis, J. Deluca, G. Lange, B. Natelson, "Functional Status, Neuropsychological Functioning, and Mood in Chronic Fatigue Syndrome (CFS): Relationship to Psychiatric Disorder," *The Journal of Nervous and Mental Disease* 191, no. 5 (2003): 324–31.

60. J. Deluca, C. Christodoulou, B. Diamond, E. Rosenstein, N. Kramer, and B. Natelson, "Working Memory Deficits in Chronic Fatigue Syndrome: Differentiating between Speed and Accuracy of Information Processing," *Journal of the International Neuropsychological Society* 10, no. 1 (2004): 101–9.

61. J. Deluca, C. Christodoulou, B. Diamond, E. Rosenstein, N. Kramer, and B. Natelson, "Working Memory Deficits in Chronic Fatigue Syndrome: Differentiating between Speed and Accuracy of Information Processing," *Journal of the International Neuropsychological Society* 10, no. 1 (2004): 101–9.

62. F. Duffy, G. McAnulty, M. McCreary, G. Cuchural, and A. Komaroff, "EEG Spectral Coherence Data Distinguish Chronic Fatigue Syndrome Patients from Healthy Controls and Depressed Patients—A Case Control Study," *BioMed Central Neurology* 11 (2011): 82.

63. X. Caseras, D. Mataix-Cols, V. Giampietro, K. Rimes, M. Brammer, F. Zelaya, T. Chalder, and E. Godfrey, "Probing the Working Memory System in Chronic Fatigue Syndrome: A Functional Magnetic Resonance Imaging Study Using the N-back Task," *Psychosomatic Medicine* 68, no. 6 (2006): 947–55.

64. X. Caseras, D. Mataix-Cols, V. Giampietro, K. Rimes, M. Brammer, F. Zelaya, T. Chalder, and E. Godfrey, "Probing the Working Memory System in Chronic Fatigue Syndrome: A Functional Magnetic Resonance Imaging Study Using the N-back Task," *Psychosomatic Medicine* 68, no. 6 (2006): 947–55; K. Claypoole, C. Noonan, R. Mahurin, J. Goldberg, T. Erickson, and D. Buchwald, "A Twin Study of Cognitive Function in Chronic Fatigue Syndrome: The Effects of Sudden Illness Onset," *Neuropsychology* 21, no. 4 (2007): 507–13; R. Mahurin, K. Claypoole, J. Goldberg, L. Arguelles, S. Ashton, and D. Buchwald, "Cognitive Processing in Monozygotic Twins Discordant for Chronic Fatigue Syndrome," *Neuropsychology* 18, no. 2 (2004): 232–39; J. Deluca, C. Christodoulou, B. Diamond, E. Rosenstein, N. Kramer, and B. Natelson, "Working Memory Deficits in Chronic Fatigue Syndrome: Differentiating be-

tween Speed and Accuracy of Information Processing," *Journal of the International Neuropsychological Society* 10, no. 1 (2004): 101–9; N. Chiaravalloti, C. Christodoulou, H. Demaree, and J. DeLuca, "Differentiating Simple versus Complex Processing Speed: Influence on New Learning and Memory Performance," *Journal of Clinical and Experimental Neuropsychology* 25, no. 4 (2003): 489–501.

65. M. Kaplan, "Neuroendocrine Abnormalities in CFS Deserve More Comprehensive Study," Chronic Neuroimmune Diseases, last updated January 1, 2014, accessed June 3, 2014, www.anapsid.org/cnd/diagnosis/neuro.html.

66. A. Kavelaars, W. Kuis, L. Knook, G. Sinnema, and C. Heijnen, "Disturbed Neuroendocrine-immune Interactions in Chronic Fatigue Syndrome," *The Journal of Clinical Endocrinology and Metabolism* 85, no. 2 (2000): 692–96.

67. D. Buchwald, M. Wener, T. Pearlman, and P. Kith, "Markers of Inflammation and Immune Activation in Chronic Fatigue and Chronic Fatigue Syndrome," *The Journal of Rheumatology* 24, no. 2 (1997): 372–76.

68. A. Kavelaars, W. Kuis, L. Knook, G. Sinnema, and C. Heijnen, "Disturbed Neuroendocrine-immune Interactions in Chronic Fatigue Syndrome," *The Journal of Clinical Endocrinology & Metabolism* 85, no. 2 (2000): 692–96.

69. J. Gaab, N. Rohleder, V. Heitz, V. Engert, T. Schad, T. Schürmeyer, and U. Ehlert, "Stress-induced Changes in LPS-induced Pro-inflammatory Cytokine Production in Chronic Fatigue Syndrome," *Psychoneuroendocrinology* 30, no. 2 (2005): 188–98.

70. M. Kaplan, "Neuroendocrine Abnormalities in CFS Deserve More Comprehensive Study," Chronic Neuroimmune Diseases, last updated January 1, 2014, accessed June 3, 2014, www.anapsid.org/cnd/diagnosis/neuro.html.

71. L. Scott, S. Medbak, and T. Dinan, "Blunted Adrenocorticotropin and Cortisol Responses to Corticotropin-releasing Hormone Stimulation in Chronic Fatigue Syndrome," *Acta Psychiatrica Scandinavica* 97, no. 6 (1998): 450–57.

72. M. Kaplan, "Neuroendocrine Abnormalities in CFS Deserve More Comprehensive Study," Chronic Neuroimmune Diseases, last updated January 1, 2014, accessed June 3, 2014, www.anapsid.org/cnd/diagnosis/neuro.html.

73. M. Kaplan, "Neuroendocrine Abnormalities in CFS Deserve More Comprehensive Study," Chronic Neuroimmune Diseases, last updated January 1, 2014, accessed June 3, 2014, www.anapsid.org/cnd/diagnosis/neuro.html.

74. T. Gerrity, D. Papanicolaou, J. Amsterdam, S. Bingham, A. Grossman, T. Hedrick, R. Herberman, G. Krueger, S. Levine, N. Mohagheghpour, R. Moore, J. Oleske, and C. Snell, "Immunologic Aspects of Chronic Fatigue Syndrome. Report on a Research Symposium Convened by The CFIDS Association of America and Co-sponsored by the U.S. Centers for Disease Control

and Prevention and the National Institutes of Health," *Neuroimmunomodulation* 11, no. 6 (2004): 351–57.

## 10. NATURAL APPROACHES TO CHRONIC FATIGUE SYNDROME

1. E. Weatherley-Jones, J. Nicholl, K. Thomas, G. Parry, M. McKendrick, S. Green, P. Stanley, and S. Lynch, "A Randomised, Controlled, Triple-blind Trial of the Efficacy of Homeopathic Treatment for Chronic Fatigue Syndrome," *Journal of Psychosomatic Research* 56, no. 2 (2004): 189–97.

2. E. Weatherley-Jones, J. Nicholl, K. Thomas, G. Parry, M. McKendrick, S. Green, P. Stanley, and S. Lynch, "A Randomised, Controlled, Triple-blind Trial of the Efficacy of Homeopathic Treatment for Chronic Fatigue Syndrome," *Journal of Psychosomatic Research* 56, no. 2 (2004): 189–97.

3. N. Porter, L. Jason, A. Boulton, N. Bothne, and B. Coleman, "Alternative Medical Interventions Used in the Treatment and Management of Myalgic Encephalomyelitis/Chronic Fatigue Syndrome and Fibromyalgia," *Journal of Alternative and Complementary Medicine* 16, no. 3 (2010): 235–49.

4. A. Hartz, S. Bentler, R. Noyes, J. Hoehns, C. Logemann, S. Sinift, Y. Butani, W. Wang, K. Brake, M. Ernst, and H. Kautzman, "Randomized Controlled Trial of Siberian Ginseng for Chronic Fatigue," *Psychological Medicine* 34, no. 1 (2004): 51–61.

5. J. Sarris, S. Moylan, D. Camfield, M. Pase, D. Mischoulon, M. Berk, F. Jacka, and I. Schweitzer, "Complementary Medicine, Exercise, Meditation, Diet, and Lifestyle Modification for Anxiety Disorders: A Review of Current Evidence," *Evidence Based Complementary and Alternative Medicine* 2012 (2012): 809653.

6. S. McDowell, H. Ferner, and R. Ferner, "The Pathophysiology of Medication Errors: How and Where They Arise," *British Journal of Clinical Pharmacology* 67, no. 6 (2009): 605–13.

7. M. Hooper, "Myalgic Encephalomyelitis: A Review with Emphasis on Key Findings in Biomedical Research," *Journal of Clinical Pathology* 60, no. 5 (2007): 466–71.

8. L. Borish, K. Schmaling, J. DiClementi, J. Streib, J. Negri, and J. Jones, "Chronic Fatigue Syndrome: Identification of Distinct Subgroups on the Basis of Allergy and Psychologic Variables," *Journal of Allergy and Clinical Immunology* 102, no. 2 (1998): 222–30.

9. J. Vercoulen, C. Swanink, J. Fennis, J. Galama, J. van der Meer, and G. Bleijenberg, "Prognosis in Chronic Fatigue Syndrome: A Prospective Study on the Natural Course," *Journal of Neurology, Neurosurgery & Psychiatry* 60, no. 5 (1996): 489–94.

10. J. Vercoulen, C. Swanink, J. Fennis, J. Galama, J. van der Meer, and G. Bleijenberg, "Prognosis in Chronic Fatigue Syndrome: A Prospective Study on the Natural Course," *Journal of Neurology, Neurosurgery & Psychiatry* 60, no. 5 (1996): 489–94.

11. A. Singh, P. Naidu, S. Gupta, and S. Kulkarni, "Effect of Natural and Synthetic Antioxidants in a Mouse Model of Chronic Fatigue Syndrome," *Journal of Medicinal Food* 5, no. 4 (2002): 211–20.

12. J. Bamidele, W. Adebimpe, and E. Oladele, "Knowledge, Attitude and Use of Alternative Medical Therapy amongst Urban Residents of Osun State, Southwestern Nigeria," *African Journal of Traditional, Complementary, and Alternative Medicines* 6, no. 3 (2009): 281–88.

13. B. Voerman, A. Visser, M. Fischer, B. Garssen, G. van Andel, and J. Bensing, "Determinants of Participation in Social Support Groups for Prostate Cancer Patients," *Psychooncology* 16, no. 12 (2007): 1092–99.

14. D. Locker, "Social Determinants of Health and Disease," in *Sociology As Applied to Medicine* (New York: Elselvier, 2008).

15. B. Van Houdenhove, E. Neerinckx, P. Onghena, A. Vingerhoets, R. Lysens, and H. Vertommen, "Daily Hassles Reported by Chronic Fatigue Syndrome and Fibromyalgia Patients in Tertiary Care: A Controlled Quantitative and Qualitative Study," *Psychotherapy and Psychosomatics* 71, no. 4 (2002): 207–13.

16. B. Van Houdenhove, E. Neerinckx, P. Onghena, A. Vingerhoets, R. Lysens, and H. Vertommen, "Daily Hassles Reported by Chronic Fatigue Syndrome and Fibromyalgia Patients in Tertiary Care: A Controlled Quantitative and Qualitative Study," *Psychotherapy and Psychosomatics* 71, no. 4 (2002): 207–13.

17. D. Chambers, A.-M. Bagnall, S. Hempel, and C. Forbes, "Interventions for the Treatment, Management and Rehabilitation of Patients with Chronic Fatigue Syndrome/Myalgic Encephalomyelitis: An Updated Systematic Review," *Journal of the Royal Society of Medicine* 99, no. 10 (2006): 506–20.

18. D. Chambers, A.-M. Bagnall, S. Hempel, and C. Forbes, "Interventions for the Treatment, Management and Rehabilitation of Patients with Chronic Fatigue Syndrome/Myalgic Encephalomyelitis: An Updated Systematic Review," *Journal of the Royal Society of Medicine* 99, no. 10 (2006): 506–20.

19. K. Schmaling, W. Smith, and D. Buchwald, "Significant Other Responses Are Associated with Fatigue and Functional Status among Patients with Chronic Fatigue Syndrome," *Psychosomatic Medicine* 62, no. 3 (2000): 444–50.

20. F. Friedberg, D. Leung, and J. Quick, "Do Support Groups Help People with Chronic Fatigue Syndrome and Fibromyalgia? A Comparison of Ac-

tive and Inactive Members," *Journal of Rheumatology* 32, no. 12 (2005): 2416–20.

21. F. Friedberg, D. Leung, and J. Quick, "Do Support Groups Help People with Chronic Fatigue Syndrome and Fibromyalgia? A Comparison of Active and Inactive Members," *Journal of Rheumatology* 32, no. 12 (2005): 2416–20.

22. J. Colby, "Special Problems of Children with Myalgic Encephalomyelitis/Chronic Fatigue Syndrome and the Enteroviral Link," *Journal of Clinical Pathology* 60, no. 2 (2007): 125–28.

23. J. Colby, "Special Problems of Children with Myalgic Encephalomyelitis/Chronic Fatigue Syndrome and the Enteroviral Link," *Journal of Clinical Pathology* 60, no. 2 (2007): 125–28.

24. J. Nijs, N. Roussel, J. Van-Oosterwijck, M. De-Kooning, K. Ickmans, F. Struyf, M. Meeus, and M. Lundberg, "Fear of Movement and Avoidance Behaviour toward Physical Activity in Chronic-Fatigue Syndrome and Fibromyalgia: State of the Art and Implications for Clinical Practice," *Clinical Rheumatology* 32, no. 8 (2013).

25. K. Schmaling, W. Smith, and D. Buchwald, "Significant Other Responses Are Associated with Fatigue and Functional Status among Patients with Chronic Fatigue Syndrome," *Psychosomatic Medicine* 62, no. 3 (2000): 444–50.

26. D. Chambers, A.-M. Bagnall, S. Hempel, and C. Forbes, "Interventions for the Treatment, Management and Rehabilitation of Patients with Chronic Fatigue Syndrome/Myalgic Encephalomyelitis: An Updated Systematic Review," *Journal of the Royal Society of Medicine* 99, no. 10 (2006): 506–20.

27. D. Chambers, A.-M. Bagnall, S. Hempel, and C. Forbes, "Interventions for the Treatment, Management and Rehabilitation of Patients with Chronic Fatigue Syndrome/Myalgic Encephalomyelitis: An Updated Systematic Review," *Journal of the Royal Society of Medicine* 99, no. 10 (2006): 506–20.

28. D. Chambers, A.-M. Bagnall, S. Hempel, and C. Forbes, "Interventions for the Treatment, Management and Rehabilitation of Patients with Chronic Fatigue Syndrome/Myalgic Encephalomyelitis: An Updated Systematic Review," *Journal of the Royal Society of Medicine* 99, no. 10 (2006).

29. A. Deale, T. Chalder, I. Marks, and S. Wessely, "Cognitive Behavior Therapy for Chronic Fatigue Syndrome: A Randomized Controlled Trial," *American Journal of Psychiatry* 154, no. 3 (1997).

30. D. Chambers, A.-M. Bagnall, S. Hempel, and C. Forbes, "Interventions for the Treatment, Management and Rehabilitation of Patients with Chronic Fatigue Syndrome/Myalgic Encephalomyelitis: An Updated Systematic Review," *Journal of the Royal Society of Medicine* 99, no. 10 (2006): 506–20.

31. D. Locker, "Social Determinants of Health and Disease," in *Sociology As Applied to Medicine* (New York: Elselvier, 2008).

32. D. Locker, "Social Determinants of Health and Disease," in *Sociology As Applied to Medicine* (New York: Elselvier, 2008).

33. D. Racciatti, J. Vecchiet, A. Ceccomancini, F. Ricci, and E. Pizzigallo, "Chronic Fatigue Syndrome Following a Toxic Exposure," *Science of the Total Environment* 270, no. 103 (2001): 27–31.

34. D. Racciatti, J. Vecchiet, A. Ceccomancini, F. Ricci, and E. Pizzigallo, "Chronic Fatigue Syndrome Following a Toxic Exposure," *Science of the Total Environment* 270, no. 103 (2001): 27–31.

35. D. Racciatti, J. Vecchiet, A. Ceccomancini, F. Ricci, and E. Pizzigallo, "Chronic Fatigue Syndrome Following a Toxic Exposure," *Science of the Total Environment* 270, no. 103 (2001): 27–31.

36. D. Racciatti, J. Vecchiet, A. Ceccomancini, F. Ricci, and E. Pizzigallo, "Chronic Fatigue Syndrome Following a Toxic Exposure," *Science of the Total Environment* 270, no. 103 (2001): 27–31.

37. E. Weatherley-Jones, J. Nicholl, K. Thomas, G. Parry, M. McKendrick, S. Green, P. Stanley, and S. Lynch, "A Randomised, Controlled, Triple-Blind Trial of the Efficacy of Homeopathic Treatment for Chronic Fatigue Syndrome," *Journal of Psychosomatic Research* 56, no. 2 (2004): 189–97; R. Awdry, "Homeopathy May Help Me," *The Journal of Alternative and Complementary Medicine* 14, no. 3 (1996): 12–16.

38. T. Alraek, M. Lee, T.-Y. Choi, H. Cao, and J. Liu, "Complementary and Alternative Medicine for Patients with Chronic Fatigue Syndrome: A Systematic Review," *BMC Complementary and Alternative Medicine* 11, no. 1 (2011): 87.

39. D. Grimes, "Proposed Mechanisms for Homeopathy Are Physically Impossible," *Focus on Alternative and Complementary Therapies* 17, no. 3 (2012): 149–55.

40. S. Kayne, *Homeopathic Pharmacy: Theory and Practice* (New York: Elsevier Health Sciences, 2006).

41. S. Kayne, *Homeopathic Pharmacy: Theory and Practice* (New York: Elsevier Health Sciences, 2006).

42. R. Hobday, S. Thomas, A. O'Donovan, M. Murphy, and A. Pinching, "Dietary Intervention in Chronic Fatigue Syndrome," *Journal of Human Nutrition and Dietetics* 21, no. 2 (2008): 141–49.

43. F. Kobayashi, H. Ogata, N. Omi, S. Nagasaka, S. Yamaguchi, M. Hibi, and K. Tokuyama, "Effect of Breakfast Skipping on Diurnal Variation of Energy Metabolism and Blood Glucose," *Obesity Research & Clinical Practice* 8, no. 3 (2014): e201–98.

44. K. Tandel, "Sugar Substitutes: Health Controversy over Perceived Benefits," *Journal of Pharmacology and Pharmacotherapeutics* 2, no. 4 (2011): 236–43.

45. K. Dykman, C. Tone, C. Ford, and R. Dykman, "The Effects of Nutritional Supplements on the Symptoms of Fibromyalgia and Chronic Fatigue Syndrome," *Integrative Physiological and Behavioral Science* 33, no. 1 (1998): 61–71.

46. G. Kumar and F. Khanum, "Neuroprotective Potential of Phytochemicals," *Pharmacognosy Reviews* 6, no. 12 (2012): 81–90.

47. A. Plioplys and S. Plioplys, "Amantadine and L-carnitine Treatment of Chronic Fatigue Syndrome," *Neuropsychobiology* 35, no. 1 (1997): 16–23.

48. M. Werbach, "Nutritional Strategies for Treating Chronic Fatigue Syndrome," *Alternative Medicine Review* 5, no. 2 (2000): 93–108.

49. A. Plioplys and S. Plioplys, "Amantadine and L-Carnitine Treatment of Chronic Fatigue Syndrome," *Neuropsychobiology* 35, no. 1 (1997): 16–23.

50. D. Chambers, A.-M. Bagnall, S. Hempel, and C. Forbes, "Interventions for the Treatment, Management and Rehabilitation of Patients with Chronic Fatigue Syndrome/Myalgic Encephalomyelitis: An Updated Systematic Review," *Journal of the Royal Society of Medicine* 99, no. 10 (2006): 506–20.

51. M. Werbach, "Nutritional Strategies for Treating Chronic Fatigue Syndrome," *Alternative Medicine Review* 5, no. 2 (2000): 93–108.

52. R. Hobday, S. Thomas, A. O'Donovan, M. Murphy, and A. Pinching, "Dietary Intervention in Chronic Fatigue Syndrome," *Journal of Human Nutrition and Dietetics* 21, no. 2 (2008): 141–49.

53. M. Werbach, "Nutritional Strategies for Treating Chronic Fatigue Syndrome," *Alternative Medicine Review* 5, no. 2 (2000): 93–108.

54. M. Werbach, "Nutritional Strategies for Treating Chronic Fatigue Syndrome," *Alternative Medicine Review* 5, no. 2 (2000): 93–108.

55. M. Werbach, "Nutritional Strategies for Treating Chronic Fatigue Syndrome," *Alternative Medicine Review* 5, no. 2 (2000): 93–108.

56. D. Maric, S. Brkic, A. Mikic, S. Tomic, T. Cebovic, and V. Turkulov, "Multivitamin Mineral Supplementation in Patients with Chronic Fatigue Syndrome," *Medical Science Monitor* 20 (2014): 47–53.

57. C. Lapp, "Q: Given the Complexities and Diversity of Symptoms of Cfids, How Do You Approach the Treatment of Cfids Patients?" (paper presented at the CFIDS Chronicle Physicians' Forum, 1991); F. Ellis and S. Nasser, "A Pilot Study of Vitamin B12 in the Treatment of Tiredness," *British Journal of Nutrition* 30, no. 2 (1973): 277–83; H. Newbold, "Vitamin B-12: Placebo or Neglected Therapeutic Tool?" *Medical Hypotheses* 28, no. 3 (1989): 155–64.

58. J. Kaslow, L. Rucker, and R. Onishi, "Liver Extract–Folic Acid–Cyanocobalamin vs. Placebo for Chronic Fatigue Syndrome," *Archives of Internal Medicine* 149, no. 11 (1989): 2501–3.

59. M. Werbach, "Nutritional Strategies for Treating Chronic Fatigue Syndrome," *Alternative Medicine Review* 5, no. 2 (2000): 93–108.

60. M. Werbach, "Nutritional Strategies for Treating Chronic Fatigue Syndrome," *Alternative Medicine Review* 5, no. 2 (2000): 93–108.

61. M. Werbach, "Nutritional Strategies for Treating Chronic Fatigue Syndrome," *Alternative Medicine Review* 5, no. 2 (2000): 93–108.

62. R. Cater II, "Chronic Intestinal Candidiasis As a Possible Etiological Factor in the Chronic Fatigue Syndrome," *Medical Hypotheses* 44, no. 6 (1995): 507–15.

63. R. Hobday, S. Thomas, A. O'Donovan, M. Murphy, and A. Pinching, "Dietary Intervention in Chronic Fatigue Syndrome," *Journal of Human Nutrition and Dietetics* 21, no. 2 (2008): 141–49.

64. L. Wilson, "Chronic Fatigue Syndrome," accessed May 13, 2014, www.drlwilson.com/Articles/chronic%20fatigue.htm.

65. M. Shilstone, *Maximum Energy for Life: A 21-Day Strategic Plan to Feel Great, Reverse the Aging Process, and Optimize Your Health* (Hoboken, NJ: John Wiley & Sons, 2003).

66. M. Timlin and M. Pereira, "Breakfast Frequency and Quality in the Etiology of Adult Obesity and Chronic Diseases," *Nutrition Reviews* 65, no. 6 (2007): 268–81.

67. M. Timlin and M. Pereira, "Breakfast Frequency and Quality in the Etiology of Adult Obesity and Chronic Diseases," *Nutrition Reviews* 65, no. 6 (2007): 268–81.

68. C. Marsh, *Prescription for Energy* (London: Thorsons, 1964).

69. M. Jackson, and D. Bruck, "Sleep Abnormalities in Chronic Fatigue Syndrome/Myalgic Encephalomyelitis: A Review," *Journal of Clinical Sleep Medicine* 8, no. 6 (2012): 719–28.

70. M. Jackson, and D. Bruck, "Sleep Abnormalities in Chronic Fatigue Syndrome/Myalgic Encephalomyelitis: A Review," *Journal of Clinical Sleep Medicine* 8, no. 6 (2012): 719–28.

## 11. PHARMACOLOGICAL APPROACHES TO CHRONIC FATIGUE SYNDROME

1. A. Fernández, A. Perez Martin, M. Izquierdo-Martínez, M. Arruti Bustillo, F. Hernández, J. Labrado, R. Díaz-Delgado Peñas, E. Gutiérrez Rivas, C.

Palacín Delgado, J. Rivera, J. Giménez, "Chronic Fatigue Syndrome: Aetiology, Diagnosis and Treatment," *BMC Psychiatry* 9, Suppl. 1 (2009): S1.

2. K. Stange, "Healing Perceptions and Relationships," *Annals of Family Medicine* 6, no. 5 (2008): 466–68.

3. L. Dall, J. Stanford, and J. Hurst, eds., *Clinical Methods: The History, Physical, and Laboratory Examinations*, 3rd ed. (Boston: Butterworths, 1990).

4. G. Morris and M. Maes, "Oxidative and Nitrosative Stress and Immune-inflammatory Pathways in Patients with Myalgic Encephalomyelitis (ME)/ Chronic Fatigue Syndrome (CFS)," *Current Neuropharmacology* 12, no. 2 (2014): 168–85.

5. C. Sostres, C. Gargallo, M. Arroyo, and A. Lanas, "Adverse Effects of Non-steroidal Anti-inflammatory Drugs (NSAIDs, Aspirin and Coxibs) on Upper Gastrointestinal Tract," *Best Practice & Research Clinical Gastroenterology* 24, no. 2 (2010): 121–32.

6. A. Kumar, R. Garg, V. Gaur, and P. Kumar, "Nitric Oxide Modulation in Protective Role of Antidepressants against Chronic Fatigue Syndrome in Mice," *Indian Journal of Pharmacology* 43, no. 3 (2011): 324–29.

7. A. Kumar, R. Garg, V. Gaur, and P. Kumar, "Nitric Oxide Modulation in Protective Role of Antidepressants against Chronic Fatigue Syndrome in Mice," *Indian Journal of Pharmacology* 43, no. 3 (2011): 324–29.

8. A. Cooper, V. Tucker, and G. Papakostas, "Resolution of Sleepiness and Fatigue: A Comparison of Bupropion and Selective Serotonin Reuptake Inhibitors in Subjects with Major Depressive Disorder Achieving Remission at Doses Approved in the European Union," *Journal of Psychopharmacology* 28, no. 2 (2014): 118–24.

9. S. Lynch, R. Seth, and S. Montgomery, "Antidepressant Therapy in the Chronic Fatigue Syndrome," *British Journal of General Practice* 41, no. 349 (1991): 339–42.

10. C. Gualtieri and L. Johnson, "Antidepressant Side Effects in Children and Adolescents," *Journal of Child and Adolescent Psychopharmacology* 16, nos. 1–2 (2006): 147–57.

11. W. Shiel, "Chronic Fatigue Syndrome: Medical Treatment," accessed July 24, 2014, www.emedicinehealth.com.

12. R. Awad, D. Levac, P. Cybulska, Z. Merali, V. Trudeau, and J. Arnason, "Effects of Traditionally Used Anxiolytic Botanicals on Enzymes of the Gamma-aminobutyric Acid (GABA) System," *Canadian Journal of Physiology and Pharmacology* 85, no. 9 (2007): 933–42.

13. D. Helton, J. Tizzano, J. Monn, D. Schoepp, and M. Kallman, "Anxiolytic and Side-effect Profile of LY354740: A Potent, Highly Selective, Orally Active Agonist for Group II Metabotropic Glutamate Receptors," *Journal of Pharmacology and Experimental Therapeutics* 284, no. 2 (1998): 651–60.

14. Z. Gotts, V. Deary, J. Newton, D. Van der Dussen, P. De Roy, and J. Ellis, "Are There Sleep-specific Phenotypes in Patients with Chronic Fatigue Syndrome? A Cross-sectional Polysomnography Analysis?" *BMJ Open* 3, no. 6 (2013): e002999.

15. A. Doble, "New Insights into the Mechanism of Action of Hypnotics," *Journal of Psychopharmacology* 13, no. 4, Suppl. 1 (1999): S11–20.

16. W. Kelly, M. Ambrose, E. Gallen, A. Houska, M. Devlin, M. Anello, R. Doyle, S. Cammon, C. Damico, L. Neri, and K. Zalewski, *Nursing Drug Handbook*, 23rd ed. (New York: Lippincott Williams and Wilkins, 2003): 14–1240.

17. R. Suhadolnik, N. Reichenbach, P. Hitzges, R. Sobol, D. Peterson, B. Henry, D. Ablashi, W. Müller, J. Schröder, and W. Carter, "Upregulation of the 2-5A Synthetase/RNase L Antiviral Pathway Associated with Chronic Fatigue Syndrome," *Clinical Infectious Diseases* 18, Suppl. 1 (1994): S96–104.

18. R. Suhadolnik, N. Reichenbach, P. Hitzges, R. Sobol, D. Peterson, B. Henry, D. Ablashi, W. Müller, J. Schröder, and W. Carter, "Upregulation of the 2-5A Synthetase/RNase L Antiviral Pathway Associated with Chronic Fatigue Syndrome," *Clinical Infectious Diseases* 18, Suppl. 1 (1994): S96–104.

19. R. Suhadolnik, N. Reichenbach, P. Hitzges, R. Sobol, D. Peterson, B. Henry, D. Ablashi, W. Müller, J. Schröder, and W. Carter, "Upregulation of the 2-5A Synthetase/RNase L Antiviral Pathway Associated with Chronic Fatigue Syndrome," *Clinical Infectious Diseases* 18, Suppl. 1 (1994): S96–104.

20. R. Razonable, "Antiviral Drugs for Viruses Other Than Human Immunodeficiency Virus," *Mayo Clinic Proceedings* 86, no. 10 (2011): 1009–26.

21. E. Iwakami, Y. Arashima, K. Kato, T. Komiya, Y. Matsukawa, T. Ikeda, Y. Arakawa, and S. Oshida, "Treatment of Chronic Fatigue Syndrome with Antibiotics: Pilot Study Assessing the Involvement of Coxiella Burnetii Infection," *Internal Medicine* 44, no. 12 (2005): 1258–63.

22. R. Hancock, "Mechanisms of Action of Newer Antibiotics for Grampositive Pathogens," *The Lancet Infectious Diseases* 5, no. 4 (2005): 209–18.

23. P. Rishi, S. Preet, and P. Kaur, "Effect of L. Plantarum Cell-free Extract and Co-trimoxazole against Salmonella Typhimurium: A Possible Adjunct Therapy," *Annals of Clinical Microbiology and Antimicrobials* 10 (2011): 9.

24. D. Dunwell, "ME/CFS and Blastocystis Spp or Dientamoeba Fragilis: An In-house Comparison," *British Journal of General Practice* 63, no. 607 (2013): 73–74.

25. S. Parija and K. Khairnar, "Detection of Excretory Entamoeba Histolytica DNA in the Urine, and Detection of E. Histolytica DNA and Lectin Antigen in the Liver Abscess Pus for the Diagnosis of Amoebic Liver Abscess," *BMC Microbiology* 7 (2007): 41.

26. I. Esfandiarpour, S. Farajzadeh, Z. Rahnama, E. Fathabadi, and A. Heshmatkhah, "Adverse Effects of Intralesional Meglumine Antimoniate and

Its Influence on Clinical Laboratory Parameters in the Treatment of Cutaneous Leishmaniasis," *International Journal of Dermatology* 51, no. 10 (2012): 1221–25.

27. I. Esfandiarpour, S. Farajzadeh, Z. Rahnama, E. Fathabadi, and A. Heshmatkhah, "Adverse Effects of Intralesional Meglumine Antimoniate and Its Influence on Clinical Laboratory Parameters in the Treatment of Cutaneous Leishmaniasis," *International Journal of Dermatology* 51, no. 10 (2012): 1221–25.

28. M. Kiebala and S. Maggirwar, "Ibudilast, a Pharmacologic Phosphodiesterase Inhibitor, Prevents Human Immunodeficiency Virus-1 Tat-mediated Activation of Microglial Cells," *PLOS One* 6, no. 4 (2011): e18633.

29. M. Kiebala and S. Maggirwar, "Ibudilast, a Pharmacologic Phosphodiesterase Inhibitor, Prevents Human Immunodeficiency Virus-1 Tat-mediated Activation of Microglial Cells," *PLOS One* 6, no. 4 (2011): e18633.

30. D. Strayer, W. Carter, B. Stouch, S. Stevens, L. Bateman, P. Cimoch, C. Lapp, D. Peterson, and W. Mitchell, "A Double-blind, Placebo-controlled, Randomized, Clinical Trial of the TLR-3 Agonist Rintatolimod in Severe Cases of Chronic Fatigue Syndrome," *PLOS One* 7, no. 3 (2012): e31334.

31. D. See and J. Tilles, "Alpha-interferon Treatment of Patients with Chronic Fatigue Syndrome," *Immunological Investigations* 25, nos. 1–2 (1996): 153–64.

32. A. Kavelaars, W. Kuis, L. Knook, G. Sinnema, and C. Heijnen, "Disturbed Neuroendocrine-immune Interactions in Chronic Fatigue Syndrome," *The Journal of Clinical Endocrinology & Metabolism* 85, no. 2 (2000): 692–96.

33. J. Smith, E. Fritz, J. Kerr, A. Cleare, S. Wessely, and D. Mattey, "Association of Chronic Fatigue Syndrome with Human Leucocyte Antigen Class II Alleles," *Journal of Clinical Pathology* 58, no. 8 (2005): 860–63.

34. O. Fluge and O. Mella, "Clinical Impact of B-cell Depletion with the Anti-CD20 Antibody Rituximab in Chronic Fatigue Syndrome: A Preliminary Case Series," *BMC Neurology* 9 (2009): 28.

35. S. Smelter, B. Bare, *Medical Surgical Nursing: Volume 1 and 2* (New York: Lippincott Williams and Wilkins, 2004) 124–211.

36. T. Chaudhry, P. Hissaria, M. Wiese, R. Heddle, F. Kette, and W. Smith, "Oral Drug Challenges in Non-steroidal Anti-inflammatory Drug-induced Urticaria, Angioedema and Anaphylaxis," *Journal of Internal Medicine* 42, no. 6 (2012): 665–71.

37. T. Chaudhry, P. Hissaria, M. Wiese, R. Heddle, F. Kette, and W. Smith, "Oral Drug Challenges in Non-steroidal Anti-inflammatory Drug-induced Urticaria, Angioedema and Anaphylaxis," *Journal of Internal Medicine* 42, no. 6 (2012): 665–71.

38. A. Grieco, A. Forgione, L. Miele, V. Vero, A. Greco, A. Gasbarrini, and G. Gasbarrini, "Fatty Liver and Drugs," *European Review for Medical and Pharmacological Sciences* 9, no. 5 (2005): 261–63.

39. T. Mathew, "Drug-induced Renal Disease," *Medical Journal of Australia* 156, no. 10 (1992): 724–28.

40. D. Venes, C. Thomas, E. Egan, N. Morelli, and A. Nell, *Taber's Cyclopedic Medical Dictionary* 19th ed. (Philadelphia: F.A. Davis Company, 2001): 333–1229.

41. A. Cleare, E. Heap, G. Malhi, S. Wessely, V. O'Keane, and J. Miell, "Low Dose Hydrocortisone in Chronic Fatigue Syndrome: A Randomised Crossover Trial," *Lancet* 353, no. 9151 (1999): 455–58.

42. A. Wilson, I. Hickie, A. Lloyd, and D. Wakefield, "The Treatment of Chronic Fatigue Syndrome: Science and Speculation," *The American Journal of Medicine* 96, no. 6 (1994): 544–50.

43. L. Arnold, P. Keck Jr., and J. Welge, "Antidepressant Treatment of Fibromyalgia: A Meta-analysis and Review," *Psychosomatics* 41, no. 2 (2000): 104–13.

44. B. Kozier, G. Erb, and K. Blais, *Fundamentals of Nursing: Concepts, Process and Practice* (Singapore: Pearson Education Asia, 2001): 352–460.

## 12. ADDRESSING THE MIND

1. E. Attree, M. Arroll, C. Dancey, C. Griffith, and A. Bansal, "Psychosocial Factors Involved in Memory and Cognitive Failures in People with Myalgic Encephalomyelitis/Chronic Fatigue Syndrome," *Psychology Research and Behavior Management* 7 (2014): 72.

2. A. Baddeley, ed., *Human Memory: Theory and Practice* (Hove, UK: Psychology Press 1997).

3. B. Carruthers, A. Jain, K. De Meirleir, D. Peterson, N. Klimas, and A. Lerner, "Myalgic Encephalomyelitis/Chronic Fatigue Syndrome: Clinical Working Case Definition, Diagnostics, and Treatment Protocols," *Journal of Chronic Fatigue Syndrome* 11, no. 1 (2003): 7–36.

4. J. Findley, R. Kerns, L. Weinberg, and R. Rosenberg, "Self-efficacy As a Psychological Moderator of Chronic Fatigue Syndrome," *Journal of Behavioral Medicine* 21, no. 4 (1998): 351–62.

5. F. Friedberg and L. Jason, *Understanding Chronic Fatigue Syndrome: An Empirical Guide to Assessment and Treatment* (Washington, DC: American Psychological Association, 1998).

6. L. Jason, E. Witter, and S. Torres-Harding, "Chronic Fatigue Syndrome, Coping, Optimism and Social Support," *Journal of Mental Health* 12, no. 2 (2003): 109–18.

7. B. Marcel, A. Komaroff, L. Faioli, R. Kornish, and M. Albert, "Cognitive Deficits in Patients with CFS," *Biological Psychiatry* 40 (1996): 535–41.

8. M. Mayer, "The Role of Severe Life Stress, Social Support and Attachment in the Onset of Chronic Fatigue Syndrome," *Dissertation Abstracts International*, 60 (2000): 3605.

9. M. Mayer, "The Role of Severe Life Stress, Social Support and Attachment in the Onset of Chronic Fatigue Syndrome," *Dissertation Abstracts International*, 60 (2000): 3605.

10. M. McDaniel and G. Einstein, *Prospective Memory: An Overview and Synthesis of an Emerging Field* (New York: Sage Publications, 2007).

11. A. Missen, W. Hollingworth, N. Eaton, and E. Crawley, "The Financial and Psychological Impacts on Mothers of Children with Chronic Fatigue Syndrome (CFS/ME)," *Child: Care, Health and Development* 38, no. 4 (2012): 505–12; J. Ormrod, *Educational Psychology: Developing Learners*, 5th ed. (Upper Saddle River, NJ: Pearson/Merrill Prentice Hall, 2006).

12. D. Pountney, "Identifying and Managing Chronic Fatigue Syndrome," *British Journal of Neuroscience Nursing* 5, no. 10 (2013): 460–62.

13. D. Pountney, "Identifying and Managing Chronic Fatigue Syndrome," *British Journal of Neuroscience Nursing* 5, no. 10 (2013): 460–62.

14. S. Van Damme, G. Crombez, B. Van Houdenhove, A. Mariman, and W. Michielsen, "Well-being in Patients with Chronic Fatigue Syndrome: The Role of Acceptance," *Journal of Psychosomatic Research* 61, no. 5 (2006): 595–99.

15. S. Van Damme, G. Crombez, B. Van Houdenhove, A. Mariman, and W. Michielsen, "Well-being in Patients with Chronic Fatigue Syndrome: The Role of Acceptance," *Journal of Psychosomatic Research* 61, no. 5 (2006): 595–99.

16. S. Van Damme, G. Crombez, B. Van Houdenhove, A. Mariman, and W. Michielsen, "Well-being in Patients with Chronic Fatigue Syndrome: The Role of Acceptance," *Journal of Psychosomatic Research* 61, no. 5 (2006): 595–99.

17. N. Ware, "Toward a Model of Social Course in Chronic Illness: The Example of Chronic Fatigue Syndrome," *Culture, Medicine, and Psychiatry* 23, no. 3 (1999): 303–31.

18. N. Ware, "Toward a Model of Social Course in Chronic Illness: The Example of Chronic Fatigue Syndrome," *Culture, Medicine, and Psychiatry* 23, no. 3 (1999): 303–31.

19. N. Ware, "Toward a Model of Social Course in Chronic Illness: The Example of Chronic Fatigue Syndrome," *Culture, Medicine, and Psychiatry* 23, no. 3 (1999): 303–31.

20. B. Saltzstein, G. Wyshak, J. Hubbuch, and J. Perry, "A Naturalistic Study of the Chronic Fatigue Syndrome among Women in Primary Care," *General Hospital Psychiatry* 20, no. 5 (1998): 307–16.

21. B. Saltzstein, G. Wyshak, J. Hubbuch, and J. Perry, "A Naturalistic Study of the Chronic Fatigue Syndrome among Women in Primary Care," *General Hospital Psychiatry* 20, no. 5 (1998): 307–16.

22. B. Saltzstein, G. Wyshak, J. Hubbuch, and J. Perry, "A Naturalistic Study of the Chronic Fatigue Syndrome among Women in Primary Care," *General Hospital Psychiatry* 20, no. 5 (1998): 307–16.

23. R. Taylor, F. Friedberg, and L. Jason, *A Clinician's Guide to Controversial Illnesses: Chronic Fatigue Syndrome, Fibromyalgia and Multiple Chemical Sensitivities* (Sarasota, FL: Professional Resource Press, 2001).

24. H. Kang, B. Natelson, C. Mahan, K. Lee, and F. Murphy, "Post-traumatic Stress Disorder and Chronic Fatigue Syndrome-like Illness among Gulf War Veterans: A Population-Based Survey of 30,000 Veterans," *American Journal of Epidemiology* 157, no. 2 (2003): 141–48.

25. H. Kang, B. Natelson, C. Mahan, K. Lee, and F. Murphy, "Post-traumatic Stress Disorder and Chronic Fatigue Syndrome-like Illness among Gulf War Veterans: A Population-based Survey of 30,000 Veterans," *American Journal of Epidemiology* 157, no. 2 (2003): 141–48.

26. H. Kang, B. Natelson, C. Mahan, K. Lee, and F. Murphy, "Post-traumatic Stress Disorder and Chronic Fatigue Syndrome-like Illness among Gulf War Veterans: A Population-based Survey of 30,000 Veterans," *American Journal of Epidemiology* 157, no. 2 (2003): 141–48.

27. C. Brodsky, "Depression and Chronic Fatigue in the Workplace: Workers' Compensation and Occupational Issues," *Primary Care* 18, no. 2 (1991): 381–96.

28. T. Sampalli, E. Berlasso, R. Fox, and M. Petter, "A Controlled Study of the Effect of a Mindfulness-based Stress Reduction Technique in Women with Multiple Chemical Sensitivity, Chronic Fatigue Syndrome, and Fibromyalgia," *Journal of Multidisciplinary Healthcare* 2 (2009): 53–59.

## 13. COLLECTIVE EFFORTS

1. A. Lloyd and H. Pender, "The Economic Impact of Chronic Fatigue Syndrome," *Medical Journal of Australia* 157, no. 9 (1992): 599–601.

2. I. Gibson, "A New Look at Chronic Fatigue Syndrome/Myalgic Encephalomyelitis," *Journal of Clinical Pathology* 60, no. 2 (2007): 120–21.

3. I. Lewis, J. Pairman, G. Spickett, and J. Newton, "Clinical Characteristics of a Novel Subgroup of Chronic Fatigue Syndrome Patients with Postural

Orthostatic Tachycardia Syndrome," *Journal of Intern Medicine* 273, no. 5 (2013): 501–10.

4. E. Del Fabbro, S. Dalal, and E. Bruera, "Symptom Control in Palliative Care—Part II: Cachexia/Anorexia and Fatigue," *Journal of Palliative Medicine* 9, no. 2 (2006): 409–21.

5. P. Santamarina-Perez, F. Eiroa-Orosa, V. Freniche, A. Moreno-Mayos, J. Alegre, N. Saez, and C. Jacas, "Length of Disorder Does Not Predict Cognitive Dysfunction in Chronic Fatigue Syndrome," *Applied Neuropsychology* 18, no. 3 (2011): 216–22.

6. M. Meeus, I. van Eupen, E. van Baarle, V. De Boeck, A. Luyckx, D. Kos, and J. Nijs, "Symptom Fluctuations and Daily Physical Activity in Patients with Chronic Fatigue Syndrome: A Case-control Study," *Archives of Physical Medicine and Rehabilitation* 92, no. 11 (2011): 1820–26.

7. C. King and L. Jason, "Improving the Diagnostic Criteria and Procedures for Chronic Fatigue Syndrome," *Biological Psychology* 68, no. 2 (2005): 87–106.

8. N. Janssen, I. Kant, G. Swaen, P. Janssen, and C. Schröer, "Fatigue As a Predictor of Sickness Absence: Results from the Maastricht Cohort Study on Fatigue at Work," *Occupational and Environmental Medicine* 60, Suppl. 1 (2003): i71-6.

9. E. Berndt, J. Bailit, M. Keller, J. Verner, and S. Finkelstein, "Health Care Use and At-work Productivity among Employees with Mental Disorders," *Health Affairs* 19, no. 4 (2000): 244–56.

10. R. Bennett, J. Jones, D. Turk, I. Russell, and L. Matallana, "An Internet Survey of 2,596 People with Fibromyalgia," *BioMedCentral (BMC) Musculoskeletal Disorders* 8 (2007): 27.

11. "National Fibromyalgia Research Association" accessed July 23, 2014, www.nfra.net.

12. The International Association for CFS/ME, "Presidential Letter," accessed July 23, 2014, www.iacfsme.org.

13. "Introduction to HHV-6," accessed June 25, 2014, www.hhv-6foundation.org.

14. "About NICE," Accessed June 29, 2014, www.nice.org.uk.

15. "Mission and Vision," accessed May 21, 2014, www.pandoraorg.net.

16. "About Us," accessed May 23, 2014, www.rmcfa.org.

17. "About Us," accessed June 12, 2014, www.wicfs-me.org.

18. L. Jason, J. Ferrari, R. Taylor, S. Slavich, and C. Stenzel, "A National Assessment of the Service, Support, and Housing Preferences by Persons with Chronic Fatigue Syndrome: Toward a Comprehensive Rehabilitation Program," *Evaluation & the Health Professions* 19, no. 2 (1996): 194–207.

19. J. Taylor, A. Gilbertson, W. Semchuk, and J. Johnson, "Effect of Verbal Encouragement on Patient Question-asking Behaviour during Medication Counselling Support Groups," *International Journal of Pharmacy Practice* 9, no. 4 (2001): 253–59.

20. J. Trabal, P. Leyes, J. Fernández-Solá, M. Forga, and J. Fernández-Huerta, "Patterns of Food Avoidance in Chronic Fatigue Syndrome: Is There a Case for Dietary Recommendations?" *Nutrición Hospitalaria* 27, no. 2 (2012): 659–62.

21. K. Phillips, L. Faul, B. Small, P. Jacobsen, S. Apte, and H. Jim, "Comparing the Retrospective Reports of Fatigue Using the Fatigue Symptom Index with Daily Diary Ratings in Women Receiving Chemotherapy for Gynecologic Cancer," *Journal of Pain and Symptom Management* 46, no. 2 (2013): 282–88.

22. J. Chan, R. Ho, C. Wang, L. Yuen, J. Sham, and C. Chan, "Effects of Qigong Exercise on Fatigue, Anxiety, and Depressive Symptoms of Patients with Chronic Fatigue Syndrome–like Disorder: A Randomized Controlled Trial," *Evidence Based Complementary and Alternative Medicine* (2013): 485341.

23. G. Richardson, D. Epstein, C. Chew-Graham, C. Dowrick, R. Bentall, R. Morriss, S. Peters, L. Riste, K. Lovell, G. Dunn, A. Wearden, "Cost-effectiveness of Supported Self-management for CFS/ME Patients in Primary Care," *BMC Family Practice* 14 (2013): 12.

24. S. Kreijkamp-Kaspers, E. Brenu, S. Marshall, D. Staines, and M. Van Driel, "Treating Chronic Fatigue Syndrome: A Study into the Scientific Evidence for Pharmacological Treatments," *Australian Family Physician* 40, no. 11 (2011): 907–12.

25. S. Chafin, N. Christenfeld, and W. Gerin, "Improving Cardiovascular Recovery from Stress with Brief Poststress Exercise," *Health Psychology* 27, Suppl. 1 (2008): S64–72.

26. K. McCully, B. Clark, J. Kent, J. Wilson, and B. Chance, "Biochemical Adaptations to Training: Implications for Resisting Muscle Fatigue," *Canadian Journal of Physiology and Pharmacology* 69, no. 2 (1991): 274–78.

27. T. Sampalli, E. Berlasso, R. Fox, and M. Petter, "A Controlled Study of the Effect of a Mindfulness-based Stress Reduction Technique in Women with Multiple Chemical Sensitivity, Chronic Fatigue Syndrome, and Fibromyalgia," *Journal of Multidisciplinary Healthcare* 2 (2009): 53–59.

28. T. Kahlon, M. Chiu, and M. Chapman, "Steam Cooking Significantly Improves in Vitro Bile Acid Binding of Collard Greens, Kale, Mustard Greens, Broccoli, Green Bell Pepper, and Cabbage," *Nutrition Research* 28, no. 6 (2008): 351–57.

# 14. CONCLUSION

1. The ME Association, "Fatigue Research Symposium," accessed May 13, 2014, www.meassociation.org.uk/research/fatigue-research-symposium.

2. Centers for Disease Control and Prevention, "Diagnosing CFS," accessed May 13, 2014, www.cdc.gov/cfs/diagnosis/index.html.

3. Massachusetts CFIDS/ME and FM Association, "What Is CFIDS/ME?" accessed May 15, 2014, www.masscfids.org/about-cfidsme.

4. Centers for Disease Control and Prevention, "CFS Case Definition," accessed May 13, 2014, www.cdc.gov/cfs/case-definition/index.html.

5. J. Wilson, "20 Things People over 20 Should Stop Doing," accessed May 13, 2014, www.jarridwilson.com/20-things-people-over-20-should-stop-doing.

6. Solving ME/CFS Initiative, "Fundraising," accessed May 15, 2014, www.solvecfs.org/get-involved/fundraising.

7. Action for ME, "International Information," accessed May 15, 2014, www.actionforme.org.uk/get-informed/international-information.

8. M. Ruiz, "Risks of Self-medication Practices," *Current Drug Safety* 5, no. 4 (2010): 315–23.

9. M. Ruiz, "Risks of Self-medication Practices," *Current Drug Safety* 5, no. 4 (2010): 315–23.

10. D. Payne, "The Importance of Prevention in Health Care," *Canadian Family Physician* 47 (2001): 2211–13.

11. Massachusetts CFIDS/ME and FM Association, "Treatment," accessed May 15, 2014, www.masscfids.org/treatment.

12. M. Reyes, R. Nisenbaum, D. Hoaglin, E. Unger, C. Emmons, B. Randall, J. Stewart, S. Abbey, J. Jones, N. Gantz, S. Minden, and W. Reeves, "Prevalence and Incidence of Chronic Fatigue Syndrome in Wichita, Kansas," *Archives of Internal Medicine* 163, no. 13 (2003): 1530–36.

13. J. Stevens and D. Stephens, "Patience," *Current Biology* 18, no. 1 (2008): R11-2.

14. H. Lewine, "When Exercise Makes You Feel Worse," accessed May 13, 2014, www.intelihealth.com/print-article/chronic-fatigue-syndrome-when-exercise-makes-you-feel-worse.

15. K. Kirk, "Confidence As a Factor in Chronic Illness Care," *Journal of Advanced Nursing* 17, no. 10 (1992): 1238–42.

# BIBLIOGRAPHY

## PREFACE

Bagnall, A. M., P. Whiting, R. Richardson, and A. J. Sowden. "Interventions for the Treatment and Management of Chronic Fatigue Syndrome/Myalgic Encephalomyelitis." *Quality & Safety in Health Care* 11, no. 3 (2002): 284–88.

Capuron, L., L. Welberg, C. Heim, D. Wagner, L. Solomon, D. Papanicolaou, R. Craddock, Miller, A., and W. Reeves. "Cognitive Dysfunction Relates to Subjective Report of Mental Fatigue in Patients with Chronic Fatigue Syndrome." *Neuropsychopharmacology* 31, no. 8 (2006): 1777–84.

Whiting, P., A. M. Bagnall, A. J. Sowden, J. E. Cornell, C. D. Mulrow, and G. Ramírez. "Interventions for the Treatment and Management of Chronic Fatigue Syndrome: A Systematic Review." *Journal of the American Medical Association* 286, no. 11 (2001): 1360–68.

## CHAPTER I

Aldrich, T. K. "Transmission Fatigue of the Rabbit Diaphragm." *Respiration Physiology* 69, no. 3 (1987): 307–19.

Heymsfield, S. B., D. Thomas, A. Bosy-Westphal, W. Shen, C. M. Peterson, and M. J. Müller. "Evolving Concepts on Adjusting Human Resting Energy Expenditure Measurements for Body Size." *Obesity Reviews* 13, no. 11 (2012): 1001–14.

Kaminski, M. V. "A New Look at Chronic Fatigue Syndrome: The Link between Antibiotics, the Intestine and Mitochondrial Dysfunction." *Mature Medicine Canada* 3 (2000): 85–89.

Meier, U., and A. M. Gressner. "Endocrine Regulation of Energy Metabolism: Review of Pathobiochemical and Clinical Chemical Aspects of Leptin, Ghrelin, Adiponectin, and Resistin." *Clinical Chemistry* 50, no. 9 (2004): 1511–25.

Rathmacher, J. A., J. C. Fuller Jr., S. M. Baier, N. N. Abumrad, H. F. Angus, and R. L. Sharp. "Adenosine-5'-Triphosphate (ATP) Supplementation Improves Low Peak Muscle Torque and Torque Fatigue during Repeated High Intensity Exercise Sets." *Journal of the International Society of Sports Nutrition* 9, no. 9 (2012): 48.

# CHAPTER 2

Anderson, V. R., L. A. Jason, and L. E. Hlavaty. "A Qualitative Natural History Study of ME/ CFS in the Community." *Health Care for Women International* 35, no. 1 (2014): 3–26.
Harvey, S. B., S. Wessely, D. Kuh, and M. Hotopf. "The Relationship between Fatigue and Psychiatric Disorders: Evidence for the Concept of Neurasthenia." *Journal of Psychosomatic Research* 66, no. 5 (2009): 445–54.
Porter, N., A. Lerch, L. A. Jason, M. Sorenson, M. A. Fletcher, and J. Herrington. "A Comparison of Immune Functionality in Viral versus Non-viral CFS Subtypes." *Behavioral Neuroscience* 8, no. 2 (2010): 1–8.
Tersteeg, I. M., F. S. Koopman, J. M. Stolwijk-Swüste, A. Beelen, and F. Nollet. "A 5-year Longitudinal Study of Fatigue in Patients with Late-onset Sequelae of Poliomyelitis." *Archives of Physical Medicine and Rehabilitation* 92, no. 6 (2011): 899–904.
Wookey, C. Review of *Post-viral Fatigue Syndrome: The Saga of Royal Free Disease*, by A. M. Ramsay. *The Journal of the Royal College of General Practitioners* 37, no. 305 (1987): 565.

# CHAPTER 3

Hampton, T. "Researchers Find Genetic Clues to Chronic Fatigue Syndrome." *Journal of the American Medical Association* 295, no. 21 (2006): 2466–67.
Scott, L. V., S. Medbak, and T. G. Dinan. "Blunted Adrenocorticotropin and Cortisol Responses to Corticotropin-releasing Hormone Stimulation in Chronic Fatigue Syndrome." *Acta Psychiatrica Scandinavica* 97, no. 6 (1998): 450–57.
Taillefer, S. S., L. J. Kirmayer, J. M. Robbins, and J. C. Lasry. "Psychological Correlates of Functional Status in Chronic Fatigue Syndrome." *Journal of Psychosomatic Research* 53, no. 6 (2002): 1097–106.
Tersteeg, I. M., F. S. Koopman, J. M. Stolwijk-Swüste, A. Beelen, and F. Nollet. "A 5-year Longitudinal Study of Fatigue in Patients with Late-onset Sequelae of Poliomyelitis." *Archives of Physical Medicine and Rehabilitation* 92, no. 6 (2011): 899–904.

# CHAPTER 4

Hardcastle, S. L., E. Brenu, S. Johnston, T. Nguyen, T. Huth, M. Kaur, S. Ramos, A. Salajegheh, D. Staines, and S. Marshall-Gradisnik. "Analysis of the Relationship between Immune Dysfunction and Symptom Severity in Patients with Chronic Fatigue Syndrome/ Myalgic Encephalomyelitis (CFS/ME)." *Journal of Clinical & Cellular Immunology* 5, no. 190 (2014): 4172.
Harrower, T. P., L. J. Findley, G. Lennox, and D. G. O'Donovan. "Pathological Findings in a Case of Severe Chronic Fatigue Syndrome." *Journal of the Neurological Sciences* 238 (2005): S512–S512.
Holmes, G. P., J. E. Kaplan, N. M. Gantz, A. L. Komaroff, L. B. Schonberger, S. E. Straus, J. F. Jones, R. E. Dubois, C. Cunningham-Rundles, and S. Pahwa. "Chronic Fatigue Syndrome: A Working Case Definition." *Annals of Internal Medicine* 108, no. 3 (1988): 387–89.
Jason, L. A., S. R. Torres-Harding, A. W. Carrico, and R. R. Taylor. "Symptom Occurrence in Persons with Chronic Fatigue Syndrome." *Biological Psychology* 59, no. 1 (2002): 15–27.
Lloyd, A. R., D. Wakefield, and I. Hickie. "Immunity and the Pathophysiology of Chronic Fatigue Syndrome." *Ciba Foundation Symposium* 173 (1993): 176–92.

# CHAPTER 5

Aaron, L. A., R. Herrell, S. Ashton, M. Belcourt, K. Schmaling, J. Goldberg, and D. Buchwald. "Comorbid Clinical Conditions in Chronic Fatigue." *Journal of General Internal Medicine* 16, no. 1 (2001): 24–31.

Kumae, T. "The Study for Prevention and Early Phase Detection of Chronic Fatigue by Spectral Analysis of Heart Rate. Part 2: Effects of Breeding Conditions and Exercise Stress." *Japanese Journal of Hygiene* 52 (1997): 233.

Maes, M., I. Mihaylova, M. Kubera, M. Uytterhoeven, N. Vrydags, and E. Bosmans. "Coenzyme Q10 Deficiency in Myalgic Encephalomyelitis/Chronic Fatigue Syndrome (ME/CFS) is Related to Fatigue, Autonomic and Neurocognitive Symptoms and Is Another Risk Factor Explaining the Early Mortality in ME/CFS Due to Cardiovascular Disorder." *Neuroendocrinology Letters* 30, no. 4 (2008): 470–76.

Majer, M., J. F. Jones, E. R. Unger, L. S. Youngblood, M. J. Decker, B. Gurbaxani, C. Heim, and W. C. Reeves. "Perception versus Polysomnographic Assessment of Sleep in CFS and Non-fatigued Control Subjects: Results from a Population-based Study." *BMC Neurology* 7, no. 1 (2007): 40.

Nijs, J., L. M. Paul, and K. Wallman. "Prevention of Symptom Exacerbations in Chronic Fatigue Syndrome Reply." *Journal of Rehabilitation Medicine* 40, no. 10 (2008): 884–85.

Nijs, J., M. Meeus, J. Van-Oosterwijck, K. Ickmans, I. Van-Eupen, and D. Kos. "Tired of Being Inactive: CNS Dysfunctions Explain Exercise Intolerance in Chronic Fatigue Syndrome." *Neuroscience Letters* 500 (2011): e14.

Ortega, F., and R. Zorzanelli. "Neuroimaging and the Case of Chronic Fatigue Syndrome." *Ciencia & Saude Coletiva* 16, no. 4 (2011): 2123–32.

Yancey, J. R., and S. M. Thomas. "Chronic Fatigue Syndrome: Diagnosis and Treatment." *American Family Physician* 86, no. 8 (2012): 741–46.

# CHAPTER 6

Ax, S., V. H. Gregg, and D. Jones. "Chronic Fatigue Syndrome: Sufferers' Evaluation of Medical Support." *Journal of the Royal Society of Medicine* 90, no. 5 (1997): 250.

Thomas, M. A., and A. P. Smith. "Primary Healthcare Provision and Chronic Fatigue Syndrome: A Survey of Patients' and General Practitioners' Beliefs." *BMC Family Practice* 6, no. 1 (2005): 49.

Wojcik, W., A. Armstrong, and R. Kanaan. "Is Chronic Fatigue Syndrome a Neurological Condition? A Survey of UK Neurologists." *Journal of Psychosomatic Research* 70, no. 6 (2011): 573–74.

# CHAPTER 7

Akagi, H., I. Klimes, and C. Bass. "Cognitive Behavioral Therapy for Chronic Fatigue Syndrome in a General Hospital—Feasible and Effective." *General Hospital Psychiatry* 23, no. 5 (2001): 254–60.

Clauson, K. A., Q. Zeng-Treitler, and S. Kandula. "Readability of Patient and Health Care Professional Targeted Dietary Supplement Leaflets Used for Diabetes and Chronic Fatigue Syndrome." *The Journal of Alternative and Complementary Medicine* 16, no. 1 (2010): 119–24.

Cox, D. L., and L. J. Findley. "The Management of Chronic Fatigue Syndrome in an Inpatient Setting: Presentation of an Approach and Perceived Outcome." *The British Journal of Occupational Therapy* 61, no. 9 (1998): 405–9.

Gilje, A. M., A. Söderlund, and K. Malterud. "Obstructions for Quality Care Experienced by Patients with Chronic Fatigue Syndrome (CFS)—A Case Study." *Patient Education and Counseling* 73, no. 1 (2008): 36–41.

Vernon, S. D., and W. C. Reeves. "The Challenge of Integrating Disparate High-content Data: Epidemiological, Clinical and Laboratory Data Collected during an In-hospital Study of Chronic Fatigue Syndrome." *Pharmacogenomics* (2006): 345–54.

Viner, R., A. Gregorowski, C. Wine, M. Bladen, D. Fisher, M. Miller, and S. El Neil. "Outpatient Rehabilitative Treatment of Chronic Fatigue Syndrome (CFS/ME)." *Archives of Disease in Childhood* 89, no. 7 (2004): 615–19.

## CHAPTER 8

Dempsey, J. A., M. Amann, L. M. Romer, and J. D. Miller. "Respiratory System Determinants of Peripheral Fatigue and Endurance Performance." *Medicine and Science in Sports and Exercise* 40, no. 3 (2008): 457–61.

Freeman, R., and A. L. Komaroff. "Does the Chronic Fatigue Syndrome Involve the Autonomic Nervous System?" *The American Journal of Medicine* 102, no. 4 (1997): 357–64.

Lakhan, S. E., and A. Kirchgessner. "Gut Inflammation in Chronic Fatigue Syndrome." *Nutrition & Metabolism* 7 (2010): 79.

Vecchiet, J., F. Cipollone, K. Falasca, A. Mezzetti, E. Pizzigallo, T. Bucciarelli, S. De Laurentis, G. Affaitati, D. De Cesare, and M. A. Giamberardino. "Relationship between Musculoskeletal Symptoms and Blood Markers of Oxidative Stress in Patients with Chronic Fatigue Syndrome." *Neuroscience Letters* 335, no. 3 (2003): 151–54.

## CHAPTER 9

DeLuca, J., S. K. Johnson, and B. H. Natelson. "Neuropsychiatric Status of Patients with Chronic Fatigue Syndrome: An Overview." *Toxicology and Industrial Health* 10, nos. 4–5 (1993): 513–22.

Levy, J. A. "Viral Studies of Chronic Fatigue Syndrome." *Clinical Infectious Diseases: An Official Publication of the Infectious Diseases Society of America* 18 (1994): S117–20.

Morris, G., and M. Maes. "A Neuro-immune Model of Myalgic Encephalomyelitis/Chronic Fatigue Syndrome." *Metabolic Brain Disease* 28, no. 4 (2013): 523–40.

Papanicolaou, D. A., J. D. Amsterdam, S. Levine, S. M. McCann, R. C. Moore, C. H. Newbrand, and G. Allen. "Neuroendocrine Aspects of Chronic Fatigue Syndrome." *Neuroimmunomodulation* 11, no. 2 (2004): 65–74.

## CHAPTER 10

Alraek, T., M. S. Lee, T.-Y. Choi, H. Cao, and J. Liu. "Complementary and Alternative Medicine for Patients with Chronic Fatigue Syndrome: A Systematic Review." *BMC Complementary and Alternative Medicine* 11, no. 1 (2011): 87.

Christopher, G., and M. Thomas. "Social Problem Solving in Chronic Fatigue Syndrome: Preliminary Findings." *Stress and Health* 25, no. 2 (2009): 161–69.

Dykman, K. D., C. Tone, C. Ford, and R. A. Dykman. "The Effects of Nutritional Supplements on the Symptoms of Fibromyalgia and Chronic Fatigue Syndrome." *Integrative Physiological and Behavioral Science* 33, no. 1 (1998): 61–71.

Knoop, H., J. Van der Meer, and G. Bleijenberg. "Guided Self-instructions for People with Chronic Fatigue Syndrome: Randomised Controlled Trial." *The British Journal of Psychiatry* 193, no. 4 (2008): 340–41.

## CHAPTER 11

Iwakami, E., Y. Arashima, K. Kato, T. Komiya, Y. Matsukawa, T. Ikeda, Y. Arakawa, and S. Oshida. "Treatment of Chronic Fatigue Syndrome with Antibiotics: Pilot Study Assessing the Involvement of Coxiella Burnetii Infection." *Internal Medicine* 44, no. 12 (2005): 1258–63.

Kreijkamp-Kaspers, S., E. W. Brenu, S. Marshall, D. Staines, and M. K. Van Driel. "Treating Chronic Fatigue Syndrome: A Study into the Scientific Evidence for Pharmacological Treatments." *Australian Family Physician* 40, no. 11 (2011): 907.

Lerner, A. M., S. Beqaj, J. T. Fitzgerald, K. Gill, C. Gill, and J. Edington. "Subset-directed Antiviral Treatment of 142 Herpesvirus Patients with Chronic Fatigue Syndrome." *Virus Adaptation and Treatment* 2 (2010): 47–57.

Snell, C. R., S. R. Stevens, and J. M. VanNess. "Chronic Fatigue Syndrome, Ampligen, and Quality of Life: A Phenomenological Perspective." *Journal of Chronic Fatigue Syndrome* 8, nos. 3–4 (2001): 117–21.

## CHAPTER 12

Assefi, N. P., T. V. Coy, D. Uslan, W. R. Smith, and D. Buchwald. "Financial, Occupational, and Personal Consequences of Disability in Patients with Chronic Fatigue Syndrome and Fibromyalgia Compared to Other Fatiguing Conditions." *The Journal of Rheumatology* 30, no. 4 (2003): 804–8.

Deluca, J., C. Christodoulou, B. J. Diamond, E. D. Rosenstein, N. Kramer, and B. H. Natelson. "Working Memory Deficits in Chronic Fatigue Syndrome: Differentiating between Speed and Accuracy of Information Processing." *Journal of the International Neuropsychological Society* 10, no. 1 (2004): 101–9.

Kang, H. K., B. H. Natelson, C. M. Mahan, K. Y. Lee, and F. M. Murphy. "Post-traumatic Stress Disorder and Chronic Fatigue Syndrome-like Illness among Gulf War Veterans: A Population-based Survey of 30,000 Veterans." *American Journal of Epidemiology* 157, no. 2 (2003): 141–48.

Stone, A. A., J. E. Broderick, L. S. Porter, and L. Krupp. "Fatigue and Mood in Chronic Fatigue Syndrome Patients: Results of a Momentary Assessment Protocol Examining Fatigue and Mood Levels and Diurnal Patterns." *Annals of Behavioral Medicine* 16, no. 3 (1994): 228–34.

Ware, N. C. "Suffering and the Social Construction of Illness: The Delegitimation of Illness Experience in Chronic Fatigue Syndrome." *Medical Anthropology Quarterly* 6, no. 4 (1992): 347–61.

## CHAPTER 13

Aylward, M. "Government's Expert Group Has Reached Consensus on Prognosis of Chronic Fatigue Syndrome." *British Medical Journal* 313, no. 7061 (1996): 885.

Friedberg, F., D. W. Leung, and J. Quick. "Do Support Groups Help People with Chronic Fatigue Syndrome and Fibromyalgia? A Comparison of Active and Inactive Members." *The Journal of Rheumatology* 32, no. 12 (2005): 2416–20.

Schröer, C., M. Janssen, L. Van Amelsvoort, H. Bosma, G. Swaen, F. Nijhuis, and J. Van-Eijk. "Organizational Characteristics As Predictors of Work Disability: A Prospective Study among Sick Employees of For-profit and Not-for-profit Organizations." *Journal of Occupational Rehabilitation* 15, no. 3 (2005): 435–45.

## CHAPTER 14

Carballo, A. M. "On Open Door to Hope for Chronic Fatigue Syndrome." *Revista de Enfermería* 33, no. 12 (2010): 4.

Chalder, T., P. Wallace, and S. Wessely. "Self-help Treatment of Chronic Fatigue in the Community: A Randomized Controlled Trial." *British Journal of Health Psychology* 2, no. 3 (1997): 189–97.

Jason, L. A., A. Witter, and S. Torres-Harding. "Chronic Fatigue Syndrome, Coping, Optimism and Social Support." *Journal of Mental Health* 12, no. 2 (2003): 109–18.

# INDEX

# ABOUT THE AUTHOR

**Naheed Ali**, MD, PhD, began writing professionally in 2005, and he has taught at colleges where he lectured on various biomedical topics. Additional information is available online at NaheedAli.com.

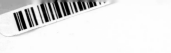

## Author's Note

Thank you for joining Grace and Noah on their journey. I hope that Summer Island's magic has touched you as it has touched me. In its fog-swept coves and quiet streets friendship runs deep, and the love of a good yarn runs even deeper.

For a detailed look at the inspiration for Jilly's amazing desserts, try Dorie Greenspan's *Paris Sweets: Great Desserts from the City's Best Pastry Shops.* Even if you don't cook, the book will seduce you. You can almost taste the *macarons* and *madeleines* melting on your tongue. Grace would definitely approve.

To learn more about the arduous responsibilities of a bomb disposal expert, look for *Bomb Squad: A Year Inside the Nation's Most Exclusive Police Unit.* Richard Esposito and Ted Gerstein offer an unforgettable glimpse into this small, select world.

I hope you will watch for more Summer Island books coming soon. One by one old friends will be pulled back home. And as seasons change, each one will face secrets and betrayals—along with the healing gift of love.

With warmest wishes,

Christina

# CHRISTINA SKYE

## A Home By The Sea

ISBN-13: 978-1-61793-225-0

A HOME BY THE SEA

**Printed in U.S.A.**

To my wonderful editors,
Tara Parsons and Tracy Martin.
Thank you for helping me bring Summer Island to life.

And to Debbie Macomber.
Thank you for all your suggestions,
wit, kindness and generosity.

# A Home
# By The Sea

# *CHAPTER ONE*

NOAH MCLEOD TOOK A DEEP BREATH. Wind gusted up the street, stabbing at his face. He hunched his shoulders, facing the icy gale. The cold air was actually a relief after the horrible day he'd just had.

It always took time to shrug off the work. You didn't forget, but at least you managed to move on. If bad dreams and explosions haunted your sleep, then you shrugged those off, too.

Slowly Noah flipped up the collar of his leather coat. He focused on the cold, slipping into the moment and letting the hard edge of duty and responsibility fade, repeating the rule he had learned years before.

*You have to move on. If you can't leave the work behind, it will drive you over the edge and one day you'll snap.*

Noah had seen it happen too often. In a job where you fought mayhem and horror on a daily basis, balance was everything. He tried to remember that rule now.

After the savage day he'd just finished, he was entitled to bury his work deep and forget about responsibility. He'd been fielding emergency calls every night for a month now, and emergency calls came to his department for just one reason.

Because everyone else had failed.

His department was the place you called when you could smell the bitter edge of your own fear. You called Noah's unit when you had an improvised explosive device or a nasty set of wires shoved into what could be a brick of Semtex. Noah was the man who always knew which wires to pull and when to back away.

Far, far away.

But tonight had been too close. He had nearly become a splatter on a concrete wall, thanks to a close encounter with a new device no one in D.C. had ever seen before. For thirty mind-blurring seconds he had looked death right between the eyes. Then he'd remembered seeing something similar in Afghanistan seven months earlier. Once Noah had seen the interior wiring, he'd made the connection. But it had been a close call.

He closed his eyes, feeling the wind pick up, rattling the windows behind him. The building where he worked was surrounded by high fences and concrete walls. For security reasons, there was no sign or business name posted. The black trucks parked outside didn't have government plates. As far as outsiders could tell, they belonged to a civilian waste-disposal company.

But the disposal Noah did was far more dangerous.

A weight dug into his shoulders as he looked up at the top window of his lab. Inside that secure room, computers were updated nightly with data about every new model of explosive device made anywhere in the world. Each morning his team pored over that data and integrated the knowledge into their disposal procedures. No detail was ignored. His team trained hard, and Noah was proud that they were the best—and that they still had their lives to prove it.

His brother hadn't been so lucky.

Frowning, Noah ran a hand through his dark hair.

*You can't go back. Matt is gone. The remote car bomb that took him is a footnote in your government training manuals now, and you all learned from it. But Matt didn't have the resources you have.*

*So he's gone. Pack it up and move on.*

It was the same conversation Noah always had about this time of night after a long, demanding shift. But how did you forget a beloved brother whose generosity and laughter had touched everyone around him? The cold sense of loss had become Noah's old friend, as familiar as his guilt. He hadn't been able to reach his brother in time to help. There had been next to nothing left of the body after the explosion.

And Noah knew *he* should have been the one who died in that explosion.

He blew out an angry breath. A big storm was headed in that night. According to the weather reports, there could be a foot of snow. Maybe more. Good thing he didn't have far to drive.

As he walked down the quiet street, Noah saw the brightly lit windows of the big townhouse on the opposite corner. He heard muted music and saw people moving inside, all diamonds and furs, dressed for a big night out. It felt odd and disconnected, like watching a movie.

Then Noah saw her.

She appeared within the frame of the window, calm and beautiful amid a throng of beautiful women. Her dark hair swung around her face and even at this distance Noah swore he could see the shimmer of her eyes. She stood right by the glass, and when she looked out light fell on the black dress she wore, brushing her high cheekbones and full mouth.

She wasn't beautiful, Noah thought. Her nose was a little short and her chin a little too long. No, not beautiful. Yet he couldn't look away.

Something about her touched him, made him feel as if his world was perfect and intact. Safe and stable, as if there was still decency and honor to be found if you looked for it.

He bit back a harsh laugh. His chosen work had stripped him of any such illusions. Any breath could be your last. Any friendly face could hold murderous deceit. He knew that cold truth from personal experience.

He felt something brush his neck. Snowflakes spiraled down in the dark.

He should be going.

But he couldn't pull his gaze from that big window.

She smiled at a man in a dark suit that looked hand tailored. She toyed with her necklace and then shook her head when a waiter offered more champagne. Orchids gleamed on a pedestal beside her. The chandelier winked over her head.

She outshone everything, in nothing but a plain black dress and a necklace with one simple pearl.

A little curve of hair brushed her neck. Noah wondered how it would feel sliding against his fingers. How her skin would warm at his slow touch.

Would she—

He jammed his hands into his pockets, suddenly aware of the night and the snow. Was he off his head? He wasn't a man to be easily distracted. He didn't fantasize about strange women he saw through a distant window. Noah enjoyed his share of hot, uncomplicated sex, and he didn't lack for willing partners in his bed. But he made sure that any woman in his arms knew that he was offering only a few hours of pleasure and laughter.

No strings. No future. No tears. He enjoyed a woman's company—but he could walk away without a backward glance.

But this woman wouldn't be easy to forget.

The knowledge made him go still. Something told Noah that this woman would trust and hope, offering her dreams and hopes in return. That trust would make her dangerous and impossible to forget. As it was, she distracted him, and she was barely visible through the window. What kind of distraction would she present if he actually met her and spoke with her?

If he touched her?

Snow brushed his neck, and Noah sighed. The storm was already pounding toward D.C. Why was he standing here, gawking like an idiot, wondering about a woman he was never going to meet?

Shift was over. He should be having a few drinks with his team by now. Maybe he'd find an easygoing woman who laughed just a little too much and wouldn't mind that Noah almost never smiled. The potential for hot, reckless sex had seemed like an excellent idea two hours ago, when he had been staring down four red wires in a cheap metal box, on his way to becoming a dead man.

"Everything okay, McLeod? No problems with your shoulder after the blast today?"

Noah swung around at the unexpected interruption. Ed Merrill, his superior, was pushing forty and carried about twenty-five extra pounds. He had just given up smoking and his temper could be volatile. Now he was frowning as he pulled a set of car keys from the pocket of his parka.

"I'm fine, sir."

The older man studied Noah intently, missing nothing. "You did all the right things. You took safe assessment and identified the device. Then you pulled back and waited for the backup team. Everything by the book."

"Yes, I got it right, sir." Noah's voice hardened. "Except the timer went wacko and spontaneously detonated, throwing me twenty feet against that concrete wall. I should have been faster—and smarter. I should have taken more precautions. I expect it in my men, so I damned well better expect it in myself." Noah cleared his throat. "Sir."

"Noted. But this is a new category of device here. You responded as well as anyone could, and you made the connection before it was too late. Rest assured, we'll do a thorough review on Monday, once forensics has gutted those components. Meanwhile, don't grind yourself up about it. Go get a beer and relax."

"Just what I was planning to do," Noah said quietly.

His superior turned up his collar against the icy wind. "Good. There won't be anything new until the tech people weigh in anyway. So go somewhere dark and smoky. Female companionship highly encouraged. It's a good night to remember you're still alive." Merrill's eyes narrowed. "Are you involved with someone?"

"No, sir."

"Good. There'll be plenty of time for commitment once your hot time is done."

Hot time meant working with live explosive devices. Hot time took all you had, all you were. Everyone on Noah's team knew the truth. You sweated and you prepared and then you did it all again the next day. Not much was left behind when you closed the door and headed home.

Without thinking, Noah turned slightly. His gaze slid back to the party in the big house across the street. The woman's hair glinted amber as she turned under the chandelier. He could almost smell her perfume as she moved, trailing a hint of something sweet but subtle. He felt a kick of hunger. Lust mixed with sharpening curiosity.

He had to meet her, just once.

"Noah, did you hear me?"

"Sorry, sir. I was just thinking about finding someplace dark and smoky."

"You keep looking at that party going on across the street. You know the owner?"

"No, sir."

Merrill tossed his keys up and down. "I do. That house is owned by a very wealthy media executive. Six magazines, four radio networks and three cable channels, last time anyone counted. And the woman in the window—someone you know?"

"No, sir."

"Someone you want to know? I could wrangle an introduction." Merrill smiled slowly. "My wife did some legal work for the owner several months back. I could walk over and pull a few strings, if you're interested in meeting her."

"Who?" Noah tried to look bored.

"The woman you've been staring at. There's snow all over your coat, in case you haven't noticed. The storm is due to hit in the next two hours, and they're saying we can expect a couple of feet. So you're going to do one of two things. You're going to get that beer or you're going to let me get you an introduction. Make up your mind. I want to be home in time to tuck my kids into bed," Merrill said gruffly.

Noah rubbed his neck. He was seriously tempted. He wanted to see her face up close and hear her laugh. Suddenly he wanted a dozen things....

*Forget it, pal. There's no place for a woman like that in your life. No room for complications or commitments. Hot time doesn't leave you anything left to share. You knew that when you signed on.*

"No need, sir. Donovan's meeting me at Wily's Place. He owes me two hundred now, after our last two games of darts. I figure I'll double that tonight." Noah managed to keep his gaze steady, away from the brightly lit house across the street. He was surprised at how hard it was.

"Fine. Go and clean up. You're entitled. But if that shoulder starts acting up, I want you into medical for evaluation immediately. Is that understood?"

"Absolutely, sir."

A sudden gust slammed over the street, hammering snow across the nearby cars.

"Good. Now get moving. Trust me, next week is going to be a three-ring circus." Merrill slid into a mud-spattered SUV that had seen too many miles in the past year. You were never off duty in Noah's unit. Explosive calls could take the team anywhere on the eastern seaboard at a moment's notice.

With a wave Merrill drove away. As the lights faded, Noah decided to walk rather than take his car. It was only two short blocks north to the small bar where his friends were waiting for him.

He refused to turn around and look back. He didn't want to see her face or the elegant line of her shoulders in that black dress. He was going to walk away and forget all about her. A woman like that could creep up on you without warning. With her calm focus and intelligence, she would keep you guessing, shaking up everything you thought was true.

And he wasn't interested in having his world kicked out from under him, no matter how beautiful her eyes or how sweet her laugh. D.C. was a big town full of pretty women. Noah would find one tonight.

Because tonight he was going to celebrate the fact that he was alive instead of a splatter on a wall.

He shoved his hands into his pockets and turned north into the swirling snow.

## CHAPTER TWO

GETTING DRUNK AND FINDING a pretty woman—that
had been his plan.

But like a lot of things in Noah's life, his plan
didn't work out the way he'd hoped. He'd gotten all
the way to the bar when he realized his cell phone
was locked in his car, parked on the street three
blocks over. Noah never used his private cell phone
at work. He carried his official pager at all times, but
with the storm coming tonight he wanted his cell in
good working order. If his family had problems, he
needed to be able to contact them.

"Hey, Noah. Where are you going, buddy?" The
door opened just as he was turning back, and light
spilled over the thin layer of blowing snow. "First
round is on the house. Second round is on me. So
what are you waiting for?" Two more men from
Noah's explosives unit appeared, peering out. Laughter and smoke and low jazz spilled into the wind.

"I forgot something, Donovan. I'll be back in ten.
Make sure you keep my seat warm and my drink
cold."

The taller man nodded. "You got it." But Joe

Donovan's eyes were troubled. He had worked with Noah since their select, top-level unit was put together, staffed by experts seconded from the FBI, the Secret Service and every branch of the military. Donovan was Noah's closest friend and he wasn't afraid to probe when the situation called for it. He moved down the stairs, speaking quietly. "That was one hell of a save today, buddy. How are you feeling?"

"Fine," Noah said tightly.

"Glad to hear it. Next week we'll have to figure out what to do when the next one appears. Because there's always another one," Donovan muttered.

"The bomb business is good these days. You know that, Joe." Noah felt the cold trail over his face and thought about how close he'd come to dying that afternoon.

"But we're good too. Yeah, we're the best." He clamped Noah on the shoulder. "And you're gonna make us even better. Now get the lead out. Didn't you hear there's the mother of all storms headed our way?"

"I heard. I won't be long."

The door opened again. Someone shouted at Joe. He gave a wave and then vanished back inside. When Noah turned around, the street was covered by two inches of snow and more was coming down in big, fluffy flakes. Noah was glad his car had four-wheel drive.

He crossed two streets, thinking about what havoc

the storm might cause. As he turned the corner, a slim figure appeared in front of the townhouse where the party looked to be in full swing. Noah's hands tightened.

She was wearing a black wool coat now, fumbling in her pocket. No scarf. No hat. No boots. Delicate evening heels that were never meant to face snow or rain.

Noah saw her drop her gloves. She picked them up and then stopped, looking uncertainly down the street. Her face was toward the light and Noah could have sworn he saw something glinting on her cheeks. Tears?

His hands tightened again. Why was she crying? Had something happened at the party? Had that man—

*Not your problem. You're supposed to be having a nice, rowdy night in a smoke-filled room, remember? Forget about her.*

Noah forced his feet on through the snow toward his old, reliable Jeep. He located his cell phone and locked up the car. Suddenly impatient, he jogged back across the street.

He turned his head. Through dancing snowflakes he saw her pass a small art gallery, open for an evening event. Then she stopped, scanning the parked cars and the nearby alley.

Noah didn't see anything but a row of garbage cans and locked cars. What was she looking for? Had she dropped something?

He tracked her prints back to the townhouse, looking at the snow. Nothing on the ground. No scarf and no fallen purse. It didn't make sense.

A snow truck growled past, wipers flapping, its big tires throwing up snow in sheets. When it passed, she was gone.

GRACE REFUSED TO FALL APART.

All she needed was one or two minutes. Time to calm down, pull herself together and take control. She was a pro at taking charge of her life, after all.

She'd pulled herself together when her mother had stopped caring about her or anything beyond the inside of a bottle. A few months later her grandmother had come down with lupus. She had died within the year. Through it all, Grace's grandfather had done everything he could to shield her from the dark realities of her life, and Grace had gone along, putting up a brave front, always optimistic and enthusiastic.

Yes, she was famous for pulling herself together. People thought she was serene and unflappable. Grace worked hard to make them believe that because she wanted to be those things.

But now as snow dusted her face, she felt the knife twist and twist again, stabbing deep. She had lost the man she loved a year earlier. After the funeral she had managed to pull her life together, helped by friends and the complex research jobs she loved. She was actually starting to feel whole and happy again.

Then she had found the letter.

Then she'd had a call from an old friend, just bursting to give her the helpful news that the man she'd loved and lost had a wife in Thailand. And there had been more gossip about other women, scattered over his far-flung travels as a UN negotiator. He had quite a record as a lover, it turned out. Yes, it had been a nice call, just a helpful update from a concerned friend.

Grace was still trying to recover from the news, and the pain was raw. Did you ever really know a person, she wondered? Or was everything just bits and pieces of a performance?

She brushed away a tear as snow crept down her collar and in the process dropped her gloves in the swirling snow. When she bent to pick them up, she heard a low, muffled sound from the row of cars across the street.

A cry?

She crossed the street, wishing she had brought her boots. Ignoring her frozen toes, she stopped to listen.

Another sound, plaintive and soft.

The noise seemed to be coming from a small alley just beyond a nearby art gallery. A cardboard box tumbled toward her, carried by the wind. When Grace grabbed it, she saw that it was empty.

The sound came again, only this time the muted

cry of pain and exhaustion tore at her heart. She plunged forward into the shadows, shivering as snow slid into her sling-back heels. Fumbling a little, she raised her small key-chain light and searched the alley.

A pair of eyes flashed against the darkness, bright in the sudden light. Grace saw a dark shape against a Dumpster near the alley's far wall. Bending down slowly, she saw a cat half covered with snow and newspapers. As the papers moved, Grace realized there were at least three kittens huddled next to their mother, all of them half-frozen in the snow. If someone didn't help them, they were going to die. She knew it without question.

Anger made her hands clench. Had someone dumped a pet here to avoid unwanted kittens? Had they hoped that the storm would solve their problem? In Oregon she had seen that kind of callousness too often. She knew the fear and pain of abandoned animals only too well.

But there was no time to be lost. The temperature was dropping and she needed something to hold the shivering animals. They wouldn't survive the storm that was already pounding the outskirts of D.C.

The big cat's eyes were dusted with snow and she seemed to struggle to move, nudging one of the kittens closer to the shelter of her body. When she saw Grace lean down, her eyes pricked forward. Then she purred softly.

Grace's heart lurched at the sound of trust and

hope. "I'll find a warm home for you, sweetie. I promise. Let's get you somewhere safe." Grace scanned the Dumpster with her light, looking for a box. But most of the trash was gone; only news-papers remained in one corner. How was she going to bundle the strays back to her car, which was four blocks away?

Frustrated, she leaned down into the Dumpster and rooted through the papers inside.

"Hello?" Snow crunched behind her. "Are you okay, ma'am?"

Grace shot to her feet. A man stood at the mouth of the alley. He wore a black leather jacket and his dark hair was dotted with snow as he walked toward her.

She cleared her throat, suddenly aware of how isolated she was here surrounded by shadows. "I'm fine." She turned around and headed toward the back door of the restaurant at the other end of the alley.

"Are you sure?"

"Absolutely." She didn't look back. She wasn't taking any chances on a stranger in a dark alley.

But the cat's low cry made her stop short. It was so cold, so lost. How could she leave them out here, even temporarily?

"Is that a cat I just heard? Out here in the snow?" The man bent down and lifted the piled newspapers, frowning at the wriggling shapes underneath. "Hell. She's got four kittens here. They're going to freeze if we don't get them inside." The man stood up, frowning. "I'll go get my car. I've got towels and a blanket in the trunk. I just hope it's not too late."

The concern in his voice was real. Grace knew she had to trust him. "If you can find a box, I'll cover them with my coat. Please hurry. The mother cat looks very weak."

"Keep your coat. I'll use mine." Carefully he shouldered off his leather jacket and added his thick wool sweater. Hand knit, Grace noted. Someone had taken great care in working those intricate cables and ribs.

She wondered if it was the work of a mother. A sister.

A wife?

Shivering, she watched him slip one leg over the Dumpster. "Do you have a box?" she asked.

"Just found one." Leaning lower, he pulled his sweater over the pile of papers, not quite touching the cat. "That should help. Now I'm going for my car. It won't take me more than a few minutes. Will you be—"

"I'll be fine. But it's getting very cold and those kittens are so small. Just *hurry.*"

An eternity seemed to pass as she waited.

Grace heard the distant sound of sirens and passing cars. Her feet were nearly numb as she hovered over the cat, talking in a reassuring tone through teeth that chattered.

Finally, car lights flared red at the front of the

alley. Grace felt a wave of relief when the man appeared, carrying a big raincoat with a towel folded inside it.

"You okay, ma'am?"

"F-fine. Just a little c-cold. This mother cat is definitely used to people. She licked my hand. So brave."

The man knelt beside her, studying her face. "You look frozen through. Why don't you go wait in the car while I round up these guys?"

Grace hesitated. He had calm, nice eyes, but she didn't know anything about him. Maybe this helpful behavior was just an act.

"Go on. It's the green Jeep. I'll drop you off on the way to the animal clinic. This snow is going to make driving slow."

His calm, take-charge attitude made Grace feel less anxious. "I'd rather help you here. I can h-hold the light while you gather them up." She held up her little key-chain light and watched approvingly. He was careful and patient as he cradled the small forms in his gloved hands and slid them under his coat. When the mother yowled, he scooped her up carefully and set her in the middle of the box, covering them all with the heavy towel, followed by his sweater and coat. "Mission accomplished. Let's get this brood moving. Meanwhile, maybe you can shine that light in front of me. I don't want to drop anyone."

Grace walked slowly, guiding him around a

mound of soggy boxes and two overturned garbage cans. Her feet were nearly numb and her hands began to shake, but she was too relieved at the rescue to care.

"Here we are. Why don't you sit in front? I'll set the whole crew on your lap while I drive."

Grace closed her eyes on a prayer of thanks. For one night at least these animals would be safe. "F-fine. I don't know who you are, but you couldn't have picked a better time to come and save us."

The man gave a low chuckle. "See if you're still thankful after you see the inside of my Jeep, ma'am."

# CHAPTER THREE

"What's a little mess between friends?" she said.

It was a mess all right. Noah cleared off an old sweatshirt from the seat so she could sit down. He had heard the faint disapproval in her tone. She wouldn't know that he'd been working for eight days straight, and this was his first real break.

He scooped a fast-food bag off the floor beneath her feet and dumped it in a holder behind him. "Sorry about this stuff."

"No problem. Everybody has to eat, Mr.—"

"McLeod. Noah." He set the kittens and their box in her lap, then slid the towel gently around them. "And some people eat better than others," he said ruefully.

"You're good with your hands."

Her voice was husky, raw with cold. Noah was certain that she was freezing. He also noted that she didn't seem to notice the chill, refusing to take care of herself until she knew the cats were safe. Once they were settled in her lap, he leaned down to crank up the heat around her feet. "Is that better?"

"Pure heaven."

He pulled out onto the deserted streets, peering through the sheeting snow. "They weren't kidding. This storm is looking bad. We could be in for a wild ride."

In the distance an ambulance whined, the sound swallowed by the gusting snow. The whole city seemed deserted, all activity stopped.

"Just as long as we're warm." She smiled, staring down at the pile of kittens, curled together warm and snug on her lap. Noah wondered if she realized that her expensive shoes were history and her elegant wool coat was streaked with mud from the Dumpster. If so, it didn't seem to bother her.

"They look okay." At least Noah hoped so.

"They're moving. That's a good sign. But we have to get them completely warm. Then we'll work on hydration," she said firmly.

Noah didn't hide his surprise. "Are you a vet, ma'am?"

"No." She smoothed one tiny, soft body, then pulled the towel back in place. "But my grandfather is. I've seen him handle abandoned animals about a thousand times, and that's what he would do. I'm Grace, by the way."

"Glad to meet you, Grace. And if anyone did the saving tonight, it was you. I'm surprised you saw them near that Dumpster."

"Just luck. I was…walking slowly. Thinking."

Her mouth tightened. She blew out a little breath.

A story there, Noah thought. But it wasn't any of his business.

He drove with extra care, alert for sliding cars and patchy ice. The snow was getting deeper, and the streets were nearly deserted except for an occasional snow truck or ambulance.

He glanced over at Grace, who was holding the box protectively at her chest. Now they had the heat covered, but what were they supposed to do for fluids? Noah was fresh out of baby bottles or eyedroppers.

But he knew someone who wasn't.

He pulled out his cell phone and hit speed dial. His older brother answered on the third ring, sounding breathless. "McLeod's. Reed here."

"Hey, big bro. I've got an emergency on my hands. Can you meet me at Dad's shop in ten minutes? And bring baby blankets—or clean towels."

There was a potent silence. Then Reed McLeod cleared his throat. "Baby blankets?"

"That's what I said, big bro."

"Do I want to know why?"

"Probably not. I don't have time to explain anyway. There's zero visibility out here and this storm is just starting. Gotta go. And be sure to bring the big car, will you? I'm not taking chances with these drifts that are forming."

"This is an emergency?"

"Yeah, it is." Noah glanced down at the kittens and frowned.

"I was just sitting down to Myra's amazing dump-lings, but I figure the story you're going to tell me will be worth it. You're usually good for a story."

He hung up before Noah could give him an earful.

Noah was a careful driver, but he barely missed getting hit three times in the whiteout. A layer of ice had formed beneath the fresh snow, and by the time he reached the meeting point at his father's shop, he was ten minutes behind schedule.

He knew that Grace was worrying about the ani-mals, though she didn't pester him with questions or complaints.

"How are your guys doing?"

"Two of them are moving around. I think they just started nursing, thank heavens. But the other two look very lethargic. The mother needs fluids. And I'm afraid that—" Her breath caught. "Wait. No way."

"What?" Noah wanted to look over at the kittens, but he didn't dare take his eyes from the road given the icy conditions. "What happened?"

"You are not going to believe this. I mean *really* not going to believe it." Grace's voice filled with a husky wave of tenderness.

The smoky sound did something odd to Noah's pulse. "Tell me, Grace."

"I thought there were four kittens. But now I can see that this cat has three kittens and one puppy."

"A puppy?" Noah swerved to avoid a Volvo, skid-ding sideways over a patch of black ice. "Damn.

Okay, now would you say that again? You can't mean—"

"I'm sure of it. The mother is treating them all the same, grooming them in turn, but I know a puppy when I see one. This looks like maybe a collie-retriever mix. He's licking my finger in search of food. At least I think it's a *he*. You're a big sweetie, aren't you, honey? So soft." Her face was radiant when she looked up. She reached over and squeezed Noah's shoulder. "I couldn't have managed this without you. How can I possibly repay you?"

As her hand skimmed his arm, Noah felt a stab of heat. He knew a few ways, but they didn't bear thinking about. *Head out of the gutter, pal.*

"Let's say you thank me by giving me at least one of these guys. Preferably two. I'd really like that puppy you're holding to be one of them. But you found them, so that's your call."

"Oh, no. I hadn't thought that far ahead. I'm only here in D.C. temporarily, so they'll need homes. Best of all would be keeping them together, at least until the little ones are older." Something crossed her face, and Noah saw worry darken her eyes. "I'll be traveling a lot for the next six months. I won't be able to take any of them with me. What am I going to do?"

"We'll work something out. They won't go back on the street." He spared time for a quick glance and saw her biting her lip. "Are you going far?"

"Chicago. Oregon. Paris. Provence. Back to Paris. Then probably Romania."

"Yep, I'd say that's far. What kind of work do you do, anyway?"

"Food research."

"Come again?" Noah slowed for a light and frowned when he felt his Jeep slide. The ice was getting worse, but he didn't want to worry her. "Is that like food technology? Artificial fragrances and additives? Because I have to tell you, I hate people who tamper with what we eat. If God had meant us to eat Red Dye #4, hydrogenated fats and square tomatoes, he would have made them that way to begin with."

Grace smiled faintly. "I'm with you. Basic is best. The kind of research I do is largely historical."

"Historical food?" Now Noah was really confused. "How historical?"

"About a thousand years. Herbs and storage skills to prevent disease. Medieval food preparation. Royal feasting rituals from Europe and Asia." She gave a wry smile. "Are you asleep yet?"

"Hell, no. That's fascinating stuff. My mom would pick your brains to learn about any of that. She might even surprise you with what she knows."

"Is she a nutritionist?"

"No. It's just a hobby of hers. Or family tradition—maybe you'd call it an obsession. She grew up in Ukraine and her family was dirt-poor, so she was hungry a lot as a child. She was homeless when she came to this country. Pretty grim times. She has great respect for a good, nourishing meal and home cooking. She taught all of us to have that."

"Your family? You cook together?"

Noah nodded. "Four brothers and one sister." He swerved again, and this time his tires spun out on a patch of ice. He eased off the brake immediately, but noticed that Grace sucked in an anxious breath. Yet even then she didn't complain.

*Strong stomach.*

Noah liked that in a woman.

"You can ask my mother for all the details when you meet her."

"Meet her? But I don't—"

Noah revved the motor, making the snow fly. The big wheels dug in hard, but they didn't move. As Noah gunned the motor again, a silver Hummer pulled out of a side street and nosed parallel to the now seriously snowbound Jeep. Grace watched the doors open and two very big men jump out.

She leaned forward, clutching her bundle of babies protectively. "Who are those men?"

"It's all right, Grace. You can relax." Noah grinned at the older man, who was wearing a big Russian fur hat. "The cavalry has just arrived."

THEY DIDN'T LOOK LIKE CAVALRY.

They didn't look like anything Grace had seen before. The younger man was blond with striking cheekbones and a tan as if he worked outside. His face was unreadable as he pulled open Noah's door.

His wary expression deepened to alarm when he saw Grace hunching protectively over the neatly wrapped bundle on her lap. "Hospital, ASAP," he snapped decisively. "Why didn't you go straight to the E.R., Noah? You passed one—"

Grace shifted in her seat. "No. I mean, it's not what you think—"

"No hospital needed. We're going home," Noah said firmly. "The women can handle it." He nodded at Grace.

"Are you crazy? If you have a baby—" Noah's brother leaned down and lifted a corner of the coat. A mewing sound filled the car. "Cats?" Reed McLeod straightened slowly, his mouth set in a wry grin. "You've got cats," he repeated. Then he yanked Noah outside into a snowbank.

A big man, looking like a jolly commissar in his big hat and long coat, watched them mock-box, jumping and shoving each other through the drifts. He shook his head. "Just ignore them," he said calmly, smiling at Grace. "They are hopeless, I am afraid. Always competing."

"I noticed," she said wryly. This had to be Noah's father. He looked like a Celtic poet, with eyes the color of a clear highland sky. Grace picked up the hint of an accent in the soft roll of his vowels. "And you must be their father."

"I must own up to that, yes. We came to help with your...babies." He gave a dry laugh. "But we will take you and Noah home now. In a real car," he added proudly.

Grace gathered the towel around her precious brood and rolled down the window a little more. "I could use some help. I've got a mother cat and four babies in this box and they're all moving. Do you think you could—"

She hadn't finished before the door opened and strong arms lifted her bundle carefully. "Wait for Noah to help you out. These drifts are already up to your knees." The tall man turned. "Noah, stop fighting with your brother and make yourself useful. Otherwise I will teach you both how to fight for real."

Ignoring his warning, Grace stepped out and hissed as her feet sank into an icy drift. "We're taking your car? The Hummer?"

"No car is better. It could drive us to Everest if necessary, but fortunately we do not have to go so far." The tall man glared sternly at his sons. "You two paper-brains, come here now. Help this nice lady before she freezes."

Looking sheepish, Noah jumped over a drift and scooped Grace up in his arms. "Sorry. There's just something about fresh snow." He gave a crooked grin. "One flake and I have to rub my brother's face in it. It's a serious character flaw. But we'll have you warm and dry shortly." He frowned as he felt Grace shiver. "Dad will have the heat cranked up to the max, count on it. He may be from Scotland, but he hates the cold."

"I don't hate the cold," Noah's father said crisply. "I just prefer to be warm and dry. Now, the lady will go in the front. You two go in back with the animals. And have a care that you don't crush any of them."

Noah settled Grace in the Hummer's front seat. Then he took the wrapped bundle from his father. "All here and accounted for." He clipped the seat belt around Grace. "Are you feeling better now?"

"Much better, thanks. How many inches are we supposed to get tonight?"

"Twenty-six, last I heard. A real bruiser of a storm." Noah's father held out a hand. "I am Alex McLeod. A pleasure to meet you."

"Grace Lindstrom. Thanks for rescuing us."

"My pleasure. I'll have us home before my Tatiana's fried dumplings get cold. It is just over the bridge and a few minutes more." He shot a measuring glance at his sons. "Mind the young ones. Turn that back heater up so they stay warm. Noah, stay in your Jeep and I will push you over to the curb where it is safe and then we will go home. Meanwhile, no more fighting, you two."

Grace hid a smile at the murmured sounds of assent. Clearly Alex McLeod ran a tight ship, but the love between the men was equally clear.

"You've met Noah. My other son is Reed. Two years older, but not much wiser." Alex nudged the Jeep carefully toward the curb, using the Hummer's big front fender. When that task was done, he gave a thumbs-up to his son.

Noah slid into the backseat beside his brother. "Nice job on the Hummer, Dad."

"Repaired under schedule and under budget," Reed said proudly. "Our contract was extended for two years. Anytime you want me to look at your fleet vehicles and give your boss a service estimate, I'd be glad to oblige."

Noah shot a glance at Grace. "I'll pass that on. Money's a little tight right now."

"Where do you work?" Grace's feet were finally starting to warm up. She tucked them under her and turned back to check on the kittens. Leaning over the seat, she folded down the edge of the towel and caught one wriggling form as it tried to escape beneath Noah's arm.

"The building near the corner."

"Down the street from the art gallery? The one with the big fence?"

He nodded.

Grace noticed he said nothing more. "I saw half a dozen trucks parked in the back. The windows were reinforced with steel bars. Are you in law enforcement?"

"I work for the government," Noah said quietly. A look passed between the three men, and he said nothing more to clarify the statement. Grace realized that he wasn't going to tell her anything else.

"Hey, get back inside here." Noah looked down and caught another kitten making a bid for freedom.

"These guys are going to be real escape artists. We may need a perimeter gate and security lights."

"Mom won't like it if they pee on her furniture, that's for sure." Noah's older brother crossed his arms, smiling a little. "But that's one scene I might like to see."

"Not in this lifetime. Your mother will know how to handle them," Alex McLeod murmured. "She raised all kinds of animals when she was a girl." His voice warmed. "Here we are, Ms. Lindstrom."

"Call me Grace, please."

"Grace, then, and a warm welcome to our house. Wait, please, so that Reed can help you over the snow."

"Reed will not," Noah said curtly. "Reed will be a good little boy and take the babies inside while I carry Grace over the snow."

"Boys. They are always boys," Alex muttered. He parked the Hummer as easily as if it had been a Prius. At the front door his wife emerged in a hooded coat that looked four sizes too big. Snow dusted her face as she moved onto the front porch. "She was worrying. She always worries." Alex's voice filled with love.

The sound made something tug at Grace's chest. There were deep emotions here. She could almost feel them tug at the air around her.

She smiled when Alex leaped out and grabbed his wife, lifting her as if she weighed nothing. "See. I brought them back safely, just as I said."

"And if you'll show some sense, you'll put me down so we can all get in before we freeze." His wife's eyes shone as Alex kissed her. "Enough of that, you big pirate. Was that a cat I heard?"

"Four of them," Noah said, scooping Grace up off the front seat. "Grace, meet my mother, Tatiana McLeod. Mom, this is Grace Lindstrom, and there are three kittens, a mother cat and a puppy inside that bundle Reed is carrying."

Grace tried to smooth her hair and tug down the hem of her black dress, which was difficult considering she was still cradled in Noah's arms. "I'm sorry to intrude on you like this, Mrs. McLeod."

"Intrude? I love guests, and unexpected ones are the best. I heard this storm could go on throughout the night so I've been cooking all afternoon. Now we are ready to eat. You can tuck your babies in before the fire. I have some old sweaters we can use for blankets."

As soon as they were inside, Tatiana bustled away, giving orders over her shoulder to her two sons.

The small house was neat as a pin, the living room filled with framed pictures. Folded afghans covered two big wing chairs and a faded chintz couch. Books sat in neat stacks on two end tables, with bookmarks inserted, and a pair of old felted wool slippers sat in front of the fireplace. All these details came to Grace as she heard the happy ring of jokes and questions swirl around her. Energy crackled everywhere, marking the bustle and arguments, measuring the depth of love and sharing in the house.

It was nothing like Grace's family. Grace had known unerring love and generosity, but her grandfather always behaved with reticence and careful restraint. Over the years silence had become natural and soothing. People didn't shove back chairs and run to the door in the Lindstrom house. Adults didn't jostle and joke, pounding each other on the back in fun. In fact, all the bustle and laughter of Noah's family made Grace keenly aware that she was an outsider.

She stared at Noah as he carried her through the living room. "You can put me down now, Noah."

"Not yet."

"Why?" Grace frowned as he carried her down a hallway covered with more family photos.

"Because I'm taking you to the kitchen. It's the warmest room of the house, and my mom has dinner waiting for us. We never keep food waiting." Noah strode into a big room with wide bay windows overlooking a small backyard. Snow had drifted up, half covering a red wooden fence and most of the branches of the apple trees ranged along one side of the yard. More snow was falling, but inside all was warmth and laughter, and the air was rich with the fragrance of caramelized onions and roasting tomatoes. Little dumplings gleamed, fat and golden, on the stove.

Grace's mouth began to water. Fried dumplings were one of her *favorite* things. And something told her that Tatiana McLeod was an amazing cook. With some luck, Grace might even leave with a few old family recipes.

Noah set her down, and she moved toward a faded wing chair near the window. "Not there," he said quietly. "It's better for you to sit over here, closer to the fire."

"Why? Is something wrong?"

For a moment he hesitated. The pain in his eyes confused Grace. Had she said the wrong thing? "Noah, I don't want to bother your family. You probably have plans for tonight. Maybe I should go."

"There is always room for one more chair at the table," he said firmly. "A guest is never turned away."

The firm tone of his voice made Grace realize this was unswerving ritual, not mere social lip service. This welcome came from old-world hospitality, faithfully preserved in this house. Even if she was an outsider, the knowledge left her feeling a little warmer, harbored against the wind that shook the windows and blanketed the yard with drifts.

This was a real family. The kind Grace used to dream about as an unhappy child. Here there would be laughter and arguments and cooking together around a big stove. Somewhere over the passing years Grace had forgotten about those childhood dreams.

"Are your feet cold?" Tatiana McLeod bustled over, drying her hands on a linen towel.

The woman's gaze was keen, and Grace felt the force of that scrutiny. "They're recovering a bit. I smell something wonderful, Mrs. McLeod."

"Call me Tatiana, please. You are smelling my *varenyky*. Dumplings, that is. You maybe call them perogies."

"I love fried dumplings. Do you use sauerkraut inside or turnips and onion? Or simply potatoes?"

"Ah, you know about making *varenyky*. I am most impressed."

"I spent some time in Poland last year. I stayed at the University of Warsaw to study for a month." Grace did not add that she had written a series of articles for a professional English cooking magazine and had won an award for her series.

"Really? You must tell me more."

"After Poland I visited the Black Sea and was lucky enough to interview the senior chef at the Hotel Odessa. He was a very nice man. He taught me all about varieties of borscht."

Noah's mother looked at Grace with outright surprise. "Not many have the good sense to appreciate borscht or our dumplings." Tatiana wiped her hands on her apron and smiled slowly. "It appears that you are one of the rare few."

Without looking, Tatiana called to her older son, who was in the process of stealing a cookie from the plate near the window. "No snacking, Reed. You will show good manners before our honored guest, please. That is understood?"

"Yes, Mama." Reed shook his head. "Although how you have eyes in the back of your head is a mystery to me."

"Years of practice, my love. There were times I needed them to survive," Tatiana said quietly. "But enough of that. The food is ready, so now we will eat."

# CHAPTER FOUR

IT WAS A SMALL ROOM, filled with the rich smells that came from slow, loving preparations. Noah's brother sat beside a petite, animated woman who was sliding a toddler into a high chair. Laughter boomed as food was passed around to the accompaniment of praise and loud arguments. Clearly, everyone had an opinion and even the brothers seemed to know a good deal about cooking. Grace hid her surprise, swept up in the conversation swirling around her. This energetic, nonstop drama was nothing like dinner with her grandfather, though she instantly felt guilty for making comparisons.

Everyone was kind, offering food and including her in the conversation.

When she had eaten eight perogies and couldn't eat one more mouthful, Grace excused herself to go check on the kittens in the adjacent den, asleep before the fire in a clean box lined with soft flannel sheets. As she stroked their warm fur, she heard Noah lean down beside her.

"Everything okay in here?"

"Just fine. The little ones are sleeping and Mom

is getting a well-deserved rest." Grace smiled as the tiny puppy looked up at Noah and thumped his tail in greeting. "I think he likes you."

"Good. Because he's definitely on my wish list. But that's your call." He picked up the puppy, his hands gentle. "You're something special, aren't you?"

Grace heard the rough tenderness in his voice. His words seemed to melt over her skin.

She pulled away from him, frowning. Angry at herself that she suddenly wanted to lean closer. "Of course you can have him. I couldn't have got them to safety without you. And it's clear that he loves you already." She scratched the puppy gently under the chin. "What are you going to call him?"

"Ivan." He saw Grace's questioning look. "As in The Terrible. Since he looks as sweet as sin." His long fingers skimmed the puppy's head.

Grace couldn't seem to look away. "Well. That's… nice," she said finally.

Noah shot her a look. "Something tells me that you aren't used to this kind of chaos. My family gets a bit noisy. At the table you looked a little shell-shocked."

"I'm not overwhelmed. And I'm not fragile." Yet, because she felt fragile at that moment, watching Noah stroke the puppy with those careful hands, Grace took a quick breath and squared her shoulders. "I can take care of myself nicely, thank you."

"I didn't say you couldn't. I said that you weren't

used to all our noise and bickering. Dad tells me it's a Ukrainian thing. My mom, on the other hand, insists it's a *Scottish* thing," he added drily. "So do you have a big family?"

Grace shook her head. "My grandfather is all. He likes things calm and orderly. Everything in its place."

Noah sat down beside her on the rug. "Sounds nice." He put the puppy carefully back in the box. "You're only staying here in D.C. temporarily, you said. What's your next assignment?"

"I have a magazine article to finish in Chicago and two workshops to teach in Oregon. Then probably three months in Paris."

Noah gave a low whistle. "Impressive. But all that travel is going to put a kink in my plan to take you out to dinner." He gave her a steady, straightforward look. "You're not involved with anyone, I hope."

She wasn't—and she didn't want to become involved. But how was she going to extricate herself without being terribly rude?

Grace ran a hand through her hair, choosing her words carefully. "I...I was involved with someone. He was English. Wonderful. We were going to be married." Her hands tightened, and she forced them to relax. "It didn't work out."

"Sorry to hear it. What happened?" Noah asked quietly.

"Isn't that a little personal?"

"Probably. But as you can see, my family doesn't

stand on ceremony. So feel free to tell me to shut up and mind my own business."

Grace looked out the window at the snow. "What happened was that his airplane was shot down while he was on a diplomatic mission in the Sudan. That was sixteen months ago."

"I'm really sorry, Grace. Losing him like that— well, it must have been horrible." Noah studied her face. "You two should have had a lot of happy years in front of you. Probably four or five kids in the works."

*In the works.*

Grace closed her eyes tightly, imagining snow swirling against the window. She had wanted children badly. She had wanted a little house with roses at the front door and a knitted afghan on every armchair. She had wanted truth and laughter and trust.

Instead—there had been a thousand deceptions.

James had destroyed their chances when he'd had his first affair. And through each following affair another piece of their future had died. And through it all Grace hadn't guessed a thing.

But she wouldn't share those details with a stranger.

"I...I'm learning to deal with the loss. I keep trying to believe that everything happens for a reason." She raised her chin, managing a smile. "Just call me Pollyanna."

"Never. I'd call you strong. Focused. And very brave," he said quietly.

He started to touch her hand, then cleared his throat and stood up quickly. A distance filled his face. Grace saw sadness drift through his eyes.

"Noah?"

He turned away as plates rattled in the kitchen. A chair slid out from the table.

"You two coming back to eat? Because I may have to finish these dumplings before they get cold," Noah's brother called out, smiling when his wife, small and gorgeous, chided him and dug her elbow into his ribs. He leaned down to kiss her, while Tatiana urged more food on both of them. Reed's daughter toddled toward him, then crowed with laughter when he held up a long noodle and made it wriggle like a worm.

It was noisy, messy and achingly seductive.

This was what a big family felt like. Grace hadn't realized there could be so much energy and emotion contained in one small room.

She felt a sudden sense of regret that she had not grown up in this kind of big, noisy family. Growing up, there had been no brothers to tease her and no sisters to confide in. There was no father to offer calm guidance and no mother to protect and steer her. After all, she had never known her father.

And her mother was mostly a string of bad memories.

Grace rubbed her forehead. None of that mattered. She was in control of her life now, perfectly content with her grandfather's love and support. She had a wonderful job doing what she loved most.

There was no room in her life for regrets.

Noah leaned over and pulled an age-softened alpaca afghan around her shoulders. "Everything okay?"

"Just daydreaming. Sorry."

"Did you like my mother's dumplings?"

"They were heavenly. I notice she added a little bit of sour cream to her dough. That's unusual, no?"

"You caught that?" Noah raised an eyebrow and leaned back against the arm of the couch. "It was a custom in her family. You really do know something about foreign food, don't you?"

Grace didn't tell him that she had traveled through ten cities in Eastern Europe, interviewing cooks all along the way. She didn't add that she was planning to write a book on worldwide varieties of dumplings someday.

She looked up as Noah's mother crossed the room, holding out a cup of hot tea. "You left this, so I made you another. It is nice and hot." Her eyes were shining. It was clear that she was delighted by the presence of her family, happy to see everyone eating well, safe here within her house. "You are well, Grace? The little cats too?"

"Wonderful."

"You must eat more! You only had one bowl of borscht and a few perogies. Even Reed's little girl, in her highchair, can eat one bowl of borscht."

"No more for me, I'm afraid. Your poppy-seed cake smells wonderful, so I have to save room for that."

"You will have the first piece then." Tatiana sat down beside her and held her hands out to the fire. "Did you enjoy your travels in that side of the world? Was there family to visit there?"

"I had a distant cousin from Slovenia. He was held to be quite a good cook. I was very little when I visited with my grandmother, so my memories are blurred. But I remember his borscht above everything. He labored over it, coaxed it and talked to it. When it was done, he served it from a big tureen in blue-and-white porcelain bowls and his finest silver. I think he would have been very happy with your version of the recipe."

"I would like to have met him. It's always good to talk about old times and recipes with someone who cares for the past. You have been back recently?"

"Three years ago. I visited Austria and Eastern Europe on a cooking internship. I didn't get to stay long in one place, but it was fascinating. I learned the common threads that make any cuisine great."

"I can tell you what those are." Tatiana swept the table with a lingering glance. "Not salt. Not the best extra-virgin olive oil. It is love that melds the flavors and tenderizes the meat. It makes the thinnest of ingredients go down with wonderful flavor. Is it not so?"

"All true. Even fine ingredients can be ruined by an angry chef or a cook trying to cut corners."

Tatiana McLeod squeezed her son's shoulder and smiled slowly. "I like this young woman. You will bring her here to dinner often, Noah. I think she could teach me some things, and that I would enjoy very much."

"It would be my pleasure, Mama, but that is for the lady to decide."

Grace had been watching the box by the fire, and suddenly she saw the towel rise and begin to creep over the sides of the box, carried by two inquisitive kittens. The puppy was right behind them, awkward and stumbling on his small, wobbly legs. "Excuse me. I see trouble."

Grace lunged to collect her charges. One of the kittens mewed and climbed up against her chest, purring loudly. Grace didn't move, swept by a feeling of contentment so rich and heavy that all movement was beyond her.

Noah grinned as he slung one arm around his mother's shoulder. "Hard to get irritated when they're so cute. But that one could be trouble. He's going to be a real explorer."

"Just like you," Tatiana said quietly. "Always moving. Always curious about every little thing. 'Why does it rain, Mama? What makes the sun set, Mama? How do you make your best borscht, Mama?'"

Noah ran a hand through his hair. "I sound like a menace."

"Not a menace. A normal and very wonderful child."

"A menace," Noah muttered, looking sheepish.

Someone called for Noah's mother, and she returned, pulling on a fresh apron as she headed through the kitchen.

As three generations of McLeods laughed and joked and argued, Grace felt a sudden longing to be home with her grandfather, eating Swedish meatballs at the kitchen table, catching up on all the news at the animal shelter and the small population of Summer Island. Peter Lindstrom wasn't growing any younger, and although he had always enjoyed perfect health, Grace knew that could change at any moment. And how could she bear that?

A hand touched Grace's shoulder. "Hey. Is everything okay? Do you need some help with your little climber?"

"No, I'm fine. They're all so incredibly cute." The littlest one snuggled against her chest, rolled onto his back and heaved out a sigh of contentment.

"They definitely know a good thing when they see one. Smart, all of them."

Noah reached down and rubbed the mother cat gently beneath the chin. She pushed at his hand, eyes slitted with pleasure, purring softly.

"They all like you, Noah. I think you make them feel safe."

"We always had at least two pets running through the house when I was growing up. Controlled chaos, my father called it. What about you?"

"We didn't have pets at home. There was no time. My grandfather was a vet, and when I was fourteen he took over the care of the county animal shelter. Then when the county's finances became rocky, he took personal responsibility for the shelter."

"He must be a very good man." Noah leaned back, braced on one elbow. "How did he manage it? Food, rent, medicine—it had to cost an arm and a leg."

"It's been difficult. Lately I think he's been drawing from his savings, but he refuses to discuss it with me or anyone else. The animal shelter is a labor of love. I help out as much as I can when I'm home, but it isn't enough. In fact, I've been thinking lately that I should choose my workshops by location. That way I can be home with him more often."

"It's a hard call, but I'm sure you'll do the right thing. Growing up with an animal shelter sounds great. How many dogs and cats did you take care of?"

"Every week was different. Some weeks we had five or six dogs and maybe a dozen cats. Some days we would have four times that many. That's when it got rough. Luckily we had lots of volunteers from Summer Island to help out."

"Summer Island? So you grew up at the beach?"

"Just a small one. The Oregon coast is very rocky

there, with cliffs right up to the water. Growing up, I thought it was the most magical place on earth. Even now after I have traveled to all kinds of beautiful places, I still think Summer Island ranks in the top five. Of course, I'm biased." She leaned back, cuddling the kitten closer to her chest. "You don't need to keep me company, Noah. Go finish your dinner. I'll be fine with my little friend here. And I really should get home before it's too late. Tomorrow I have an important project to prepare for."

Noah shook his head. "I'm afraid you aren't going anywhere tonight. They've just issued a county-wide safety alert. No one should be out on the streets tonight except in an emergency. There are collisions all over the state from the whiteout, and the security personnel have their hands full." He glanced at his watch. "My mother is making up a bed for you here in the den. Anytime you want to sleep, let me know." He cleared his throat. "She was going to give you my old room, but Reed, his wife and their daughter are going to sleep up there. The temperature is supposed to drop and there have been intermittent power outages, but we'll be fine. When my father built this house, my mother insisted on having two fireplaces so that we'd be prepared for all kinds of storms. That was another remnant of her tough childhood back in Ukraine. Things are different for her now, but I don't think you ever forget."

It was so tempting to relax. If she stayed, she

would be drawn into all this bustle and warmth and generosity. And then there was Noah himself.

Grace was honest enough to admit that he intrigued her. He was calm and casual, but she felt the weight of authority in his words. He handled problems without loud talk or fuss. Something told her he had a great deal of practice taking care of problems.

What kind, she didn't know, but she wanted to. She wanted to know everything about him.

And that kind of curiosity was dangerous. She wasn't going to get serious about another man until she healed from the first.

Yet Grace couldn't ignore the sweet tug of temptation. If she wasn't careful, she might forget all her good intentions. Here among this loud, close family, it would be so easy to relax.

She stood up, feeling a desperate need to be away from the warmth and belonging. "That's very kind of you, but I can't stay here. Maybe I can find a cab."

"No cabs running. Everything is shut down tight. Sorry, Grace, but we'll make you comfortable here. Plus I know my mom is itching to ask you more about your visits to Eastern Europe. She's never been back, you see. All her family is gone now."

"I'm sorry to hear that. But really, Noah, I need to go. I have a project to finish tonight. And I want to call my grandfather. If he hears about the storm, he'll be worried about me."

Wind hissed around the house, rattling the windows.

The lights flickered, and then the room plunged into darkness as the power went out.

## *CHAPTER FIVE*

TATIANA BEGAN CALLING crisp orders from the kitchen. "Reed, please find the flashlight and batteries in the top drawer of the kitchen cabinet. Alex, my love, there are more blankets in the guest room closet. I have hot water already boiled, but we will need the Thermos bottles. I also have marshmallows and chocolate, to make those things you boys loved so much in Boy Scouts. Shores, you called them."

"S'mores, Mom. And that sounds great." Noah rubbed his hands together. "The power should go off more often."

Reed appeared at the door, holding a flashlight. "So, bro, let's go get the sticks and marshmallows."

"You're on."

Twenty minutes later, Grace was downing her third heavenly mixture of perfectly roasted marshmallow, graham cracker and melted chocolate. She didn't even have to move. With the kitten on her lap, Noah held up cooked morsels for her to eat from his fingers. She had to admit, the whole experience was more than a little hedonistic. The brush of his hands and rich tastes made her feel wonderfully decadent.

Noah tucked the blanket around her on the couch. Candles flickered in the kitchen and then footsteps moved away up the stairs. The house grew quiet as the snow swirled outside the window. With the power gone, Grace's sense of being enclosed in a cocoon was complete. The flicker and snap of the fire lulled her to sleep, along with the warmth of the little kitten curled up on her lap. She yawned and smiled sheepishly. "I think the day has finally caught up with me."

"Get some rest. I'll keep an eye on these bad boys. Once the weather settles down in the morning, my dad and I will get you home in the Hummer."

"I appreciate this generous hospitality."

"I'm happy you're here, Grace." Noah studied her face in the firelight. "I feel calm when I'm around you. I can't quite explain it." He leaned back, scratching one of the kittens. "So how about dinner tomorrow, assuming that the roads are clear?"

"I...I don't think I can."

"Then what about Friday?" The other kittens stirred. A sleepy head rose and big dark eyes looked from Grace to Noah.

"I don't think this is a good idea."

"It's just dinner. Everybody has to eat, remember? And since you brought these amazing animals into my life, now we're both responsible. You're going to need my help to take care of them."

He was right. Grace had taken on more responsibility than she expected in that alley tonight. But she had to make the situation clear. "I'm feeling over-whelmed, Noah. I didn't expect any of this. And just so you understand, I'm not considering a relation-ship."

His eyebrows rose. "All I asked for was a simple meal together. No need to make it complicated."

But it *was* complicated. She had spent eight years with a man she thought she adored. A man who seemed above reproach, dedicating his life to help-ing others find reconciliation under hostile circum-stances. If you couldn't trust a man like that, who *could* you trust?

Grace forced the bad memories down before they could swirl up. "I'm sorry, but no."

"So our timing is wrong. At least agree to a snow-ball fight." He raised his palms. "Nothing compli-cated in that."

He made it so easy for her to feel safe and com-fortable, but Grace refused to give in to that gor-geous smile. "Really? I'm not quite buying that."

Noah lifted the restless kitten from her lap, tuck-ing it back into the warm spot next to its mother, where it immediately began to nurse. "If there's one thing I've learned in life, it's the importance of taking opportunities when they're offered. Life has its own timetable, and if we look away or hesitate or blink, a moment can pass. Things can change." His voice hardened. "People can be lost forever."

Grace heard the sadness again. This time it held something like remorse.

She was surprised at how much she wanted to ask him what he had lost and why. There she went, getting pulled in again. Questions could take her places she didn't want to go.

Instead, she blurted out an answer that neither one of them expected.

"Fine. I accept your challenge. Tomorrow at 10:00 a.m. in the backyard. But we have to have some rules. Time limits and number of rounds per bout. I like things to be spelled out," she said firmly.

He leaned back, smiling faintly. "Three rounds or the first one to declare defeat. Five minutes max per round."

"Accepted."

He looked more pleased than he should have as he pulled her blanket up around her shoulders. Side by side they watched snow dust the windows while the fire crackled. His shoulder was warm against hers and Grace felt strength radiate from his body. His presence seemed to anchor her.

She yawned and found herself wondering how his hands would feel on her bare skin. What if he turned and brushed his lips over hers?

Quickly, the flow of her imagination turned dangerous. She sat up straighter and forced her tangled thoughts away from hot images of Noah kissing her.

Touching her.

*Impossible.* Stiffly, she picked up a pillow and blanket and lay down on the couch. She *wasn't* getting involved.

"Good night, Noah."

She heard his soft laugh. "'Night, Grace. Sleep well."

"I will." She caught back a yawn. "And a friendly warning. This snowball fight of ours isn't going three rounds. It will only go one." Grace yawned again and closed her eyes. "I give it about three minutes. And then you are *so* going down, Noah McLeod," she murmured.

As she pulled the blanket around her, Grace felt him slide a second pillow under her head. "Wanna bet?" he whispered.

SOMETHING WAS HAPPENING.

Noah stood in the doorway, frowning. He had told her it wasn't complicated, but that was a lie.

The complications might have begun when he had seen her all but climb into that Dumpster, oblivious to her elegant evening heels and silk dress. They might have started when she had cradled the hungry kittens, looking fierce and protective. Then she had surveyed his crowded, noisy dining room, and he had seen her face fill with the ache of longing.

It didn't make sense, but Noah felt he could read her emotions, even though she worked hard to hide them. To others she would appear cool and controlled, but he saw the way her fingers clenched and her shoulders tightened. She faced life head-on, strong and stubborn, and she loved what she did. He knew that much. But he wanted to know everything about her. And he wanted to share parts of himself he *never* shared.

He turned away, angry at the urge to sit across from her. Not to touch, but simply to watch her sleep.

And that kind of longing was dangerous. The work he did left no room for emotions that could confuse and distract him. When you had three seconds to make a life-or-death choice of half a dozen wires, you had to have a clear mind.

You had to be able to walk away. That had been Noah's personal rule for as long as he could remember. It had never been a terrible sacrifice—until now.

He blew out a quiet breath, listening to the snow at the window. The wind was whining and the noise had disturbed the mother cat, who sat up alertly.

"It's okay, Mom. You and the kids are gonna be fine."

A sound from the couch made him turn. He caught Grace's pillow as she shoved it free in her sleep. She was a restless sleeper, twisting under the covers. Several times her lips shaped words that Noah couldn't understand. Clearly, she was fighting old battles in her sleep.

Carefully, he slid her pillow back in place, listening to the hiss and pop of the fire. He should have been sleepy, but he was fully alert, aware of every noise and movement in the quiet house. Most of all he was aware of Grace sleeping so close.

He smelled her faint perfume and heard every

breath she took. And the force of his awareness left him irritated.

A shadow fell over the floor. Noah realized his mother was holding up a dish towel and looking at him from the doorway.

Quietly, he crossed to the kitchen and closed the door so their noise wouldn't wake Grace. "Dish duty again?"

"I'll dry. You will wash. You're very good at that. I trained all my sons very well," Tatiana said with calm pride. "She is nice, Noah. I like her very much. But there is pain in her eyes. What did you say her job was?"

"I'm still trying to figure that out. I think she writes magazine articles and does historical research on food, but we haven't gotten that far. I only met her tonight, and that was completely by accident."

His mother's eyes narrowed. "A very wise man once told me there are no accidents. Only fate, my son. It is never wise to fight the touch of fate. But just the same, I hope you will be...safe."

"Safe? I don't understand."

Tatiana frowned at him. "Probably not. But I see what I see. I hope you will find the right woman. One who makes your steps light with happiness."

"Don't worry about me. I take the days as they come. No attachments means no regrets."

"For now. But not always. Someday I wish..." She touched his cheek and then rolled her eyes. "How like an interfering mother I sound. You will please ignore me."

"You're a hard person to ignore."

"That is a very nice thing to say." Tatiana hesitated. "I had a call from Matthew's wife today." She seemed to shape her words carefully. "They will not be coming for New Year's. They will not be coming here for Valentine's Day or Easter, either. She told me they've purchased a house."

"Where? Virginia?"

"That's what I thought. But no. Miranda is going to take my granddaughter across the country to Oregon. I had to look it up on a map. So far away. We will never see them." Tatiana's voice wavered.

Noah slid his arm around her trembling shoulders.

She had hidden her pain all during dinner, he realized. She had put on a good face. Now she could hide it no longer.

"You should have said something before this."

"And ruin our first meal together in weeks? I'm not so weak. I will not let her steal our granddaughter out of our lives. Sophie has the right to know who her father was. How brave your brother was and how strong he was and how hard he worked. *To serve and protect.* He was so proud of his work," Tatiana said with husky pride. "Sophie has the right to know her father's family. And I will fight Miranda to make this so. I swear it with all my heart. She will not take her away and cut us off." Her voice broke. "I have not told your father, my love. It will break his heart.

He loves Sophie so much. His first grandchild," she whispered.

"We all love Sophie," Noah said gruffly. The sadness of losing his brother in the line of fire was still a fresh wound. Now were they to lose all contact with his young daughter? "What about her classes at school? Her friends?"

"Her mother insists she'll have an equally good education in Oregon. She has already requested the transfer of Sophie's files and enrolled her in a private school there. I think—I think that she has planned this for a long time, maybe right after Matthew's death. But she never gave any clue. Such a woman, she is." Tatiana took a harsh breath and forced a smile. "She thinks it is for the best perhaps. Maybe...maybe our family reminds her of all she has lost. I know that she did love Matthew once. Before the long hours made her bitter." Noah's mother looked at him and shook her head. "I think that Miranda is more worried about herself than anything else." Tatiana looked away.

Noah realized that his mother looked tired and frail. The knowledge shocked him. He had always thought that her strength would never fail. She had been the toughest one of his family, steeled by a childhood of deprivation, war and loss.

But the day that she had lost her youngest son had been a nightmare that would walk with her always. A D.C. policeman, Matt had answered a midnight call and then received the full blast of a car bomb.

That explosion should have happened to *him,* Noah thought angrily. He was the one trained to deal with improvised explosive devices, not Matt. His team should have been dispatched to handle the device.

Due to a misreading of the situation, the wrong agency had been called in.

And gregarious, optimistic Matthew McLeod had been torn apart by a wall of destruction that hammered past at 26,000 feet per second. He had died instantly. The shadow of his loss would hang over them always.

"Mom, leave the dishes. I'll finish them," Noah said gruffly. "You should go and rest."

"Nonsense. If I can't dry a few pans and forks, what good am I? Now enough of this dark talk. Tell me about how you found this woman and her kittens."

Noah put another pan into the hot soapy water. "She was rifling around in a Dumpster, ruining her evening clothes and not caring a bit. She looked— fearless," he said thoughtfully. "As stubborn as she was frozen."

"Stubborn? This would be good. And fearless, you say?" Tatiana picked up another wet plate, looking thoughtful. "I like very much that she rescued five creatures who had no one else to help them." She looked at her son.

Noah met her gaze. "It was just an accidental

meeting, Mom. We aren't—involved. I barely know her."

"And yet you would like to know her, yes?"

"Liking doesn't change anything. She's just visiting D.C. and I don't have time in my life now for anything that's serious. End of story."

Tatiana pulled a clean plate from his hands. "You can't hide from feelings and attachments forever, Noah. We all lost something too precious to imagine when Matthew died." Her eyes shimmered. "He would not want us to live in the shadows of pain and loss. That was not your brother's way."

"I know. But I can't forget and I won't forgive."

Tatiana's eyes glistened with tears. "He wants us to start." She put her hands flat on the counter, closing her eyes. "He would want us all to look forward instead of back." She took a long breath. "Somehow we must try. Now leave the last pan, my love. We will have some tea and the rest of the poppy-seed cake while you tell me what *really* happened to you today at that job you never discuss." Her eyes narrowed. "Do you think I did not notice how your right shoulder hurts you or you rub your wrist? You did something brave and I think that you were hurt."

Noah muttered under his breath. "I slipped on an icy step, Mom. Nothing brave or serious about that. My job is usually boring." He shrugged. "It's not like on TV. Mostly we sit and look at computers."

"You are sure? You would not lie to me?" She stood very still.

Yet again Noah thought how fragile his mother had become in the year since his brother's death. "Of course I'm sure. I was grabbing for my pager and I didn't watch where I was walking. I landed on my arm, looking like a fool. End of story." He carried his mother's tea to the table and then went back for his own.

"I see. But next time you will be more careful, please, and watch where you walk." She stared out at the snow, still falling hard. "And when you—look at your computers, you will also be careful. *Promise* me this," she said fiercely.

"I will be. McLeod's honor."

"Good." Tatiana squeezed Noah's hand hard and took a deep breath. "Now finish that cake before your father comes looking for it. He always knows when there is one piece left, and I must help his willpower a little."

WIND WHISPERED AGAINST the windows, driving snow against the glass. The house was quiet except for the hiss and pop of the fire that was still going in the room next door.

Tatiana McLeod was not afraid of silence or the dark. She welcomed the shadows as a friend. Only then would she see her lost son.

*Matthew?*

She stared at his old chair, empty near the window. Always empty.

The house was quiet yet full of small sounds. The

settling of walls. Sleepy breaths that sounded against the snap of the fire. Even the restless kittens were finally asleep.

Tatiana stood in the dark kitchen, listening to all of it. This was hers, her oldest dream. This was the home that she had made by fierce effort, drawing her family around her, keeping them safe at all costs.

Except she had not kept her youngest son safe.

Matthew was gone, lost to the twisted fury of a man given over to hatred. He had graduated from the police academy at the top of his class and married two weeks later. His daughter, Sophie, was the light of his life and the joy of his parents. But his wife, society girl Miranda Dillon, had hated his job, hated the duty he took so seriously. Again and again she had tried to make him leave to work for her father in his huge plumbing fixtures business.

Matthew had always sidestepped the argument. On that one subject he would not bend.

Now his pampered widow was taking Sophie away with no concern for Matthew's family or what it would do to the little girl.

Tatiana clenched her fists in anger. She had to hold back her fury and the pain of her losses. She wouldn't let her family be torn apart. She would keep them safe, even if she had to...

*Always so stubborn.*

The words were soft, almost her imagination. But three times she had heard them in the haunting months since Matthew's death.

"I've had to be stubborn." To make a family was simple. To keep it together was the hard thing.

A breeze touched her cheek. There might have been a glimmer of light near the stove.

*You work too hard, Mother. You always did.*

She signed, closing her eyes as a sudden warmth filled the air around her. *I miss you terribly, Matthew.*

*It will be better. You'll see.*

"Will it?" Her muscles clenched with anger that followed in the wake of sadness. "Why *you?* Why not someone evil? Or why not take me instead? You had your whole life to live."

Her shoulders shook.

*Shh.*

Again she felt a current of wind on her face. *Everything happens for a reason. Now I see this all so clearly.*

"Well, I don't! I can't understand at all—and I can't forgive, either. Now your wife, cunning and quiet, plans to take your little daughter away, too." Tatiana's voice broke. "Far away, Matthew. From us and your memory."

*She is doing what she thinks is best, Mother.*

"Really? I thought she was doing what was easiest. She wants to make Sophie forget you. I hate her."

As Tatiana's fists clenched in terrible anger, she knew the mistake she had made. He was silent then. He was always silent when she said something bitter or angry. It was as if he was held in a gentler place and these darker emotions could not touch him there. So he simply slipped away.

Tatiana closed her eyes, hunched over the table. She leaned down to touch the chair where her son had always sat—until the night he was killed. "Stay, Matthew. I won't—that is, I'll try to find some affection for your widow. I'll try to understand why she is doing this cruel thing. But I won't let her cut Sophie off from you and us. We're in her blood, too. Miranda and I will have to come to some kind of compromise."

She felt a stirring of air touch her cheek. It might have been the movement of a hand passing in the darkness.

With her eyes closed, Tatiana heard her son's beloved voice beside her. *She's caught in darkness right now.* The words were a mere whisper. *She has lost me and she's lost her hope and she's lost the world along with it. Give her time, Mama. You are so strong...and she is not.*

The wind stirred again, like a gentle hand at her shoulder.

And then he was gone.

Tatiana knew in an instant, because the kitchen suddenly felt silent and cold. Now the darkness was only darkness.

She was alone. No spirits walked to ease her sadness.

Strong? Yes, she had always been the strong one. She had fought for her family since the icy morning when she had woken up in Ukraine huddled next to her grandmother and four sisters with one quilt between them. Tatiana had sworn she would make a better life. She had sworn to see that her family never went hungry. And she had vowed to pass on the memories and traditions of the homeland she loved, despite its years of war and unrest.

She had done all those things, through the blood and sweat of her body and her fierce will.

But she was strong no longer. The blow of losing her youngest son had bent her double like a birch tree in a spring storm, snapping her in two. Her family might believe she was strong. Her friends might marvel and offer compliments.

But inside, Tatiana's tears gathered into silver rivers. And she was broken, bent by the weight of sadness just like the ruined trees she remembered from her girlhood.

# CHAPTER SIX

*Two weeks later*

HE HAD CALLED HER TWICE. He had texted her once.

Grace hadn't returned any messages. She told herself it was better this way. More practical for both of them.

After all, what could come of a few dates? Hesitant pauses. Awkward conversations. Groping in the dark and then an embarrassed refusal?

*No.* She had to have peace and order in her life, and her heart told her that Noah would upset her careful efforts at recovery. She had learned one thing over the past year: *you had to be strong before you learned to be vulnerable.*

Two weeks had passed since she had found the kittens—and met Noah. They had feinted through their snowball fight to the hilarity of Noah's family. At first Noah had held back, but Grace wasn't afraid to fight dirty, shoving snow down his collar, pulling his feet out from under him, rubbing snow in his face. With the noisy laughter of his family rolling in her ears, she had been declared the winner at the start of round three, by unanimous vote. Noah had taken his defeat well, but hours later, standing on the driveway after he had returned Grace to her townhouse, he had taken his consolation prize.

The long, slow kiss began as snow fell gently, brushing their faces. He had murmured her name while his hand rose, cupping her cheeks. Then he turned her face up to his and tasted her mouth slowly. The hunger had slammed over her instantly. Grace had thought she remembered how it felt to be kissed and know the swift heat of desire, but her experiences with James hadn't really prepared her for Noah.

The rich, earthy feelings that followed his kiss had left Grace giddy and confused. They caught her when she least expected it, fogging all her senses and her normal caution.

And she needed to stay cautious and in control. She had been out of balance too long with James. She was getting her life back now. Once things had quieted down, she would call Noah.

Her computer, books and notebooks were stacked neatly on the table. She had an important meeting tomorrow, but she was well prepared. Yet the thought bothered her: Was that all she had in her life—work and meetings?

Suddenly restless, she grabbed her coat and gloves to take a walk. Maybe the brisk air would clear her tangled thoughts.

She closed and locked her door, then pulled on an

old knitted scarf. It was a simple lace stitch, nothing complicated, but it would always be special because it was the first lace she had ever knitted. You remembered the first times most, she thought wryly.

A car raced past and slush sprayed around her boots, but Grace trudged on, glad to be outside. At least her preparations were done. All she had to do was sell her idea. That wouldn't be easy because the competition for this particular project would be keen.

Lights flickered in the twilight. A car angled to the curb and stopped. A Jeep, Grace realized as the driver's-side door opened.

"What does it take to get a call returned, an executive order?" Noah jumped out and shoved his hands in his pockets. "You must be busy these days."

Grace took a deep breath. He looked good—even better than she remembered. Snow dusted his broad shoulders as he studied her without moving. "You forgot these the other night."

He dug out a plastic bag with Grace's favorite red fingerless gloves. "Mom wanted me to tell you. Since you didn't return my calls, I decided to swing by." His eyes were wary. "And since you haven't asked, I'll tell you that the mom and all the kittens are doing fine. Puppy, too."

"Noah, I—" Grace flushed. "I'm sorry. I *should* have called. That was very rude of me. And you know that I can't thank you enough for keeping the cats."

"Hey, don't apologize. You made it clear when

you said you didn't want to get involved. As for the cats, we love them. The puppy is great." He shrugged. "So I'll be getting back. It's been a busy week."

"Noah, wait. *Please.*" Grace put a hand on his arm and felt the muscles flex sharply. "Look at me."

After a moment his dark eyes settled on her face, focused but completely unreadable. "I'm looking. But what is there to say?"

She felt his muscles tense again and noticed there was a cut above his eyebrow that hadn't been there before. "What happened to your face?" Without thinking, she touched the healing skin gently.

"Cut it shaving," he said tightly. "So what did you want to tell me, Grace?"

She felt low and cravenly, embarrassed at her behavior. "Look, I'm just trying to do the right thing. I didn't *plan* to meet someone. I didn't want to get involved when I'm still tangled up inside." Grace looked down at her fingers, opened on his arm. "And then I met you. I saw how gentle and careful you were with the kittens and how far you went to make me feel comfortable with your family. And suddenly—" She stopped, feeling heat fill her face. But she owed him an explanation—and an apology. "Suddenly *you* were there, and I was being pulled in, caught up in emotions I couldn't understand or trust. I couldn't stay aloof or in control around you. So I chose not to call or have any contact. That was my decision, and it was very badly done. I hope you'll forgive me."

"There's nothing to forgive," Noah said tightly. "You were protecting yourself in the only way you could. You were being practical."

"I wish it were that simple," Grace said. "I should have explained and then trusted you to understand. I took the cowardly way out."

Some of the wariness left his eyes. "Yes, you should have trusted me. Because I do understand." His eyes darkened. "And I suppose if I ask you to go for a walk, you'll say no."

She didn't want to say no.

Surely she could handle a few minutes in his company without coming unglued. "I'd say yes, actually." She hesitated, then slid her arm through his. "And you can tell me about the cats. I miss them." She took a breath. "After that you can explain what really happened to your face. I don't believe your story for a second."

THEY WALKED FOR FIFTEEN minutes, sometimes talking, sometimes silent. At first Grace felt uncomfortable and self-conscious, but slowly the silences grew more comfortable, like the kind between old friends. Feeling comfortable like this didn't make sense.

But maybe not everything *had* to make sense.

"So I want to know all the details about the little guys. Are they healthy? Growing a lot?"

"My mother has been giving them a special mix

of broth and egg yolks. She swears it will help them grow. All I know is it smells nauseating. Then yesterday my father took Ivan the Terrible for a short walk on the back patio." He gave a dry laugh. "Don't worry. It was only for a few minutes, just enough to give the little guy a chance to work on his muscles. He's the most uncoordinated animal I've ever seen."

As they walked it began to snow lightly. Grace watched car lights glow red in the twilight as commuters headed home or out to dinner or to the ballet and opera. It was all so different from the quiet harbor community where she'd grown up in Oregon. Back on Summer Island there were no secrets, no blessed anonymity. Everyone knew everyone else's business.

She had been thrilled to escape to culinary school in New York and then head on to the Cordon Bleu in Paris. The world had called to her and her year of study at the Sorbonne had been heaven. When work brought her here to Washington, she found the same kind of anonymity, and she had felt right at home.

Except lately her trust level was at rock bottom. Since learning about James, she questioned every statement and every motive, her own as well as everyone else's. She searched for odd nuances and tallied up whatever didn't make sense.

That kind of negativity drained you fast, she had discovered. It left you only half alive.

As she studied the hard angles of Noah's face captured in the light of passing cars, Grace realized that right now at this moment, one place felt safe. Noah had a knack for paying complete attention to those around him. When you talked, he listened as if no one else existed or mattered. It was a novel and very heady experience, she discovered.

Not that it changed anything. Tonight was a pleasant adventure, nothing more.

"You want to talk about him?" Noah was watching her, his eyes grave.

"Him?"

"Your fiancé. You were thinking about him just now, weren't you?"

"Yes, but how did you—"

"Your eyes. You looked like someone had kicked you in the chest and you were choking," Noah said roughly.

Had he really seen all that in her face? If so, was her pain so visible to everyone around her?

Grace felt a wave of nausea. The truth was that all of James's friends had known what he was doing. Only *she* had been blind to the scattered signs. They were apart for weeks while he was working, so it had been easy to miss the other demands on his time and emotions.

But over the long months Grace had stopped hating him. She had even stopped hating herself for missing the signs until he was dead. And now she was moving forward. She wasn't going to let bad memories destroy her trust and hope. She wanted her life back.

She took a shaky breath, trying to smile. "That easy to read, am I?"

"Maybe not by others. But you're doing it again," Noah said quietly. "That struggle to breathe. The tension in your hands. Talk to me, Grace."

Memories of loss made her throat tighten. She hadn't talked about the dark details with anyone, not even her closest friends. Definitely not with her grandfather, who would have been horrified by James's behavior. "I—I can't."

"Talking will help."

"What does it matter? He's gone. All the damage is done." She felt tears burn suddenly. "Before he died he slept with half of my friends. Maybe *all* of them. What did I know?"

"The fool," Noah's voice was hard. "The cold-blooded idiot." A muscle clenched at his jaw. "A man would have to be blind—and very sick to hurt you that way. He hurt himself, too, even if he couldn't see it." He took her hand, helping her climb over a mound of snow at the edge of a driveway. They walked for a while, neither speaking. "So how did you find out?" Noah finally asked.

"The first clue? I was going through some of his old clothes after he passed away, and I found a letter in the pocket. There was no stamp. He was always a little forgetful that way." Grace stared down the street, reliving that moment of her searing disbelief. "I was certain it was a mistake, so certain that some friend of his had given him the letter to drop off.

Just a favor, right? Then a mutual friend, who happened to be the woman he'd written the love letter to, called me in Paris." Grace had to stop and concentrate on the words. "She was devastated. She let it slip that he had been with her the day before the crash. He had visited her at least once a month. She said she was...pregnant. She hadn't told him yet." Grace blew out a shaky breath. "I couldn't help her. I couldn't console her. I should have, but I couldn't say a word of sympathy. I was still sure it was a mistake." The street blurred suddenly. "It had to be some other James. Not *my* James. It just wasn't possible." Grace stumbled. Dimly, she felt Noah's hand grip her waist. "Not the man I was going to marry as soon as his humanitarian missions in the Sudan were done."

The bitterness rose and tried to take control, but she fought it back. It was getting easier every day. She was finally starting to move on.

If she could just let the memories go.

She rubbed her neck and glanced at Noah. His hand was still on her waist, offering silent support. "So there it is, the whole sad cliché."

"You're no cliché. And you'll get through this."

"I'm working on it, believe me." She stood taller, feeling the cold wind bite against her wet cheeks. Some days she even thought she *was* over it. There had been too many tears, Grace thought. *No more of them.*

"You're a very good listener, by the way."

"I try."

"And you certainly succeed. I haven't told that to anyone." She chewed on her lip and dug for a tissue in her pocket. "So now it's your turn. Tell me what really happened to your face."

"I told you. I—"

"Yeah, right. Like I believe that. You're the steadiest, most coordinated man I've ever met." Grace eyed him without blinking. "You said you work for the government."

After a moment Noah nodded.

"And?"

"And nothing."

"Because you can't talk about it?"

Noah released her waist and studied the street. "That's right."

Grace blew out a little breath. More secrets. She'd had enough of them, thanks to James. But these secrets were different. They were meant to protect, not harm. That was important.

"So…did someone attack you? Was it dangerous?"

Noah said nothing.

"Did you have to kill someone?" she asked quietly.

His eyes cut to hers. She thought she saw wariness. "What if I did? Would you walk away?"

She heard his anger, but something told her he was baiting her. "Maybe I should. I don't have a high threshold for secrets these days, Noah."

After a long time some of his tension faded. "Understandable." He rubbed his wrist, frowning.

Something made Grace reach over and push up his cuff. Before he could react, she saw a band of bluish bruises and a long cut along the top of his hand. "You fell," she said quietly. "It must have hurt."

Noah stepped back and smoothed his cuff down. "Not so bad." He rolled one shoulder slowly. "As these things go."

She had a thousand questions, a thousand frightening images of Noah lying bloody on a street, surrounded by ambulances. "So do you...fall...often? At this job you can't discuss for an agency you can't mention?"

"Does it matter?" His eyes were focused on her now, his body still and very controlled.

"Yes. It shouldn't. I—don't want it to matter. I don't have any room in my life for a new set of secrets, Noah. But suddenly you're here and you make me feel so...safe. As if things are fresh and I can actually think about starting over." She leaned closer and brushed snow off his collar. Her hand rose, opening over his jaw. "That scares the hell out of me," she said hoarsely.

His covered her hand with his. "Make that two of us."

"You? I can't see *you* being afraid of anything. You're always so calm, so focused. Nothing gets past you."

"You believe that? Only a fool or a dead man feels no fear. A healthy dose of worry can save your life in a bad place."

"And you know about bad places? Because your life has been in danger?"

"I didn't say that."

"You didn't have to." Grace swallowed. "Noah, exactly what kind of work—"

"I can't tell you, Grace. I can't tell you or my family or my friends. That's the bottom line. And if that bothers you too much—"

"It does." She looked up at him. "But I can live with it."

Noah's eyebrow rose. "Don't look now, but we might actually be making some progress."

Grace couldn't help smiling as Noah reached behind her and turned up her collar. Snow drifted down and swirled around them and somehow the normal, average night felt a little magical.

"Could be," she whispered.

## CHAPTER SEVEN

WITHOUT A WORD Noah took her hand and tugged her down the street. He stopped at a window filled with cupcakes, pastry, ice cream and brightly colored gelato. Grace was mortified when her stomach growled loudly. "Here? For dessert? But I haven't eaten dinner yet."

"Tonight, why not live dangerously? Have dessert first. I take you for a pistachio with chocolate sprinkles kind of girl." One eyebrow rose. "Am I right?"

It ruffled Grace's feathers that he had pegged her perfectly. "Why?"

"Pistachios because they are rich but subtle and have an unusual color. Chocolate—well, because you're alive and it's there."

She couldn't let him be smug. "Maybe. But not tonight. I'll try cappuccino fudge raisin. Or maybe a lemon gelato."

"Sounds tempting." Noah frowned as she shivered. "Is it too cold out here?"

"No. I love this. I've missed snow. Come to think of it, I really miss the water, too." She felt a little tug at her heart, remembering foggy dawns gathering

driftwood with her grandmother and sunset camp-
fires roasting marshmallows on the beach. Growing
up in Oregon, there were things she had hated about
Summer Island. But now, as an adult, Grace saw just
how special her childhood had been, perched on a
quiet island beside the ocean. Not that it was perfect.
Not given the mother who usually had no clue that
Grace existed, drifting from bar to bar in an alcoholic haze.

But Grace had found a home on Summer Island
and an extended family of close-knit friends there.
Grace wouldn't trade that childhood for any other.
Suddenly, she missed it all, missed it so fiercely that
longing backed up in her throat until she couldn't
breathe.

"What's wrong?"

"I was just thinking about the town in Oregon
where I grew up. It's nothing like Washington. It's
very small and everybody knows everyone else's
business. But the sun burns over the water every
afternoon and at dawn the fog creeps in with a gray
hush off the ocean...." She shook her head, sighing.
"I just realized how much I miss it."

"How long since you've been back to visit?"

Frowning, Grace replayed her hectic schedule of
the past twelve months. "Over a year. I didn't even
realize it." She ran a hand through her hair. "I've
seen my grandfather during that time, of course. We
try to meet up every six months, sometimes in Portland or maybe Seattle or San Francisco. He adores

San Francisco. And it's important for him to get away from his work. He never wants to take time off, but running an animal shelter—doing it with very little money and a mostly volunteer staff—can be draining. Someone has to keep an eye on him. I need to go home before long and do just that." She made a promise to herself. After she finished in Chicago, she had workshops scheduled in Portland. Then she would drive to Summer Island before leaving for Paris.

She shivered, feeling a sense of premonition. Life had taught her it was a bad idea to take anything for granted.

"You're freezing." Noah pulled her scarf up higher at her neck.

Grace felt the warmth of his hands wrap around her, as real and substantial as he was. "A little."

"Let's go get that ice cream."

"Not yet." She turned, studying the lines of his face. "I have a confession to make. I wasn't entirely honest earlier. Since that night at your house, I've been thinking about my future. About a serious relationship. But…I don't want to mess up again, Noah. I know there's chemistry here. I can feel the sparks."

He nodded slowly, then turned her palm up, kissing the tender curve of her wrist. "And?"

"I don't know. Or maybe I don't *want* to know."

His tongue touched the center of her palm. Grace shivered.

She closed her eyes. "Noah, I can't think when you do that."

"No kidding. When you touched my arm, I forgot my middle name."

"What is it?"

"Never mind. Something tells me that you'll make a little sound right before I kiss you." A muscle worked at his jaw.

Grace's heart pounded. Frustration gnawed. "Noah—where is this going?"

"Don't know," he said huskily. "But it sure feels good."

He pulled her slowly closer. His body was warm against hers.

Then he kissed her, slow and deep, and Grace thought she was lifted right off the ground, floating in a haze of hunger.

He made her remember all her sunny, young dreams of heroes, and all of her grown-up fantasies of dark seduction. She wanted to trust him completely. She wanted to feel alive, entirely free in his arms.

It had been so long since she could trust that way.

Noah's thumb slid across her lips and her heart drummed in sharp answer.

"What are you thinking about, right this moment?"

Her head slanted back. "About things I thought I'd forgotten. About heroes."

*About trust,* she thought.

"Not James?"

"Not even a little." Grace was surprised to realize it was true. Right now...that was just a name. But before she could explain that to Noah, Grace heard a child's sudden, rising laughter. Two figures crossed the street, and the little girl pointed at the ice-cream shop. When she turned, her face was to the light and Grace heard Noah mutter sharply.

With an excited laugh, the little girl rocketed over the sidewalk and launched her small body into Noah's arms. "Uncle Noah! It's snowing. My feet are wet. I love the snow. Are you cold? Where's your hat? Do you want some ice cream? I *missed* you."

In a burst of questions, the dark-haired little beauty looked up at Noah, hugging him tight.

Grace felt something squeeze in her chest as Noah's big hand slid over the girl's hair. The look on his face was a study in love and contained conflict. "You bet. I love the snow, honey. And we're just going to get some ice cream. We were going to have our dessert first tonight. What do you think of *that?*"

"Dessert first?" The girl's eyes lit with excitement. "Really?" She glanced at her mother, who was striding toward her with a grim look.

Grace noticed long blond hair and an expensive cashmere coat. High heels and supple leather gloves. There was no mistaking the woman's anger.

"Sophie, I've told you *never* to run away from me like that. It is very, very bad."

"I know, Mommy. But it was just Uncle Noah. I can see him, can't I?" The child gave Noah another hug and laid her head against his waist. "I haven't seen him in days!"

"Now Sophie, that's hardly true. You saw him just last month," her mother said tightly. "But if we don't hurry, we won't be home in time to read that new book you got."

"Oh." The girl's eyes darkened. She was caught by indecision. "But maybe we could have dessert first, too. Just like Uncle Noah," she said wistfully.

"Absolutely not. We'll eat when we get home. I was going to get a cake to take back, but now there isn't time." Her mother glanced at Noah and then looked away, turning up her collar. "Most people eat dessert in its proper order," she said curtly. She reached out for the girl's hand. "Let Uncle Noah get on with his plans for the evening. You don't want to be a bother, do you?"

"Sophie's never a bother." Noah's voice was very controlled and precise. "Sophie is a treasure, right, honey?" He smiled down at the little girl who was holding his arm so tightly. "And I'm in no rush. Why don't I treat the two of you to a milkshake, Miranda? Then I can introduce you to my friend Grace."

"We haven't time." The tall blonde gathered up her child, glaring up as more snow fell. "We are already running late." She looked at Grace, and then back at Noah, summoning a thin smile. "But of course, thank you for asking. Maybe some other time."

"When?" Noah's voice grew more harsh. "Next week?" he murmured, so that only Miranda heard. "Next month? Oh, I forgot. You won't be here next month. You'll be on the West Coast, won't you, Miranda?"

The tall woman glanced at her daughter, all effort at politeness forgotten. "Noah, stop it. I—I'll call you this week and talk. I know that Sophie would like to come for ice cream." Her voice wavered a little, then hardened. "Yes, this week." Her voice rose. "So we'll call you then, Noah. Right, honey?"

The little girl's forehead creased. She looked at her mother in confusion. "But we're here now, Mommy. Why can't we go inside with Uncle Noah *now?* I don't understand."

"Because I don't—because it's almost your bedtime, Sophie. And you know that your stomach hurts if you eat sweets too late at night." Miranda buttoned the top button of her daughter's coat and took her arm firmly. "Lovely to see you, Noah. And you, Grace. I'll…call." As she pulled Sophie away, the little girl's lips quivered.

She began to cry, rigid in the snow. "I want to see Uncle Noah. I want to stay, Mommy. I don't want to go home. Daddy won't be there," she said on a soft, strangled sob. "It's been so long and I *miss* him."

Grace caught a sharp breath, feeling the girl's raw pain.

"Hey, don't cry, Sophie. It's going to be fine. Really. I'll get you tomorrow and we'll come back here for ice cream. Then I can read to you from that new book you like. How about that?" Noah knelt in the snow, drying Sophie's eyes with a tissue. "It will be a date."

"Really? Can I go, Mommy? Please?"

"I don't think—" Miranda looked at her daughter's pleading, tearstained face and sighed. "Oh, very well. If Noah calls first and you aren't too tired." She stared at Noah, her mouth flat. "Because his schedule may change, darling. He's a very busy man," she said coldly.

"I'll be there, Miranda," he said.

"Will you? Or will you get a call someplace that needs you?"

Grace saw Noah flinch and realized they were in very deep waters.

"I'll be there. Count on it, Sophie."

"Yay! And I *won't* be tired! I'll take a long nap and be all dressed and ready to go!" The girl danced in a little circle. "I can't wait!"

"Sophie, you're going to fall if you don't stop that." Miranda gripped her daughter's hand. "And we'll all freeze if we stand out here in the snow much longer." With a little nod at Noah, Miranda turned Sophie and nudged her down the sidewalk. "We'll see you soon."

She didn't look back.

But Sophie kept turning to wave all the way up the street until they vanished around the corner.

NOAH DIDN'T MOVE, his shoulders tense as he stared up the street. Finally he ran a hand through his hair. "You probably don't want to ask about that." He looked at Grace, his face set in bleak lines. "That was my brother's wife. There have been problems with her lately. You see…my brother is dead. We're all trying to sort things out, and it's not going well."

"I'm sorry, Noah." Grace slid her hand into his. "I'm *so* sorry…. She seems like a lovely little girl."

"Yeah, she is. Smart as a whip, but very vulnerable right now." He stared into the dancing snowflakes, watching a black Volvo pull away from the curb, vanishing into the night. "Sophie is great. But her mother…"

"You don't have to talk about this."

"Talking is good. Aren't you going to toss that suggestion back in my face?" he said. He shoved his hands deep into his pockets. "But talking doesn't help you forget. Or forgive." He shook his head. "No more about Miranda. I promised you some ice cream, and I always keep my promises."

But the lightness between them was gone now. Noah listened, but there were lines in his forehead. Even when he smiled, Grace thought there was something distant in his eyes. By the time they walked outside, he had barely touched his double espresso cone.

"Maybe I should go back now," Grace said quietly.

He looked at the melting ice cream and tossed it into a nearby garbage can. "Give me a few minutes, okay? We're all taking my brother's death hard. He was the youngest, the one who saw the good in everyone. He never complained, just gave you his total support." Noah ran a hand across his face. "Now he's gone and his wife wants to take his daughter all the way across the country to live. We'll never see Sophie then. It's as if Miranda wants to erase everything about us—and make sure that Sophie does, too."

"It's...heartbreaking." Grace's voice was husky. "I can't begin to imagine how that must hurt you."

"Yeah, it hurts plenty. But we'll work it out. My parents were very involved in raising Sophie while Miranda developed her real estate business. Now that Matt is gone—" Noah's voice hardened. "Now everything is changed, but she can't just cut our family out of Sophie's life. We'll take her to court if it comes to that. I hope it won't."

He stopped. "And I'm talking about it again. Kick me, will you?" He managed a wisp of a smile. "I promised you a nice night. So what can I do for penance?"

"None required. Really, Noah." Grace was glad to distract him. It looked as if he needed some serious distraction after that awful encounter. "But I don't want to go home yet, either. Maybe we can find a bookstore. I've been looking for a gift for my friend's birthday."

"You got it. What kind of book?"

Grace cleared her throat. "A knitting book. She's amazingly talented. I think she'd like a book of traditional lace patterns."

She waited for the yawn. The blank look.

Instead, Noah nodded thoughtfully. "Sounds like a great gift. And I think you're in luck." He took her arm. "Two blocks over. My mom used to shop there. Come on."

## CHAPTER EIGHT

NOAH PULLED HER through the snow, working from memory. Up ahead he saw the decorated windows of a small shop, as beautiful as an art gallery. Bright balls of yarn gleamed inside as he read the hand-painted letters on the picture window.

*Eat. Drink. Knit.*

"Found it."

Grace didn't answer. He realized that she was digging in her pocket and staring at a pair of intricately patterned gloves.

"Something wrong?"

"I thought of another project. I was going to make a pair of these for a friend back in Summer Island. She's a middling knitter, too, but she never makes anything for herself, and I know she would like them. Then I ran out of yarn. Look—there in the right side of the window. The exact yarn I need." She glanced up at him and gnawed at her bottom lip, sounding resigned. "So that would make two things to look for. Would you mind?"

An alarm bell went off in Noah's head. She was

too serious for a simple request like this. So what if she had two things to look for?

The English Creep, Noah thought grimly. Grace had asked him to stop for something and he had been surly.

Noah hated the man even more now, if that was possible. And if he had dared to lay a hand on Grace, mocking or threatening her, Noah would—

What could he do? The man was dead, and there was nothing anyone on earth could do to punish him now. As his anger cooled, Noah realized that Grace had too much self-respect and intelligence to stick around someone who abused her. He decided it was probably a pattern of condescending jokes and careless derision. And that was still bad enough to make his temper rise.

Grace was staring at him uncertainly. The wariness in her eyes made him bite down a curse.

One thing was certain. Tonight Noah was going to smooth away every negative memory that James had left behind.

"Not a problem. I'm very curious about this dark hobby of yours. My mother used to do a lot of knitting and crocheting and I've been thinking it would be good for her to start again. Maybe you can help me pick out some yarn and a project, something fairly easy. They make patterns for things, right?"

Instantly, Grace's face lit up. Noah had to draw a sharp breath at the radiance and energy that filled her eyes. She wasn't jaw-dropping gorgeous. You felt her presence and her intelligence, not her beauty. Noah had definitely dated more beautiful women. And yet right now, with the snow dusting her hair and color swirling through her cheeks, she was the most striking woman in the world.

She gave a husky laugh. "Patterns? Oh, they make patterns, my friend. Thousands of them. You're in very good hands with me. Let's go." She took his arm and pulled him toward the door into the elegant, welcoming store. "Get ready to take a walk on the wild side."

HER EXCITEMENT WAS INFECTIOUS. Noah was caught up in her laughter and her pure joy in helping him find absolutely the right project for his mother. But she really wasn't kidding about it being wild. As he walked along aisles jammed full of little balls in a thousand colors, he felt as if he'd entered a strange, alternate universe. This wasn't yarn the way *he* thought of it.

He flipped over the tag on a ball of eye-popping coral yarn. "Soy? And angora? That's rabbit fur, right? They mix soy and rabbit fur? How do they do that?"

He was totally confused now.

"Sustainability and choices are what people want today. You name it, they've tried it. Sugar, banana leaf, bamboo, even milk."

"No kidding. What happened to good old wool?"

"Still here. But now it can be mixed with cotton

or bamboo or silk. Let me show you." Grace moved quickly, a woman with a mission. Noah liked the thoughtful way she ran her hand over a rainbow display of yarns and then settled on three balls of blushing peach. "This is what I need for those gloves. They're alpaca mixed with silk. Feel how smooth."

There was a shine in her eyes. She radiated like a kid at Christmas.

"Very nice. But I don't know if she would like this."

"This project for your mother." She hesitated. "It might be expensive..." Her voice trailed off. "Good yarn will be more than you expect. I just thought you should know, in case you want to change your mind."

There it was again. The uncertainty and wariness. Noah watched her gnaw her lip and was sure that the English Creep was to blame.

"So there may be sticker shock? I'm game, but I don't have a clue." He peered around him. "Where do we start?"

Grace smiled slowly. "Well, does she knit or crochet?"

"Both," he answered easily. Grace stared up at him, looking surprised by his certainty.

"I know the difference," he said with a lift of his brows. "You knit with sticks. You crochet with that short kind of hook."

"Two needles, long and straight like this, for knitting." Grace held up a pair made of dark, polished wood. "For crochet a hook, shorter and curved at the end like this." She pointed to a nearby display.

"Needles," Noah said with a nod. He had seen his mother use metal ones.

"Okay, so she's a knitter. Now what kind of things does she like to make? Clothing? A blanket or an afghan? Socks or slippers? Or maybe a nice scarf?"

Noah rubbed the back of his neck. As a boy, he remembered his mother kicking off her shoes after dinner, settling down in a big wing chair, and pulling yarn from the basket near her feet. He remembered handmade socks at Christmas and sweaters at birthdays. Funny, his mother hadn't gone for anything tame or sedate. Everything she made had been a riot of color and texture. She was as fearless in her hobby as she was in her life, he realized now with the eyes of an adult.

"She always made us socks at Christmas, but the last thing I saw her working on was a blanket. It was sky-blue with squares. Lots of texture. Sorry, but I can't tell you much beyond than that."

"No, that's good. So she liked that color of blue?"

"She likes anything with deep, rich colors. One year we all got lime-green socks. The next year it was purple hats." Noah frowned at a sudden rush of memories. Every Christmas his family gathered together, joking and jostling and catching up on news while they opened presents. One year their socks were all dyed with Kool-Aid, his mother had explained proudly. His younger brother, Matt, had pulled his sock onto the dog's tail, and they had tumbled over laughing as their big Lab raced through the house, tail high, sock waving. Matt had said—

Sadness hit Noah like a body blow.

Matt was gone. They'd never laugh together again. There would be no more pranks, no more snowball fights.

No more anything.

Grace cleared her throat. "Is something wrong?"

He summoned a smile. The only way to deal with loss was to get on with living. His job helped. Noah knew that every day he had a chance to save someone else from dying the way Matt had died.

"I'm good. Let's go for the bright colors. She likes deep blue and sky-blue. Maybe some paler greens. Almost silver—whatever that's called."

"You've got an excellent eye. That will make a wonderful mix. Now for a pattern." Grace twined her fingers through his, leading him down one aisle and up another. She stopped in front of a bookcase that was jammed with yarn, sorted in shades from light to dark. "Let's choose three or four colors to take with us. That will help when we look at patterns."

Noah saw a perfect color of blue. He knew his mother would like this one because it was on her favorite set of china. Idly, he flipped over the tag—and whistled. "Twelve dollars? That's the price for *one* of these? So how many does it take to make a blanket? Five or six maybe?"

"More than that." Grace glanced at the printed tag wrapped around the ball of yarn. "At this yardage, even a small blanket would take a dozen."

Noah did a quick calculation and whistled again. "So this is going to get expensive. You were right. Well, if you can't splurge on your mother, what kind of son are you? Let's go for it. Twelve it is."

Grace squeezed his arm. Something came and went in her eyes. "I think she's going to love this yarn. Now for a pattern." She picked up a book, flipped through the pages and then held it out. "What do you think of this one?"

"I don't know. It looks pretty complicated."

"Actually, each block is knit separately. You sew them together at the end. The sewing is probably the worst part."

Noah looked at the different textures and wavy squares. "She'd like this. It reminds me of something she made a long time ago. I think her mother and sister had started work on a marriage quilt. They were collecting squares like these. Then she told me the soldiers came. All their blocks got left behind. She's always regretted that." He nodded. "Yes, this is the one. But why don't I get just two sample colors. I'll buy her a gift card so that she can choose other colors if she doesn't like mine."

"We can give you a gift card in any amount." Footsteps tapped closer. A tall woman in a striking lace shawl nodded approvingly at the pattern Noah was holding. "I couldn't help but overhear, and I think your mother is a very lucky person. Does she need knitting needles, too?"

"Beats me."

The owner chuckled. "You can wait on that. She may prefer metal or wood, or she may have a set stashed away." The woman studied Grace. "I've seen you here before, I think."

Grace nodded. "I've been in a few times. You have a lovely store."

The owner beamed. "Why don't you drop by on Wednesday night? Our knitting group meets upstairs. I provide tea and coffee. Everyone brings a different dessert." The owner raised an eyebrow at Noah. "Maybe your mother would like to come, too."

"I'll ask her. Thanks."

"Fine. Now, I'll get this all rung up for you. What I need to know is the amount of the gift card, sir."

Noah thought of the pain and loss he had seen in his mother's eyes. Maybe this would help. In fact, he should have thought of it sooner. "Make it an even hundred."

Grace raised an eyebrow. "Be still, my beating heart," she murmured.

Noah made a mental note to remember the name of the yarn shop. It was a nice place and well organized, but who knew that a few balls of yarn could make a woman go dreamy-eyed like this? In a smooth movement he took the yarn Grace was holding and handed it to the store owner. "Add this in, too."

"Noah, you don't have to—"

"That's right, I don't. Now be quiet and let me make you smile."

She started to say something else. Then she shook her head. "You're a dangerous man, you know that?"

More dangerous than she knew, Noah thought. He was fighting a losing battle. If he didn't touch her in the next five minutes, he might not survive.

SNOW STILL DRIFTED down gently as Noah took the bag of yarn and tugged Grace outside.

Grace felt oddly giddy as the door closed behind them. Noah hadn't laughed at her request to visit the yarn shop. In fact, she was fairly certain he had enjoyed himself.

She was intensely aware of his broad shoulders as they brushed hers on the narrow sidewalk. Without any warning all that restless awareness turned sharp and focused. She hadn't expected to feel this race of yearning. She could tell by the tension in his face that Noah felt it, too.

She felt his hand open and press into her back. Silently, Noah drew her closer. She heard the drum of her heart.

He didn't push her, sliding one hand slowly through her hair. Grace felt that touch all the way to her toes. Her cheeks were hot and she took a sharp breath, trying to be sane and in control, all the things she prided herself on.

His mouth brushed the line of her jaw, the curve of her cheek. Suddenly, control fled.

Their bodies were close, and she wasn't quite ready when his mouth came down on hers, searching and open. He didn't take. He didn't demand. He simply offered her the promise of pleasure and belonging.

She closed her eyes, feeling his mouth skim hers. His body was hard, but his hands were very gentle, and Grace wanted to pull him closer until she found the warm muscles beneath his clothes.

Here in the darkness she felt the strangest mix of safety and danger. To touch him was dangerous, challenging her need for balance and order. Yet on some deep level, Grace knew that she could trust this man completely.

The problem was whether she could trust herself—or her very vulnerable heart.

She opened her hands on his chest. Instantly, Noah went still. A muscle clenched at his jaw.

Grace felt the taut line of his body. He was very aroused. But he didn't move, didn't push her response.

She wasn't confused now, only maddened by the need to feel his mouth again. Breathlessly, she pulled his head down to hers and whispered his name. When his mouth opened on hers, slow and hungry, Grace let herself fall into a sheer dive of pleasure.

Her fingers opened, sliding beneath his jacket. She heard his breath catch. Blindly, she rose, brushing the corners of his mouth as she tasted him slowly. She hadn't expected the heat or the need. She had never been reckless or blinded by hunger in a man's arms like this.

Now Grace was all those things. She wanted to laugh, but she could barely breathe as Noah wrapped his arms around her. She was crushed against him on a public street, her heart slamming and her knees shaking, and she didn't care a bit. She didn't have a word for the storm of emotions whirling through her. When he kissed her again, Grace gave up looking for one.

She touched his face, feeling breathless and strong and impossibly alive, as if everything else in her life had been no more than a pale rehearsal for this moment.

"Noah, I—" She stopped as a shrill beep came from his pocket.

Noah frowned, digging in his pocket. "Sorry." He slid out a pager, flipped it open on his palm and glanced at the screen. For long seconds he didn't move, his face unreadable. Grace felt the intensity of his focus, swept off to whatever world was waiting on the other end of that message.

She saw the moment that the smile left his eyes. He took a deep breath. "Damn." He touched her face. "I have to go. I'm sorry, Grace, but it's—important." He stabbed a hand through his hair. "Why don't I call my father and have him take you home? I'll walk you back to the yarn store. You can wait for him there."

He was distant. Grace could see that he was already immersed in whatever work had summoned him. And she was certain there was danger involved. She thought of the bruises on his hand. The long welt. "You'll be careful?" She didn't ask for details. She wasn't sure she wanted any.

"Always."

She nodded slowly. "There's no need to bother your father. I'll just catch a cab. If I walk over two blocks, there's always a line at the hotel."

"Out of the question. You're not walking anywhere alone tonight," Noah said flatly. "And I won't have you taking a cab. If I had more time, I'd drop you off myself." His eyes narrowed as the pager rang again.

He scanned the text screen while he pulled out his cell phone. "Dad? Yeah, it's Noah. Look, I've got a favor to ask. Grace is here. We were just taking a walk, but I have to go."

Noah listened for a moment. "You would? Thanks, Dad. That would be great. I'll tell her." Noah slid his phone back into his pocket. "He should be here in fifteen minutes. I'll walk you back to the store."

NOAH CRANKED UP the heat and took a long drink from the water bottle he always kept in the front seat of his Jeep. His first page had read four-one-four. Level-four risk. Level-four explosives involved.

Very dangerous.

He stared at the traffic racing past and thought about Grace's eyes, so bright with life and humor. She had stunned him with the tentative force of her kiss and the trembling pressure of her hands on his chest.

He had seen the joy die when he got the page to leave.

Their first kiss had changed things, Noah thought wryly. Where the night would have led them, he hadn't a clue. Now he'd never know.

He glared out at the snow. No point in getting angry. The job came first.

When the light changed, he plunged into the stream of evening traffic headed east. Downtown.

No regrets. Regrets were cold stones in an empty cup.

This was what he was. This was what he did. And at least tonight the right man was going out to handle the explosives. A man who knew the risks and accepted them.

Not like Matt.

It was the one thing Noah could be grateful for as his pager beeped again and the threat level shot up to a six.

## CHAPTER NINE

AFTER NOAH LEFT, Grace wandered aimlessly.

Shelves of soft yarn offered no distraction now. She kept thinking where he might be, telling herself there was no reason to worry. She didn't know what he did, beyond being called out on short notice. He worked for the government, but that description could apply to any number of jobs.

Grace massaged a knot of tension in her forehead. Noah would tell her when he was ready—if he could. She respected the need for secrecy.

But waiting for news left her jumpy. She would have gone to find a cab except that she had told Noah she would stay and wait for his father.

She leafed through a knitting book, pretending to look at the pages. Every few minutes she checked her watch. At least Noah's mother would soon have his gift. Losing a son had to be unimaginable, but she prayed that the knitting project would distract and comfort her. Grace remembered her own bad times, when the slide of smooth wool and the click of wooden needles had brought her solace, along with happy memories of quiet afternoons knitting with her grandmother.

The big Hummer appeared exactly when predicted, and Alex McLeod jumped over the snow, scooping up her bags like a man half his age.

"I'm sorry to trouble you, but Noah insisted."

"And well he should. I'm happy to drive you back. I hope we can make a stop at home on the way." Noah's father helped her inside and glanced down at her bags. "Nice things in there?"

"Yarn for a project. They had the exact color I needed. Several magazines, too."

Alex nodded slowly. "Tatiana used to knit. She hasn't picked up anything lately." He frowned at the crowded streets, nudging the big Hummer around snowdrifts from the recent storm. "Frankly, I wish she'd start up again. She needs it now. She still broods about our son."

"Noah told me about him," Grace said quietly. "I'm so sorry. It's such a loss."

"A loss no father should ever know," Alex said tightly. "I still hear his laugh and turn around, expecting to see him behind me." His hand tightened on the wheel. "But Tatiana feels it worst of all. She won't talk about it, though. Frankly, I don't think she should be alone tonight. Not to brood and remember." He glanced at Grace, choosing his words carefully. "She likes you, Grace. If you would come and spend a few hours with us, you would be doing me—and Noah—a great favor."

"I'd love to come. Your wife is a wonderful cook and I warn you, I'm going to pry out all her secrets. In fact, that's what I love about food and cooking. There's always more to learn. Even the best recipe is never finished, but always waiting for a new touch from a master's hand."

"With that kind of energy you must be very good at your job. Maybe on the way you can tell me a little more about this work you do. It's some kind of research?"

"Mostly, I write about historical cooking, how breads were made and foods were preserved. Traditional kinds of herb use and fermentation." Grace was describing her next project when her cell phone rang. She saw the Oregon area code but didn't recognize the number.

"Sorry. I should take this." Grace hurriedly dug out her cell phone, wondering who was calling.

A deep voice boomed out. "You're a hard person to track down, Grace. I've called you three times, twice at your apartment. No luck."

"Gage! Sorry to miss your calls. Are you in D.C. now?"

"Stopping over on the way home. I lost your cell number, then tried Caro, but they're expecting a big storm. The reception has been rotten. It took me an hour to get through."

Lieutenant Gage Grayson was married to Grace's closest friend back on Summer Island. The girls had been inseparable growing up, supporters during bad times and a general cheering section over the years. Gage was finishing a tour of duty in Afghanistan and due home shortly. "So you're headed home? That's wonderful. Caro will be wild. I wish I could be there."

"Still working too hard, are you? Caro says she hasn't seen you for months."

"Guilty, I'm afraid. So much food, so little time. But I'm planning to be back in Oregon in two weeks. Will you be there?" Grace heard the sound of voices and airport gate numbers being announced in the background.

"I'm not sure. But I know I've got my first night planned. Caro beside me, *Casablanca* on the tube and a fire at full blaze. Wait—hold on Grace. They just made a flight change."

She heard the phone shift, and then more muffled announcements. When Gage came back, the line was filled with voices. "I was hoping to meet you for coffee, but I'll be boarding in twenty minutes. I was able to hop an earlier connection. Sorry."

"Hey, don't apologize. Just jump in your seat and get home. I know a woman who can't wait to see you. A dog and cat, too."

"Yeah, I miss them all. So—everything's really okay with you? I mean, I was sorry to hear about your fiancé's death. I hope things are going better now."

"Yes." Grace took a deep breath. "It was...rocky for a while. But it's better." It finally felt better, she realized. She could talk about James without flinching. "Now go get that flight, Marine. And give all my love to Caro. Plus check in on my grandfather, would you? Remind him I'll be there before the end of the month."

"Will do, Grace. There's nothing wrong with Peter, is there? He's not sick, I hope."

"No, he's fine. He just doesn't know how to slow down. I worry about him."

"Understood. I'll do a full reconnoiter and have Caro call you with the details. We'll be putting in some time helping out at the shelter, too. How does that sound?"

"Just wonderful. Thanks so much, Gage. And—just take care, okay? Everyone on Summer Island has you in their thoughts."

"Thanks." Emotion tightened his voice. "I appreciate all your help and support. It means a lot, to me and my men. Those knitted helmet liners were snatched up faster than ammo, by the way. Now I really should go. Don't want to lose my flight after coming halfway around the world."

"Go. Be safe." Grace heard more bustle and then the line went dead. She continued to hold the phone, thinking of Caro and the wonderful reunion she would have with her husband. If any two people deserved happiness, they did.

Alex glanced over at her. "Everything okay?"

"It was the husband of my best friend. He's on his way home from Afghanistan. The Marines."

"Glad to hear he's got some leave coming. Sounds like everyone is close where you live. Summer Island, was it?"

"That's the place—and yes, we are close. I just wish I could get back there more often." She ran a hand through her hair. "Lately, all I seem to do is travel. Still, I can't complain. I have my dream job and I savor every second of it."

Alex gave her a searching look. "But you miss your friends back in Oregon. And you worry about your grandfather."

"He's always been healthy as an ox, but he's getting on in years. Yes, I worry about him. He works way too hard." Grace watched the slow, snarled traffic crawl. "But he won't stop."

"Men are like that. My suggestion—if you'll pardon an interfering man—is to tell him you worry about him. That might just slow him down. He'll care about how you feel, Grace."

"Maybe. But I know how much he loves those animals of his." She smiled at Alex. "Probably as much as you love your cars. I imagine you work twelve-hour days."

"I suppose I'm just as guilty. I'm trying to give more work to Reed. Since losing Matt, I want to be home with Tatiana. She worries about all of us." He hesitated. "About Noah, especially."

Grace watched Alex's hands tighten on the wheel. "Is it…very dangerous, this work of his?"

She knew she shouldn't ask, but somehow the words slipped out.

"Dangerous? I guess that depends on who you ask."

"I'm asking you, Mr. McLeod."

"Alex," he corrected. "I'll tell you what I know. Mind you, it isn't a whole lot." His eyes narrowed. "His work is hard and the hours are long. He has a great deal of responsibility." He took a slow breath. "And yes...it can be dangerous. But most of the time it's routine and it's tedious, nothing more than that. So we are going to pray hard that tonight is one of the routine nights." He forced a smile. "Since I can't say more than that, why don't we talk about you? I have an ulterior motive, you see." He rubbed his neck. "My wife is feeling restless lately. I admit, I goaded her to ask for the recipe for that whole-grain bread you mentioned, but she was too proud to ask."

"Of course I can show her. We could make some this weekend, if you like."

"Actually, I had a better idea." Alex gave a guilty smile. "I hoped you might start tonight. My wife should have everything you need at the house."

"You are tricky, aren't you? You planned for me to come. But that's fine. It will keep our thoughts off...other things."

*Like Noah.*

They would all be thinking about Noah—and whether he was safe.

"Just turn here, could you? I'll run in and get some things from my apartment first."

While Alex turned around, Grace ran inside for her notes on the newest bread recipe she was testing. When she came out, a man stepped out from between two cars, blocking her way. He lifted a big camera and moved in on her face, the camera whirring loudly.

"Wh—what are you doing?" Grace blinked, frozen in the glare of his powerful flash. "Who are you?" She heard Alex call her name. The door of the Hummer opened.

The man with the camera moved back to include Alex in the photo as he emerged from the car. "I'm nobody."

"Back off," Alex growled.

The man sidestepped as Alex moved protectively in front of Grace. "Free country, pal." But he wasn't prepared for the powerful hand that gripped his shoulder or the quick way Alex covered the lens of the camera with his palm.

"*Hey*—you can't do that."

"Do what?" Alex said calmly. "I tripped on some ice. You just happened to be in the way."

"Like hell, you b—"

The camera went flying as Alex spun the man around and pushed him against a parked truck. "The lady asked you a question. Who are you?"

Muttering, the man took a swing at Alex but missed.

"Name," Alex said, his voice hard and cold.

"W-Wilson. Henry."

"Who do you work for?"

"No one, damn it. I'm strictly freelance."

Alex frowned, "Why are you interested in the lady? Who were you going to sell these photos to?"

"None of your f—"

"Language." In one deft move Alex lifted the man up over the Hummer's hood, feet dangling. "Answer the question politely."

The man named the largest newspaper chain in the country, spitting out each word.

"Now isn't that interesting?"

"But why me?" Grace demanded. "No one cares where I go or what I do."

The man on the hood snorted. "They damned well care about James Marfield though. Someone at the paper is doing an in-depth exposé about failures of world diplomacy. Whatever the hell that means," the man snarled. "Your James is number one on the list."

Grace took in a strangled breath. Not more of James's shadows.

"Forget this job," Alex said curtly. "If the lady tells me you've been bothering her again, I will find you and make these suggestions in a more concrete way. Do we understand each other?"

"Y-yes." The man fell back with a curse when Alex released him. He grabbed his camera from the snow and scowled. "Thanks for ruining my new Nikon."

"Anytime," Alex said pleasantly. "Call it a professional hazard. Freelancing can be dangerous."

"Yeah, be a smart-ass now. But I won't be the only one who's following her. There's a big contract for photos on this story. They want info about Marfield." He glared at Grace and laughed harshly. "About his private life, too. Get ready for life in the fishbowl, honey," he called as he ran across the street.

Grace stood stiffly. Anger choked her at this invasion of her privacy. "I—I'm sorry about that."

"It's not your fault, Grace. I'm just glad to help."

"You're pretty tough, aren't you? I see where Noah gets it."

"I don't allow my family or friends to be harassed, if that's what you mean." Alex picked up the gloves that Grace had dropped and knocked snow off the soft pink merino.

"You're—not going to ask me what he meant?"

"No. You'll tell me if you want to. And if not, there's no point in asking you anyway."

Grace took the gloves he was holding out to her. "The strong, silent type. Another trait that Noah inherited." She shoved her hands in her pocket and looked down at the outline of the camera where it had dropped in the snow. "James Marfield was my fiancé. He died in a plane crash. One year, four months and nineteen days ago," she said quietly. "He was smart, funny, intense and generous. He had traveled everywhere. I thought he was the best thing that ever happened to me. How wrong can a person be?" she said softly.

Alex held open the door to the Hummer. "Let's go home."

As they drove through the darkness, she told Noah's father all the rest, about James's lies and lovers. About a probable baby. When she finished she felt drained.

"Noah knows about all this, but not about the reporter. I'd like to tell him that myself, if you don't mind."

"Of course."

"I was...so naive. I believed all that traveling James did was for his humanitarian causes. And he really did so much good. People simply trusted him." She ran a trembling hand across her eyes. "Even now his memory...hurts."

"Don't blame yourself," Alex said sternly. "It's never wrong to trust. He's the one to blame, and only him."

"On some level I believe that. And truly it's getting better. Some days I don't think about him at all."

"This reporter may make life very uncomfortable. These people will dig and dig until they find something sensational enough to sell papers and books."

"Then I see a lot of big hats and sunglasses in my future." Grace laughed tightly. "Luckily I won't be in D.C. much longer."

"We'll miss you." Alex reached out and squeezed her shoulder. "In the little time we've known you,

you've touched our lives, Grace. I thought you should know that. But I hope you won't be gone forever." He smiled cockily. "Otherwise I might have to mount a research expedition of my own."

Emotion tightened her throat as Grace studied that tough, honest face. "No, I won't disappear forever."

"Promise?"

"I promise you."

"Good. Because friends and family are all that really matter in life. Age has taught me that." His lips curved. "And now get ready for a bread inquisition. If I know my Tatiana, she will be waiting at the door right now with apron in hand."

*Port of Baltimore, 8:35 p.m.*

IT WASN'T LIKE TV. There were no sirens, no throngs of police cars or bustling SWAT teams. When Noah's unit was dispatched, they moved with a low profile and unmarked vehicles. The sleek chopper that had brought him from D.C. looked like an ordinary commercial issue.

But it wasn't. As Noah pulled on his Kevlar suit, he watched the grim, determined faces around him. Each person was totally focused on a specific threat assessment. The sense of danger was tangible. His target lay somewhere in the big shipping crates just inside the doors of the anonymous warehouse ahead.

Noah's boss strode up, secure cell phone glued

to his ear, gathering updated intelligence about the shipper, source location and probable explosive devices sealed inside.

"Robot inoperative. There's some kind of lead lining on the crates. No X-rays available. But we're definitely picking up explosive vapor. Ten minutes ago the bomb dogs signaled for Semtex vapor signatures and ammonium nitrate." The big man's eyes narrowed. "Are you sure you're up for this, McLeod? Your hands took a beating yesterday during that circuit fire. I can pull Kelly in to handle this."

Thomas Kelly had a wife and two kids, with a third on the way. He had good hands but only half the experience Noah did.

"Negative, sir. I'm suited and ready. Time may be critical here."

After a moment Noah's superior nodded. "It's all yours then. Keep your eye on the ball."

Noah nodded and stared down the empty vista of cement in front of the warehouse door. Sounds seemed to recede until all he heard was the heavy thump of his heartbeat inside his protective suit. He shook his head, shoving down errant thoughts of Grace, his parents and all the things he wanted to do before he died.

Sweat trickled into his eyes beneath the heavy helmet. Already the 100-pound bomb suit weighed on his shoulders. He felt a rush of adrenaline.

No one moved as he started the long walk toward the warehouse.

"I'm here, Matt," he whispered. "Take a little walk with me, bro. This one feels bad."

## CHAPTER TEN

TATIANA OPENED THE FRONT DOOR, her hair in disarray and flour streaking her cheek. "You talked her into coming, Alex. I'm so glad. Please come in, Grace."

Alex smiled at his wife. "That's not all I talked her into, my love." He walked past her, looking smug.

Tatiana glanced at the bag Grace carried. "She is going to knit?"

"No, she is going to teach us how to make that wonderful peasant bread from France. And then she is going to knit while the dough is rising."

"Really?" Tatiana clapped her hands in delight. "I have tried many ways, with all kinds of flour and all kinds of starter. It is always nice but not special. No chewy center. I am about to give up, and then you mention knowing the recipe, and I am so happy. I have a pot of tea ready and I have just finished a fresh poppy-seed cake."

"Perfect. You can trade me your cake recipe for my bread recipe." As Grace set down her purse, a pair of knitting needles poked out. "But first I'd like to see the kittens and Ivan. I miss them all. And after that, if you do feel like knitting…"

Tatiana gnawed at her lip. "I was thinking to start again, just a simple scarf. I have forgotten so much. I don't remember how to make the first stitches. Me, who knitted my first hat when I was four!"

"I can show you all that. I have a feeling you'll be flying through the rows inside an hour." Grace smiled as Alex took out beige cooking aprons for all three of them.

He rolled up his sleeves. "So I should get the package of yeast, right?"

"Actually, no." Grace held up her bag. "Trade secret. This is a natural fruit-based starter. Not sourdough or commercial yeast. This is the special sauce." Grace took off her coat. "Ready to rock and roll?"

FORTY-FIVE MINUTES LATER Tatiana had three pages of notes, and her first loaves of bread dough curing. The bread was French, but based on an old Italian recipe Grace had learned in Florence. She had noticed Tatiana's growing tension, and her darting glances at the wall clock. When that happened, Grace launched into a new detail of bread making.

They were about to stop for tea when the phone rang. Tatiana shot out of her chair, dropping the big wooden spoon from her hands. Her face was stark white.

"Answer it." She took a hard breath. "Something

is wrong. Alex, I can feel the weight. Too many shadows." Her hands shook. She closed her eyes, leaning rigidly against the counter. "Please, God," she whispered. "No more bad news…"

Alex pulled her against his chest and squeezed her. He murmured something in her ear, a look of unspeakable tenderness in his eyes. But Grace saw the tension in his shoulders and knew that Alex was fighting his own battle with fear as he turned to pick up the phone.

Without thinking, Grace moved beside Tatiana while Alex answered.

Tatiana's fingers locked on Grace's arm. If it was bad news…

Instead of fear, Grace summoned an image of Noah laughing as he ground snow down her collar. Then another memory of Noah tucking the puppy under his jacket.

*Nothing can happen to him,* she thought fiercely. *Please.*

Noah's father cleared his throat. "Yes? He told you to call? I see. He will be busy then. Yes, I understand."

Grace leaned forward, straining to catch every syllable.

"When he is done, yes. Thank you for calling. It is…good to have news," he finished gruffly.

Alex put down the phone and looked at the two women. By now, Grace had her arm around Tatiana's shoulders, while Tatiana's hands opened and closed on Grace's other arm.

"He is safe?" The words were a hoarse whisper. "Noah—he is not hurt?"

"He's fine, Tatiana. It was busy for a while. Now they're clearing up the last odds and ends. He will call when he can. For now he wanted us to know that all is well."

It wasn't a *routine* night, Grace thought, shivering. Alex's face registered that clearly.

How did they bear this terrible waiting and uncertainty? How did they go on, week after week, knowing that one night he could leave and never come back? Grace thought about how much courage that took.

She wasn't sure she had it.

Silence fell. Then Tatiana's shoulders squared. "Now we will have tea. We will eat cake and watch our dough rise and we will not think of shadows." She smiled slowly at Alex. "Tonight we will use our best china, too. We will celebrate life and family." A bit of her old spirit returned and she flashed an impish glance at Grace. "And excellent crusty bread too, I think."

THEY DID JUST AS TATIANA wished. They had tea and cake and talked about dumplings. They argued about travel and politics and olive oil. With encouragement from Grace, Tatiana started to knit again, muttering when the stitches were crooked and tight.

"Bah, it is terrible, this. Once my needles would fly. I could make a whole sock in a night." She shook her head. "But I will work hard. It helps to have a good teacher."

"It will come back. In a week you'll be burning through a set of socks again."

"Not in a week, I think. But soon." Tatiana took a long breath and rolled her shoulders, looking down at her old metal needles. "I forgot how the wool feels in my fingers. How the needles glide. So calm it makes me. Thank you for this gift of helping me remember." She patted Grace's hand and stood up. "Time to check on the bread."

Time seemed to slip into a pleasant blur. Grace gave Tatiana instructions while she continued to knit. All of them laughed when Alex appeared with a puppy under one arm and three wriggling kittens under the other.

"Now everyone is here. Come and visit with Grace, you unruly lot."

Grace hugged the warm, furry bodies one by one, caught in almost tangible sense of calm and belonging.

But she didn't *really* belong here. It would be dangerous to become too attached to this brave, stubborn family. She barely knew Noah. Who knew what the future would bring? Grace tried to stay polite but detached even though her heart demanded that she listen and trust.

*Not yet.*

Love didn't grow in a day, she thought tiredly. She was asking for heartache if she believed that.

The phone rang again. Tatiana flew to the desk, scattering flour in her path. "Yes?" She gripped the phone, staring out into the falling snow. "You are fine? Yes? Thank heaven. And you will be done before long? No?" Her eyes clouded. "All night." But she forced a smile. "My son, the important man. Yes, Grace is here with us. We are making bread from her recipe. Very clever it is, too. So you must finish and come home while it is hot from the oven." She listened for a few minutes, then nodded and said something in Ukrainian. After that she held out the phone to Grace. "He wishes to speak with you." With a quick smile Tatiana whisked Alex out of the room, leaving Grace alone.

"Noah?"

"Right here. Thanks for sharing your recipe. My mom is over the moon."

"She's a wonderful student." Grace hesitated. "Is it— Are you very busy?" She wanted to say *safe,* but she refused to give voice to cold possibilities.

"Things are a little tight. Several people are away at a conference, so the rest of us are playing catch-up. And it's snowing again. How about a snowball fight when I'm done here?"

"You're on, pal."

Grace heard the deep growl of a truck motor. Noah covered the phone, answering a question she couldn't hear. When he was done, he sounded rushed. "I'd better go. But tell my mom and dad I'll be in touch. And *tell them not to worry,*" he added firmly. There were more voices nearby. He spoke to someone, then returned. "Gotta go. I'll be thinking about our snowball fight," he said quietly. "About how your mouth tastes in the snow."

Heat swirled through her body. Grace swallowed hard. "Finish up there. Then come find out," she whispered.

But the line was already dead.

SOMEHOW, BETWEEN TENDING dough and helping Tatiana rediscover the intricacies of casting on stitches and pattern reading, the night flew past. It was almost one o'clock when Alex caught her yawning.

"Sorry. But I think I'd better go. The rest of your dough will be fine in the refrigerator until morning."

Tatiana took her hands. "Why don't you stay here tonight? You could sleep in Noah's old bed." She glanced shrewdly at Grace. "I think you must be a little curious, no?"

Grace blushed, which made both Alex and Tatiana laugh. "It's too much trouble. And I have to be up very early," she said quickly.

"No problem. Alex and I are always early to wake. Alex can drop you wherever you like. Can't you, my love?"

"Of course." He refilled Grace's plate. "Have more cake."

Grace looked from one to the other. "You aren't going to let me talk my way out, are you?"

"No," the two said together.

"And think how you will have more time with the kittens," Tatiana said quickly.

"Low blow," Grace muttered. But she had to admit that she was curious about Noah's old bedroom. "I'll stay. Thank you for the invitation and for a wonderful evening."

"So polite." Tatiana smiled broadly at her husband. "Yes, always perfect manners. I wish I could have seen her digging in that Dumpster to save her kittens, Alex. Noah called her unforgettable." Tatiana picked up her knitting needles and chuckled. "I believe only someone very special could take our son's breath away," she added wisely.

Grace had the clear feeling that she had been outmanned and outgunned by a champion. When Tatiana brought in one of the kittens to sleep in Grace's lap while she knitted, Grace was sure of it.

THE HOUSE WAS QUIET.

The fire had died down and everyone was asleep. Grace stared up at the ceiling, warm and cocooned beneath a down quilt in the upstairs bedroom that had once belonged to Noah.

It felt odd and impossibly intimate to be curled up beneath the soft blankets where Noah once slept. She thought of Noah here in these sheets, dreaming.

*I'll be thinking about how your mouth tastes in
the snow.*

Through the window she watched a single star
winking above the trees. She wondered if Noah had
seen the same star, bright and glinting, as a young
boy. There were so many things she didn't know
about him, so many puzzles to be solved. But Grace
dimly realized one thing.

Her feelings for him were nothing like what she
had felt for James. This emotion between them
was deep and unpredictably complex. It didn't require words or need constant confirmation. She
didn't know where their relationship would go. She
couldn't see how they would make anything work
with their busy lives set so far apart.

What if it wasn't meant to be serious? What if her
heart ended up tied in knots, torn painfully in two
again?

Maybe, a quiet voice whispered, getting hurt was
the price you paid to know you were alive.

AFTER ALEX MCLEOD finished checking the house
and putting out the fire, he walked slowly up to bed.
He found his wife where she usually was, reading or
working in her big wing chair. Her back was turned
to the door while she muttered over her knitting,
but when he came closer, Alex saw that her fingers
were tense.

Cold tears slid in streams down her cheeks.

"Tatiana, what's wrong?"

She jumped a little, then leaned forward, trying to hide her face. "I couldn't sleep. Just restless. You know how I am."

"Yes, I do know." Alex sat down beside her, turning her face up gently. "You were crying. Why didn't you come to me?"

"Because it's my fault. Because it's me who can't forget. Why should I keep bothering you again and again?"

"Why? Because I love you. Because I want to know when you're in pain. Because years ago we promised to share everything, the pain and fear just as much as the happiness and laughter."

"I know. And I should have come to you tonight. But I hate to be helpless, caught up in these constant, helpless feelings that never stop. I was never weak before. How much everything is changed after Matt."

"Come to me. Two people can share the pain better than one. Promise me you will not sit like this and cry alone."

"I promise." She managed the ghost of a smile. "Really. Now let's go to bed. It's cold and I need to feel your arms around me."

"Not yet. I want to see something first."

"Now? What is it?"

He shook his head, wrapping a well-loved afghan around her shoulders. Then he took her hand, guiding her quietly down the long hallway. They stopped outside Noah's old room, where Grace was sound asleep.

Smiling, Alex stepped back and pointed inside. Tatiana peeked around the door into the room, lit only by the dim hall light.

But the light was enough to make out the bed.

Tatiana covered her mouth, biting back a laugh at the sight before her.

The mother cat was stretched out across Grace's feet, drowsy and contented. Around her the three kittens lay curled into tight balls, purring happily. Each one was tucked into another, all three strung together like fluffy commas.

Nearby, the puppy had burrowed under the covers, with his body stretched full length and his feet in the air. His head was nestled on Grace's shoulder.

Tatiana gave a quiet sigh of contentment, sliding an arm around her husband's waist. The two stood, listening to the sounds of the house shifting and the soft purring of the kittens and the gentle panting of the puppy.

In the silence they walked back to their room, hand in hand.

"Animals know who to trust." Tatiana studied her husband's strong face. "It is hard to fool them. They find the place they feel most safe." She gripped Alex's hand. "She is the one for Noah. I feel it, Alex. And yet...she could hurt him in a terrible way."

"I see that, too." He brushed the hair off his wife's

cheek. "But that must be his choice to make. And hers. When did young people ever listen to advice, anyway?"

Then he caught her up and carried her to bed. Neither one spoke after that. Their hearts were full and their bodies met with the warm knowledge of long experience in a place where desire burned fresh, never dimmed.

# *CHAPTER ELEVEN*

*Four in the morning*

AT LEAST TONIGHT there was a happy ending, Noah thought.

He looked across at his personal war zone.

Hardware, timers and wires covered every inch of his desk, carefully removed from their crates. The team around him was working frantically to isolate and categorize every detail of these new weapons that had hit American soil. The crates had been tracked from a container ship inbound from Malaysia in the successful conclusion of a yearlong sting operation by combined U.S. and British intelligence. Thanks to faulty construction, one of the devices had leaked during transit. The circuits had been dangerously unstable by the time Noah opened the crate. But he had isolated the power source, rendering the device safe before it discharged.

His boss opened the door at the far end of the lab. "Roll it up, everybody. We're off as of tonight."

"But I still have two more devices to examine, sir." The voice came from behind Noah.

"Not now you don't. It's no longer our assignment. Everything is going over to Quantico. Pack it up."

Despite low muttering, the tired group complied. No one was surprised. Here in the lab Noah and his team provided initial assessment of hazardous materials, along with best methods of containment and control. But within twenty-four hours forensic materials and hardware were turned over to the FBI labs for full analysis.

It was over.

Noah pushed back from the crowded desk and rubbed the cramped muscles in his shoulder, watching people tag the last of their work and then file out. In the past seven hours he had downed five cups of bad coffee, one dry tuna sandwich and a cardboard corn muffin, courtesy of the vending machines down the hall. The memory wasn't pleasant.

He thought about the fresh bread Grace and his mother were making and his stomach growled.

"Yeah, me, too." His boss grabbed his coat and gloves and glanced at the now-deserted room. "Someday they won't need us. Someday men will stop trying to butcher and maim each other in every way possible." The graying security expert sighed and flipped off the lights. "At least that's what I keep telling myself."

Noah didn't hold out a lot of hope in that area. Men always seemed to find new tools of destruction. He grabbed his jacket and followed his boss down the hall. Through the narrow window at the end of the corridor a gray sky bloomed, tinged with pink. Almost dawn.

He pulled out his cell phone and typed a quick text message. All clear. Tell Mom.

Noah knew that Alex always slept with his phone nearby, in case one of his sons called. Within seconds his father replied.

Thx. Get some rest. BTW Grace is here. She's asleep in your bed....

And then his father typed in a smiley emoticon.

Noah shook his head. The world was changing way too fast when your father texted you with a smiley face, he thought wryly.

Outside he headed straight to his Jeep. First stop—his apartment for a hot shower. He would be at his parents' place in an hour. With luck he could weasel some of that bread and a mound of scrambled eggs along with freshly brewed coffee. No one made hair-straightening black coffee like his dad did.

Noah smiled slowly.

The coffee could wait. First he wanted a long, hot kiss as he coaxed Grace awake slowly in his bed.

SOMETHING TOUCHED GRACE'S cheek. She stretched lazily, muttering. Something skimmed her nose. A warm, searching mouth slid over hers until she ached. She felt her brain fog.

What a perfect dream.

It had to be a dream, she told herself.

How else to explain this unfamiliar heat and need that flashed up like starlight, just on the edge of control.

No, not unfamiliar. *Noah...*

She rolled over and breathed the word in a rough sigh, twisting in the warm quilt.

Then she shivered. Warm breath on her cheek. Callused hands on her hair.

"Richard? Or is it you, Tony?"

*"Neither."* Noah pulled back the covers, sliding down beside her.

Grace had to laugh when she saw the irritated glint in his eyes. "A joke. Of course I knew. Even asleep, I knew," she whispered breathlessly.

Warm hands slid down her arms and under her knit shirt. Slowly, expertly, they opened on her breasts. Grace sucked in a sharp breath, hit by a wave of pleasure.

"Noah, what are you—"

"Temporary insanity. I plead guilty. Want me to go?"

She closed her eyes, feeling his hands still. She tried to clear her head. "I can't think straight," she rasped. "What if your parents—"

"Both of them are downstairs starting breakfast. They won't be up for at least thirty minutes. My mother's determined to get another loaf of bread baked just right for you." He was watching her intently. "I probably shouldn't be here."

Her heart pounded. "Probably not."

"I can't seem to stay away," he said roughly. "I've never felt like this."

Grace knew just what he meant.

When had she ached like this? When had she ever felt this giddy rush of freedom?

Never.

She closed her eyes on a sigh. Her whole body hummed, intensely alive. She had never realized what it felt like to ache, trembling beneath careful hands while she simply...let go.

Was this really happening? Was she actually in Noah's house, in his bed, while his parents made breakfast one floor away?

"Wait," she whispered. She sat up slowly, feeling the attraction tighten between them. So easy to fall, she thought. But she took a deep breath and tried to focus. "I want this. It should be so simple to touch and trust. But it's not. I care too much to pretend with you, Noah." Her fingers opened and twined through his. "I don't want halfway or maybe or close enough. If we do this, it will change everything." She felt her heart stabbed by the understanding in his eyes. "You see?"

"I do. And you're right. There's nothing safe about feeling this much." Awareness snapped between them as he looked at their linked fingers. Something came and went in his face. "It wouldn't be simple to touch you. I'm sure of that." He sounded tired. Slowly he brought her hand to his mouth and kissed her palm. "I wish we were different. I wish...a lot of things."

She felt his arms tighten.

Then Grace felt him pull the covers around her and stand up. He kissed her forehead.

He cleared his throat. The room felt unbearably cold when he closed the door behind him.

Grace heard Noah tell his father that she was asleep and he didn't want to wake her. Their footsteps moved away toward the stairs.

She pulled the quilt over her head, feeling her face flame. What had nearly happened? She lay rigid, listening to the slam of her heart. She was *never* reckless like this. She made careful choices after calm deliberation. Growing up in the wreckage of a childhood littered by the memories of her mother's drinking and irresponsibility, Grace knew just how much pain bad choices could bring.

And they had been on the edge of something terribly reckless. Noah's father had been right in the hallway. What if he or Tatiana had walked in on them? She stifled a groan at the thought.

She had to go. She had to walk out of Noah's house and start being calm and sensible again. She was going to clear her head and stop acting like...

Like a woman opening her heart, too long in shadows.

Her eyes closed. Her fingers gripped the quilt. It was the right thing to do.

But like most of the *right things* you did in life, this one was going to hurt very badly.

HE CAUGHT HER AT THE FRONT door while she tugged on her coat.

"Hey. I'm just about to cut you a slice of that bread my mother's been fussing over for the last hour." His eyes narrowed when Grace didn't answer him. "What's wrong?"

"Wrong? Where do I start? That—the thing that just happened upstairs was wrong," she breathed. "And next time it might not stop. You're worth more than that, Noah. We both are."

His eyes never left her face. "Don't run away, Grace. You're smarter and tougher than that."

"Am I?" She rubbed the painful knot burning over her heart. "If I were as smart as you think, things would never have gotten this complicated. You confuse me, Noah. You awe me, too. The way you make me feel…it's too much. I have a lot of *okay* in my life, not reckless and wonderful."

He smiled at that. The tenderness in his eyes hit her like pure sunlight. It almost made her reconsider. But she couldn't back away from what was right. They'd both regret it later.

"Fine. We'll take some time, slow things down. I'll give you a day or month to get used to reckless and wonderful. I can be patient, but…"

"There had to be a but."

He cupped her cheeks gently. "But I'm not letting you vanish. Not until we know *exactly* what we have here." His arms slid around her waist. He pulled her closer. "And I'm not going to make it easy for you to forget me."

He kissed her, slow and thorough with aching tenderness. Grace felt her heart dive straight to the bottom of her chest. "You don't give an inch, do you?"

"So I'm told."

"And you also like to bend the rules, I see."

"When it's necessary, yes. Because I plan to win, Grace. I plan for us to win together. The way I see it, life is about being strong enough—maybe stubborn enough—to open a door and take a gift when it's offered. Too often you don't get a second chance," he said fiercely.

With a sigh she slanted her forehead against his. She could feel his heart pounding where their bodies met. "You make this sound so easy. But it's not. I'm not spontaneous or casual. I think. I worry. My friends say, 'I worry, therefore I am.'"

"You think I don't? You think this is *casual* for me? Honey, nobody said it was going to be easy or casual." His voice was harsh. "Exactly the opposite. But what happens when I touch you is a gift, and right now a voice is telling me that we're just getting started. Do you trust me enough to believe that?"

"It's life I don't trust," she whispered. "Things

like this don't happen to me. I live a sane, organized, predictable life. I *like* it that way," she insisted breathlessly. "At least I thought I did."

Noah lifted her hand, studying their entwined fingers. "It's good to be a little reckless. Sometimes you need to eat dessert first," he whispered.

Behind them dishes rattled in the kitchen.

"Stay. Have breakfast." His eyes were grave. "It would mean a lot to my mother. To all of us. Even you can be reckless for forty-five minutes, right?"

Grace closed her eyes, feeling all her good intentions drift out the window. "Okay. But no playing dirty. Give me one week to sort things out. And while I do, hands off."

"It's a deal." He started to kiss her and then raised his palms in the air. "Your rules. For now, hands off." His eyes darkened. "You have exactly one week."

THE BREAD WAS A MARVEL, rich and chewy with a golden crust. Tatiana glowed at Grace's praise. Not surprisingly, the men finished off every chewy crumb within minutes.

It was clear that Noah's parents were curious about their developing relationship, but they were far too polite to ask questions. Their good-natured joking with Noah only made Grace realize what family meant and how much she would give up if she stuck to her plan.

Before she had finished her first cup of tea, her

cell phone alarm chimed loudly. She blanched. "Oh, no—I forgot my big appointment and I can't be late. Not today." She shot to her feet. "I—forgive me for being so rude. I really have to go."

Alex stood up. "I can drop you on my way to work."

"Thanks, Dad, but I have it." Noah gulped down his coffee and followed Grace to the door. "I'm off today."

"Noah, I need to stop at home and change. Do my hair. Makeup." She shrugged. "I can't believe I forgot." What kind of effect did the man *have* on her? She shouldn't have stayed the night before, but the evening had been so wonderful.

She shook her head in irritation. "This is definitely a panty hose day. I'll be rushed so you don't need to wait."

"Not a problem. I'll take you wherever." Noah grabbed his gloves—and a loaf of warm bread for the road. "Let's move. You can give me directions in the car."

As THEY DROVE, Grace told him where she was going.

He blinked. "*There?* The White House? That's your appointment?"

"Right. Now you see why I can't be late."

"Why didn't you say anything?"

"It's not a done deal. The competition is major so I didn't want to talk about it."

"Are you kidding? You'll get it." Noah drummed

his fingers on the wheel. "But explain it again. What's a digital, collaborative cookbook?"

"The French cultural attaché will be there along with the head White House chef. This is the final interview," Grace said tensely. "The project is to create a huge cooking reference offered for the English-speaking market. It will have full recipes, videos of cooking techniques, interviews with key chefs in France who have visited here. There will be history, travel advice, food-shopping tips. Everything! *The White House Cooking Series.*" She caught a breath. "This is so big, Noah. The biggest thing I've ever done." Grace looked at her hands and saw that they were trembling. "And with the White House chef involved, we'll have access to just about anyone. Look at me. I'm a wreck. How am I going to be *any* good? And I barely have an hour to get ready," she rasped.

"You'll do it, honey." Noah's voice was utterly calm. "Practice your pitch on me while we drive. And don't worry, I'll get you there in time." His mouth curved. "I know the back routes."

SHE FINISHED DRYING her hair while her cell phone and computer charged. Her best black suit steamed in the bathroom while the shower ran. As Noah made a pot of strong coffee, Grace added her final makeup.

"Don't I get to see the panty hose?" he murmured. "Lingerie would be nice, too."

"Out." Laughing, Grace shooed him from the sunny bedroom of the apartment she was renting during her D.C. stay. She stepped into discreet black pumps and eyed her reflection in the mirror.

Slowly, her confidence began to return. *The White House Cooking Series* was a huge project, but she had prepped for almost a year. She had researched all the major French cookbooks and followed every important French cooking blog. She had researched historic state dinners back to the American Revolution. She knew five of the seven chefs in France who would be interviewed for the project.

The project would be a key cultural collaboration.

She straightened the small strand of pearls at her neck and opened the door.

Noah let out a low breath. "Nice before, but now you're amazing. You look calm and smart and absolutely gorgeous." He glanced at his watch. "Finish your coffee. I've got your computer at the door. It's charged and packed."

"Thank you for this, Noah." Just seeing him grin gave her a new wave of confidence.

He held open the door. "Better move."

HE SPED HER DOWN BACK ALLEYS and across warehouse lots that Grace didn't know existed. He cut through parks and around a university loading dock. They made it to 1600 Pennsylvania Avenue with ten minutes to spare.

Noah parked and held open her door, radiating pride. "Go knock them dead, honey."

## CHAPTER TWELVE

*Three hours later*

GRACE STOOD ON THE STREET corner.

Dazed, she watched traffic stream past. Her hands shook. She took a hard breath, pulled out her cell phone and dialed Noah.

He answered on the first ring. "All done?"

She felt dizzy. Truck horns blasted and she tried to focus.

"Grace? Talk to me. How did the meeting go?"

She couldn't answer, watching the unending snarl of traffic but not really seeing any of it. The interviews had been long and grueling, details upon details. They had probed her training, career background and personal goals, even her private life. She hadn't realized exactly how high-profile this project was going to be.

She rubbed her face, jittery from too many questions and too much coffee. Jittery from having her life poked and analyzed for three long hours. "Intense. Very intense."

"Where are you?"

"Near 18th Street."

"I'll come pick you up."

She cleared her throat. "I—I can't, Noah."

"Why? I'll just be ten minutes. Wait for me."

"No." She said the word slowly. A taxi slammed on its brakes and Grace winced. "I can't because... I got it." She whispered the words, still not able to process the news. "Noah?"

"I couldn't hear you, Grace. Say that again."

"I—I got it. I'll be working on the series!"

"That's great! Congratulations. I knew you were brilliant and this seals it. So when do we celebrate?"

"Tonight. My place. I'll supply the champagne and you supply...the heat."

She wanted to shout. She wanted to cry and dance a crazy jig in the snow. Most of all she wanted to grab Noah and kiss him speechless. But she didn't have time for any of it.

"Noah, they want to start immediately. The hours will be killing, and now I have to leave for France in five days. I want to go see my grandfather first and then visit two libraries while I'm back in Oregon. I'm not sure when I'll be back after that."

This time it was Noah who didn't answer.

"Noah, are you there?"

"I'm here, Grace. This sounds like a huge project. An opportunity like this doesn't come every day. I completely get that. But we can still find time somehow. Hold on." Grace heard muffled sounds, and then he was back. "What time tonight?"

"Seven. No, make it seven-thirty."

"Got it."

Another car horn sounded, just to her right. Grace looked over and caught a breath when Noah stopped in front of her. She ran to the car and slid inside. "How did you get here so fast?"

"I was doing an errand around the corner." He leaned across the seat, kissed her hard, then pulled back into traffic. "I'm pretty damned proud of you, Grace Lindstrom. Just for the record."

She sat back with a sigh. For long seconds she simply squeezed Noah's hand. It was a massive project and there would be at least a dozen people looking over her shoulder, checking details and questioning her recipes every step of the way. The time frame was a killer, but it would be the most exciting thing she had ever done. She had to carry it off—not because of money or ego, but because she could really showcase the rich history of cooking here at the White House—and even before the country's formal founding. She couldn't *wait* to start.

Grace leaned over and kissed Noah's cheek, then smoothed away the lipstick mark. "Just for the record, big guy? I highly doubt that you were 'doing an errand around the corner.' But we'll let that pass because I'm so glad to see you." She looked down and smiled. "I'm still jittery. But it's going to be amazing, Noah. They have access to all kinds of archives, both here and in France. There will be complete digital footage made of every recipe, with great tips and techniques that will be posted online, available exclusively to those who buy the book and DVD. We're going back as far as General Lafayette and the American Revolution, including the first contacts between our countries. The research is going to be fascinating. Nothing watered down, either."

He nodded, his eyes on the snarled traffic. "Just the kind of thing you can do in your sleep. They chose the right person."

"But it's scary." Grace pressed a hand to her chest. "I keep telling myself that I can handle all this. Book, DVD and audio. It's the new world, a cooking revolution. I can't believe I'm going to be watching it happen."

"Not watching. *Making* it happen," Noah said. "You're going to knock this one out of the park. Mark my words." He reached over and pulled her hand to his mouth, kissing her palm. "And I am going to tell everyone that I knew you when."

"Don't talk that way. This won't change me or my life beyond making for a crazy twelve months. And...we'll find time, if you can just be flexible." It took courage for Grace to ask, to open herself to rejection. "My life is going to be crazy when this gets rolling. Will you wait for me? Not for a week, but months while I travel."

He bit the soft skin at the base of her thumb. "I can wait," he murmured. "Not forever, but a few months should be fine." His beeper chimed as he eased his car into a parking spot.

Grace looked up, surprised to see that she was back at her apartment. How did he do that so well? She had never liked to drive in city traffic, and D.C. was known to drive grown men to tears at rush hour. "I—I don't know what to say, Noah. Thank you. Just—thank you."

"Thanks not needed or wanted. Now get going. You've got important work to do. *Vive la Révolution,*" he quipped. He walked around the car and held open her door. "But remember we've got a date tonight." He skimmed one finger along her cheek, waited a moment and pulled her into his arms. "I'm bending our rules," he murmured, kissing her slowly with a focused intensity that sent little warnings through her body. "Tonight, I'm bringing all the heat we can handle. We'll see where it takes us and then reconsider your rules."

He would always affect her this way, Grace thought. He would make her feel beautiful and desirable, but he didn't pressure her for a response. He didn't need to push because he took her as she was, not as an extension of some image he wanted to project about himself. He didn't need that kind of shallow ego boost.

He was strong, not like James. Never like James.

At her door, Grace looked back. Noah gave her a nod and a little wave.

Some instinct made Grace turn back and reach

through the open window. She pulled him down, kissing him with sudden urgency, struck with a harsh sense of passing time. In a second everything could change. She didn't let go, not even when her heart began to pound and his breath thickened. "Noah, be careful. Whatever you do, please be careful. And I'll be thinking about tonight," she whispered.

"So will I. Now get moving. The food revolution is about to start, and you don't want to be late."

FIVE O'CLOCK CAME AND WENT.

Six, too.

When Grace glanced at her watch, she was stunned to see that it was almost seven. She closed her research folders with a snap and stretched. Her muscles ached from sitting too long and a headache hammered from too much coffee. As a further complication, she had dropped her cell phone in the snow that afternoon, and by the time she dug it out, it was ruined. Tomorrow she had to get a replacement. Grace didn't know how she'd fit that errand into her jammed schedule.

Meanwhile, she had twenty-two new emails waiting, all of them connected to the new project. She had met the two editors and had a rough outline of the variety of dishes to be included. In a stroke of luck she had located a handwritten note from George Washington praising General Lafayette's chef.

She needed a break.

Rubbing the tense muscles at her neck, she went to check her refrigerator.

Baby organic lettuce. Sundried tomatoes. Two grapefruits.

Hardly fare to feed a hungry man. Where was Alton Brown when you needed him? Gnawing at her lip, she checked her pantry and made some quick calculations. There was a small Greek grocery at the corner, where she could buy what she needed for a rich, chipotle-flavored chili. While that was simmering, she would make double chocolate brownies with Grand Marnier icing. Definitely whipped cream for the top.

Feeling better, she skimmed her emails and signed off.

Twenty minutes to go. Time to switch gears.

Grace ran a hand through her tumbled hair and grabbed her coat. Cowboy chili to the rescue. What red-blooded man didn't like steamy layers of chipotle and roasted tomatoes, with a hint of espresso at the base?

IT WAS A RACE, BUT THE CHILI was nearly done and the brownies were just going into the oven when her doorbell chimed. Grace took a step back and pressed a hand to her chest at the sight of Noah, lean and dangerous in thigh-hugging worn blue jeans and a black turtleneck that fit his muscular chest like a dream.

Her heart turned over as he handed her a bunch

of scarlet roses and then a bunch of white ones. "I couldn't decide so I got both." He leaned down to nibble the curve of her ear. "You look wonderful."

"Actually, I look tired. And I've got food in the oven. Don't distract me, you hunk."

"I can smell it. Something smoky and hot. It almost smells like..." He sniffed. "Is that coffee?"

"Chili simmered with coffee, chocolate and three kinds of beans. An old family recipe. Not exactly Swedish, but it was my grandmother's best creation. Chocolate brownies for desert."

"How did you manage all of that?"

"Lindstrom's rules—always have a Plan B. Thank heavens there's a little grocery around the corner, and I knew they stocked just what I needed." She took his coat and found a glass pitcher for the roses.

"That smells incredible." He walked to the kitchen, watching her stir the chili. "I guess it won't make your White House series."

"Not too much cowboy chili at the Cordon Bleu," she murmured.

"They don't know what they're missing. So what does your family think of this new job?"

"There's just me and my grandfather now. My grandmother died six years ago. Lupus complications. I called him earlier, but he was out. I'll try again later."

"And your mother?" Noah asked quietly.

It was the first time he'd asked for details about her family. Grace sensed the reason—that they were moving to something deeper. He wanted her to know that. He was giving her a chance to agree to the implications.

Or not.

"My mother is dead. She died in a car accident a long time ago." Grace took a deep breath, methodically arranging the roses in a vase. She thought of the flowers at the church that rainy winter day so many years before.

The roses she had tossed into her mother's grave.

She had been dry-eyed, not filled with sorrow or loss. Just relieved that her mother was gone. There would be no more drunken phone calls, no pleas for money or angry shouting at her grandparents.

Grace took a sudden wrenching breath. "The truth is, I hated her. Even the day she was buried, I hated her. That makes me a very twisted daughter," she whispered.

Noah touched her shoulder. "I'm sorry, Grace. We don't have to discuss this."

"Yes, we do. It's time I told you the things I never mention. Whatever happens, I want this thing between us to be real and strong, Noah. That means with warts and shadows included." Her shoulders hunched and she looked him straight in the eyes. "My parents were both alcoholics. My father left when I was seven. My mother wasn't so bad then, but after he left she fell apart. By the time I was eleven she'd been in and out of rehab half a dozen times. My grandparents kept hoping it would stick, but it never did. Then one day she left. Just walked out for coffee and cigarettes and never came back. I was alone in Portland and I had no money or food. I called my grandfather and he came for me. He didn't say a word against her and didn't ask any questions, just took me out to the car. We went straight to a restaurant and I remember how good my sandwich tasted. Ketchup was a miracle. Onions were a prayer. I…I hadn't eaten in three days. She hadn't left any money." Grace rubbed her eyes slowly. "He told me to pack what I wanted and then he drove me home to Summer Island. I never went back to her." She paced the room restlessly. "Summer Island was the first place I'd lived where I didn't have to worry that she'd come out to the school bus with a can of beer in her hand or answer the door with her blouse all unbuttoned and nothing on underneath. I didn't have to worry where she was drinking or who she was with."

"And in spite of all that, you still loved her," Noah said quietly.

"What makes you say that?"

"It's what children do. It's what makes us human. It's the warts and the shadows, honey. Like it or not, family's in the blood."

After a long time Grace sighed. "I did love her. I still have faint memories of her laughing as she pulled me in some kind of red wagon. We had a little dog then, called Buster. I loved that dog, but never knew what happened to him. Maybe he went to a friend or maybe he ran away. All I knew is that I cried every night for weeks, asking God for another dog, but I never got one. I asked for a different mother, too." Grace rubbed her eyes. "Why am I telling you all this? We're supposed to be having a romantic dinner."

"It's important. Family is always with us. While we breathe, we remember."

"I guess you're right." Grace frowned at the bleak memories. "But my real life began on Summer Island. For the first time I had friends and a room of my own. My grandparents helped me start over, and I can't ever repay them for that. They always told me that whatever I wanted to do, I would succeed. I never heard the word *no* growing up with them. I love them so much."

Noah nodded. "I know the type. That makes us both very lucky."

"I want the kind of love my grandparents had, Noah. I've seen the mistakes and how badly life can go wrong. I don't want that," Grace said slowly.

"It's a journey, honey. Thing can go wrong. People can be weak and make mistakes. You just move ahead."

A timer chimed in the kitchen. "That's the brownies." Grace ran a hand through her hair and then pointed to a chilled bottle. "No more sad family history. Let's have some champagne.'"

When Noah saw the label, he whistled.

"You're worth it. Whatever happens, this has been amazing."

He pulled her into his arms. "It's not nearly over yet, Grace." His mouth skimmed her ear, her cheek. Against all her intentions Grace felt her heart turn over. Would it be so dangerous to trust him, to follow her heart down this crazy, wonderful path?

Boots echoed outside in the hallway. The doorbell chimed. Frowning, Grace peeked out the security hole. "Yes?"

"FS Express. I've got a delivery for Grace Lindstrom."

"From whom?"

"Paragon Productions. I need a signature."

The man carried in three boxes, waiting while Grace signed for each one. When she was done, he sniffed the air. "Man, those brownies smell good. Too bad I'm on a diet."

When he was gone, Grace opened the boxes, which were filled with files, old documents and photographs. The letter from her new editor noted possible directions for the first part of the book, as well as questions about each section. All sensible and helpful.

Except that Grace was supposed to go through three boxes of material in twenty-four hours. She sat down slowly and blew out a breath, the letter in her lap.

"Not good?"

"Not good. They want me to dig through all of

this in twenty-four hours. How can I do that?" She looked at Noah, feeling her joy fade. "I wanted this night to be special."

"Hey, you still have to eat. We can do that. Then you can attack these boxes. We'll see how the rest works out."

"I don't think—"

The doorbell chimed again. Grace shook her head. "Please not another box," she muttered.

But a different man stood outside. Grace recognized the manager of her building.

"Sorry to bother you, Ms. Lindstrom." The man looked worried. "I just got a call from someone named Carolina Grayson. She says she's been trying to reach your cell phone all day."

"It's broken. I have to—" Grace stopped. "What's wrong? Why did she call? It's not Gage or my grandfather, is it?"

He held out a sheet of paper. "She said to give you this number and tell you to call her as soon as possible. That's all I know."

Grace felt Noah behind her, his strong grip on her shoulder. "There's a calling code for long distance somewhere." Grace tried to think, her mind racing. "I have to call my friend Caro. I need the calling code. It's here somewhere."

"Use my cell." Noah pressed his phone into her hand. "Don't waste time looking."

Grace's hands shook so much she almost dropped the phone. She tried to dial, then felt Noah ease the phone from her fingers. "Give me the number. I'll do this while you drink some of that champagne and try to relax."

Grace took the phone, waiting impatiently, relieved when she heard her friend's voice. "Caro, it's Grace. I just got your message. Sorry, but my cell phone is broken. What's happened?"

"Thank heaven I found you, Grace. They finally located this number at your grandfather's office. I didn't want to bother you, but Gage is with him now."

"With my grandfather? I don't understand." Grace felt dizzy. "Why? What's wrong?"

"He's been hurt, Grace. He and Gage are on the way to the hospital. I'm leaving in a few minutes, but I had to find you first. I—I think you need to come home right away. Your grandfather is—he's in bad shape."

# CHAPTER THIRTEEN

GRACE'S TRIP TO OREGON was a nightmare, blurred by worry and exhaustion. Because of her last-minute arrangements she had to change planes twice. By the time she reached the Portland airport, she was dead on her feet.

She had left a message for Noah, then left a message at her new job, explaining that she would be gone for at least five days because of a family emergency. Until she got a new cell, she was forced to use a pay-as-you go phone as her contact number, along with her grandfather's home number. From what she had learned from her friend Caro, Grace knew she would be spending most of her time at the hospital.

The medical report had left her chilled. *Broken ribs. Possible punctured lung. Lacerations on the left hand and leg and trauma to the head.*

No one knew what had happened. Her grandfather frequently worked late at the animal shelter, doing whatever tasks needed to be tackled. Given their lack of staff, it wasn't surprising that he had been alone the night before. Caro said it looked as if a heavy supply bookshelf had overturned, knocking him down and pinning him to the floor. When one of his volunteers showed up at ten the next morning, the elderly vet was delirious from cold, trauma and blood loss. At the hospital one resident speculated that he might have had a stroke and knocked the shelf over as he fell.

They were currently doing a battery of tests, and only the thought that Caro and her husband were at the hospital kept Grace calm during the last leg of her journey. She couldn't bear to imagine her grandfather waking up alone, in pain and confused.

As she drove her rental car from the airport though midnight streets, Grace felt guilt wash over her. Staring into the darkness, she prayed for her grandfather. He was all that mattered now.

GRACE WAS FIGHTING exhaustion when she finally reached the hospital. Stiff and disoriented, she was searching for the intensive care unit when she felt a hand on her shoulder.

Deep mahogany eyes probed her face. "You look like you're going to crash any second, Grace. Sit down while I get you something to drink."

Lt. Gage Grayson was as handsome as ever. Grace had seen him twice since he had married her best friend. He looked thinner since the last time she had visited, and there were deeper lines on his sunburned forehead. Grace felt awful that he had spent his precious leave time here at the hospital instead of at home with Caro.

"Thank you for being here, Gage. I was so worried. Am so worried," she finished. She sat down, then stood up almost immediately, pacing the narrow hall. "Where is he?"

"Just down there. He's asleep now." Gage bought her a bottle of cold juice and sat down beside her. "Better?"

She managed to nod even though it wasn't better and it wouldn't be remotely better until she knew every detail of her grandfather's condition. "How is he, Gage?"

"He's come around twice, but only for a few minutes. No visitors allowed until morning. The doctor came by at eight and said he'd be back early tomorrow. We'll get more information then. There isn't a lot you can do here tonight, Grace. Caro and I have a room in the motel across the street. Why don't you go over and get some rest? I'll be here if he wakes up."

"That's—" Grace swallowed a lump in her throat. "That's so generous of you." Her eyes burned with sudden tears. "You go. I want to stay here tonight." She squeezed Gage's hand. "And thank you again for all that you and Caro have done. I hate taking up your precious time together while you're on leave."

"Forget about that. I owe your grandfather more than I can ever repay. He took in my pets when I had nowhere to turn. He's a good man." He crossed his arms, frowning. "You should rest. You'll be no good to him if you're run-down and exhausted."

"I can't leave," she said hoarsely. "I need to be close in case..." She didn't finish. She couldn't bear to say the words aloud.

"There won't be any 'in case.' Your grandfather is going to be fine," Gage said gruffly. "He's got more strength and willpower than any man I know."

"He can definitely be stubborn. I'm very glad for that now. But I still don't understand what happened. Was it a stroke?"

"Hard to say until the test results are back. We'll know soon."

She nodded, trying to relax, but her mind kept whirling from possibility to possibility. "What about the animal shelter?"

"We've got volunteers lined up. Everyone in town wants to pitch in. You don't need to worry about that."

"That's the first thing my grandfather will ask me. You know how devoted he is to his animals."

Gage smiled. "Yeah, I got that message loud and clear. And I know it weighs on him. But he didn't want you to worry about any of this." Gage shook his head. "In fact, he made us promise not to call you. He didn't want you upset."

"Upset?" Grace shot to her feet, pacing again. "That's just crazy. Of course I had to know."

"That's what we thought. Caro called as soon as she could. But Caro says he was too proud to admit he needed help. In the last months the shelter has been understaffed and work has been piling up. It might have become more than he could handle."

"He should have told me," Grace said. "I would have come home to help. All he had to do was tell me." More waves of guilt hit. If she had come home sooner none of this would have happened.

Her fault.

She sank into a lumpy chair next to Gage, staring down the hall. "I should have been here to check on things. I should have seen what was going on."

"Hey." Gage gripped her shoulder. "Don't start guilting about this. He's a tough old bird, and the last thing he would have wanted was you hovering around, fussing over him. You were right where he wanted you, off in D.C. carrying on with your life and making a success. Do you know how often he bragged about you to Caro and the staff at the shelter?"

Grace closed her eyes. "I should have called him more often. I should have heard how tired he was when he called me."

"No one here saw anything. I doubt that you could have, either. But what's done is done. No point making yourself sick over what you can't change." Gage looked up as footsteps rapped down the hall.

A tall woman sprinted toward them, her dark hair flying and her purse swinging from side to side. She wore plain black clogs and a long gray sweater over leggings that hugged her slender curves. Her deep blue eyes widened when she saw Grace.

"You made it. I'm so glad Caro tracked you down."

"Jilly." Grace whispered her friend's name and then reached out for the physical comfort that came from someone who felt like family, someone who knew your oldest secrets and deepest fears. They had been friends since the age of twelve, when Jilly had first moved to Summer Island with her foster family. Like Grace, Jilly had worked hard to find stability in her life. She had followed her dreams. Now she was an up-and-coming chef in Arizona.

"Honey, you need to eat something. You look terrible." Jilly shot a look at Gage. "Is anything open? Maybe a sandwich, do you think?"

He gave a little two-finger salute. "I'll go reconnoiter."

Grace closed her eyes, leaning on Jilly's shoulder. "He's been so good to do all this. But he and Caro should be at home. His leave won't last much longer, will it?"

"Don't bother to argue, because I've tried. They would rather be here helping. Just like I would. Now close your eyes and lie down here on the couch. I'm going to find you a blanket."

"But I—"

Jilly simply ignored her, striding around the corner.

When she returned, she was carrying a big crocheted afghan and a plate with a sugar doughnut. "First you eat. Then you're going to rest. I knew you'd refuse to leave until you saw your grandfather, but at least you're going to sleep. I'll be here. And don't argue with me on this," Jilly said fiercely. "I can take you in a fight, Lindstrom. Just remember that."

Grace yawned, overwhelmed with worry. But there was comfort in her friend's brisk energy. Jilly had always been the doer, filled with a thousand ideas and the energy to try all of them. Clearly, she still raced through life, taking every corner on two wheels. "Okay, but just for an hour. It feels as if I've been traveling for days."

"Eat the doughnut. It's crappy, but it will fill you up."

Grace forced down the sweet, sticky pastry and then drank from the water bottle Jilly produced from her big leather tote. She blinked back tears as Jilly smoothed the afghan over her. "It's so good to see you again. I've missed all of you."

"As if I wouldn't come," her friend snapped. "I love your grandfather. He's as cool as they get." Jilly smiled crookedly. "You, I'm not so sure about, gadding all over Europe and never coming home to see us. And I'm still waiting for that French *macaron* recipe you promised me. Now quit talking, stretch out and close your eyes. Stat," she said firmly. "I'll come get you if there is any news."

Grace curled up on the long couch. "Just an hour...." she whispered.

And then she gave in to the dark grip of exhaustion.

GAGE WALKED DOWN the hall from the elevator carrying two tuna sandwiches and a hard-boiled egg.

"Asleep yet?"

"Finally," Jilly whispered.

"She's as tough as her grandfather."

"Tell me about it."

Gage put the food down on the table next to Grace, for when she woke up. Then he followed Jilly down the hall, where their voices wouldn't wake Grace. "She can't see him until morning. Make her go rest."

"Not happening. She's too stubborn. But I'll take over here. I've got a thermos of coffee in my bag and a new romantic suspense. I'll be fine. You need to go across the street and take care of your wife."

Gage looked undecided. "Are you sure that—"

"I'll be fine. Get going. Caro needs you now. And you should get some sleep, too. You have to be feeling a bit of jet lag."

Gage glanced back at Grace. "You're sure you can do this, Jilly? With the hours you've been keeping down at the café…"

"I slept this afternoon. I'm just fine. Now *go.*" She smiled, giving him a little shove toward the elevator. "And give Caro my love. Then tell her to get ready, because I've got a lot of things to discuss with the two of you tomorrow."

Gage ran a hand across his neck. "About that thing?"

"Yeah." Jilly smiled. "About that thing."

Noises came and noises went.

Shoes squeaked and tapped. Carts clattered.

Grace slept through it all, caught in cold, blurred dreams of bad things she couldn't quite see. The old memories of childhood crept out, mocking and shrill. Warning her that everything could be stripped away in a second.

Beside her, Jilly stood watch, a silent and unyielding guardian.

By two in the morning the floor was quiet. Families had gone home and the late medications had been dispensed. Hall lights were dimmed outside rooms with patients caught in fitful dreams.

Down the hall from the ICU, Jilly kept her vigil near Grace. She glared at anyone talking loudly, making them move away so that Grace could sleep. As the hours ticked past, she drank her way through four cups of single-origin organic dark-roast coffee and two hundred pages of the newest release from her favorite author. Her energy level had always been off the charts, so an all-nighter was no problem. Jilly wasn't much of a knitter. Unlike her friends, she didn't pull out needles for solace. She had never gotten the hang of string and points, though she had tried hard. She would never admit it, but her friends' skill at needlework completely amazed and intimidated her.

Jilly simply wasn't the crafty type. Not that it was a loss. She would have been laughable in lace or soft, clingy angora. She generally gave up makeup and hair products to make time for an extra fifteen minutes of sleep and an early-morning run.

She had a rangy, athletic body that usually stayed hidden beneath the crisp jacket and comfy knit tank tops that she wore as a busy chef. She didn't inspire overblown love poems or romance in the men she dated. It was more likely that they treated her like a comfortable old friend. And Jilly liked that just fine. Why complicate life by adding grand passions or sloppy emotional entanglements? Her single goal in life was to become the best chef west of New York City. With that prize achieved, she intended to bank a few million dollars with a restaurant and a branded food franchise based on organic Southwestern specialty foods. In the eight years since she had enrolled in cooking school in Arizona, Jilly had set her feet firmly on the path to that goal. She already had a gourmet salsa line sold in several high-end Scottsdale resorts, with more due soon. And with a new restaurant in the works, sleep had become a limited commodity.

But loyalty outweighed ambition. Friends would always come first.

When Caro had called her with the news about Peter Lindstrom, Jilly had cut short an important business meeting and flown home to Oregon. She was here for the duration, determined to help Grace and the tall, quiet man who had done so much for Summer Island without ever asking anything in return. Dr. Lindstrom was a hero to Jilly—and to most of the people in the close-knit town. He had given Jilly her first pet rabbit. Then he had let her work after school as a volunteer at the animal shelter. A few months later he had appeared at her door carrying an abandoned golden retriever pup.

It was love at first sight. The two had gone everywhere, best friends and companions. Samson had eased Jilly's rough road through adolescence, when everything Jilly did seemed to be the wrong thing. She had never been part of the popular crowd, and she had never had many dates. She preferred to spend her spare time helping at the animal shelter and reading up on cooking at the Summer Island Library.

When she had lost Samson, all the joy had been sucked out of her life. For weeks the world seemed to close in on her, and even her friends couldn't cut through her depression. Then Dr. Lindstrom had rescued her again.

This time her solace had come in a tiny package of white fur, wet nose and big clumsy feet. The Samoyed puppy had been hit by a car and left behind on an isolated road. The vet had operated and set a fractured bone, and after a slow recovery, the restless white ball could totter around awkwardly. But he was still badly frightened of people, and Dr. Lindstrom had warned her that the puppy would be a challenge.

Jilly never turned down a challenge. She kept her new friend active and trained him carefully. She had made him part of her busy life while she scouted locations for her future restaurant and products for her line of organic food. They had traveled up and down the coast by car a dozen times, and now her friend Duffy knew an impressive set of commands.

The puppy was outside in Jilly's SUV at that moment, chewing on his favorite rope toy while Jilly stood hospital duty. Every hour she snuck outside and took him for a wild run, crossing the road and sprinting along the beach to his delighted barking.

She stood up, stretching. Two interns walked by and eyed her tall, slim body.

Jilly was oblivious. Tough and cynical, she had no time for sex and she didn't believe in romance, which in her eyes pretty much covered all the possibilities. She wasn't elegant and smart like her friend Grace; she wasn't brilliant and dedicated like her friend Caro. Growing up as a foster child had left Jilly with few illusions. She was glad that she had found a foster home on Summer Island and happier still when she reached her majority so she could be off on her own. The only people that really mattered in her life were her friends, Dr. Lindstrom and the brilliant local chef who had been her career mentor during high school. Sally McGill could work magic with French pastry and had a thriving career teaching expensive retreats at her cliff-side estate overlooking the harbor. Throughout high school Jilly had helped at those weekend retreats and in Sally's big kitchen Jilly had found her first real glimpse of a family.

Sally didn't coddle her. She was rude, red-haired and had a razor edge to her wit. Her temper kept most people at bay, but she and Jilly had sized each other up as friends within minutes of meeting. Now they could work side by side for hours, never talking yet perfectly happy.

Sally had pushed Jilly to go to culinary school, and Sally had become her first investor, though Jilly had found half a dozen more, thanks to her contacts from cooking school. She pinched herself every morning, unable to believe that her oldest dreams were actually starting to take shape.

Jilly finished her thermos of coffee and pushed away thoughts of all the work that was building up in her absence. For one wild minute she actually thought about digging up the unfinished scarf she had been trying to knit for the past year.

Instead, she stood up and stretched. Her clumsy efforts would only leave her muttering in frustration.

Pacing the hall, she thought about the future. Grace was what counted now. Caro and Grace and their oldest friend Olivia had gotten Jilly through an

awful adolescence and a high school experience that
rated somewhere between traumatic and agonizing.

Jilly could never repay them for that.

Friends always came first.

## CHAPTER FOURTEEN

HER MOUTH BURNED.

Someone was banging a pan near her head.

Grace sat up with a start, squinting at a bank of fluorescent lights. She was disoriented as an orderly pushed a cart of bedpans down the hall.

A hospital hall.

Her grandfather was here.

The memories fell like stones. She shoved off a pink afghan and looked around for Gage or her friend Jilly. Suddenly she saw the swing of long arms and the gleam of wild black hair.

Jilly waved at her, carrying a huge leather tote bag and a worn piece of rope. "My puppy is out in the car. We take a nice brisk run every hour." Jilly ran a hand through her hair and gave up trying to smooth down its chaotic waves. "You look better after your nap. I think you'll survive."

"Thanks to you." Grace bit into a protein bar that Jilly had pulled out of her bag. "Has the doctor come by yet?"

"Not for another hour. And you won't be able to see your grandfather until he clears it, so you may as well relax. We could go up to the cafeteria for coffee."

"No, I'll wait. Thanks again for coming, Jilly. And for staying."

They sat together, silent, remembering other times of loss and worry. Then Jilly turned, frowning at her friend. "Wait a minute. What happened with that big project you told me about? It was a digital cookbook, something to do with the White House, right?"

Grace nodded.

"Well, did you get it?"

"I'm not sure." Grace hesitated. She didn't want to answer questions now, when her grandfather's illness changed everything.

"I thought you had a big interview coming up."

"I did." The lie came before Grace could think. "I...haven't heard yet."

"Well, you've got my vote."

Grace shrugged. "It will be very hands-on, and you know I like lots of freedom to follow my research." She studied her friend critically, noting the circles under Jilly's eyes. "You've been working too hard. You're not smoking again, are you?"

"That's one bad habit I finally kicked. But things are hectic. I'm finally looking for restaurant space and it's a pretty heady experience. I warn you, I'm going to pick your brain clean about layout, suppliers and overhead models."

"Pick away. I'll help you any way that I can. And congratulations on making the big leap." Grace squeezed her friend's hand. "You always wanted to have a restaurant, ever since that day in fourth grade when you made us all line up, put on aprons, and copy you while you made pretend chocolate chip cookies."

Jilly rolled her eyes. "What a little ass I was. How could you three stand me ordering you around?"

"Because we were friends. Always and ever, remember? The girls of Summer Island."

"I remember. It's the one *good* memory I have of growing up." Jilly frowned. "Are you really okay—I mean about James?"

"It's getting easier." Grace didn't want to talk about that, either. Anxiously, she glanced at the wall clock, calculating how long until the doctor made his morning rounds. She needed answers.

"Stop worrying. Gage said your grandfather looked good last night. He recognized Gage, too. That's a great sign."

"I can't relax until I've seen him. I want him to know I'm here, that he's not alone."

"He won't ever be alone. Too many people on Summer Island love your grandfather." Jilly handed Grace a bottle of orange juice from the nearby vending machine. "Drink that. All of it," she ordered.

"Still giving orders," Grace muttered. They both looked up as Gage stepped out of the elevator, handsome in a denim shirt and worn jeans with scuffed cowboy boots.

"That is one seriously handsome chunk of man-hood," Jilly said appraisingly. "Great biceps."

Grace bit back a laugh. "Shh. Don't embarrass the man." Then her breath caught as Gage's wife stepped off the elevator, pregnant and glowing.

"Caro, you didn't tell me!"

"I wanted it to be a surprise." Caro leaned against her husband, then slid one hand gently over her rounded stomach. "I'm eating everything in sight that isn't nailed down. Last night I actually got a craving for capers and chocolate milk." She shook her head. "I get tired at the strangest times now. But Gage has a tight rein on my nesting urges at the new house."

"What new house?"

Caro smiled. "We bought the Dragon Cottage. We got an amazing deal or we couldn't have swung it. Unfortunately, it's in pretty bad shape."

"You always loved that old cottage," Grace mused. "I'm so glad for you. Can I come visit while I'm here?"

"Absolutely. I may assign you some paint scrap-ing, I warn you." Abruptly, Caro cleared her throat. "I'm so sorry about your grandfather, Grace. He hasn't been sick a day before this. None of us saw this coming."

The words helped to heal Grace's guilt just a little.

She turned as the elevator chimed again. A doctor moved past, speaking quietly on a cell phone. Caro nodded to Grace and they followed him down the hall toward the intensive care unit.

"YOU'RE HIS GRANDDAUGHTER, correct?"

Grace nodded, gripping Jilly's arm.

"I'm glad you're here. I'm afraid you can only have five minutes with him. He may not be conscious."

"I understand. But my grandfather didn't have a history of high blood pressure or heart disease. I don't understand what happened."

"We're still doing tests to see if there is evidence of a stroke. Meanwhile, he has a punctured lung and two broken ribs. They have to heal completely before he is mobile again."

"How long will that take?"

"Time predictions are always tricky, Ms. Lindstrom. If everything goes well and if he responds to our treatment, it could be a month or it could be three months. That will be up to his body and his will to recover."

Grace nodded slowly. It was going to be a long process. *This changes everything,* she thought. *He needs me right here beside him.*

She waited impatiently for the nurse to finish inside. "Remember. Five minutes and no more," the doctor reminded her. "We can talk when you're done." Then he strode off to answer a page.

Grace took a breath and walked inside the small room.

Equipment beeped. An IV line hung from a pole near the bed. Her heart squeezed when she saw her grandfather. He had always been the healthiest man she knew, tall and tanned, outdoors every moment he could find.

Now Peter Lindstrom was pale, his eyes closed, and Grace realized she had never seen him at rest. Her grandfather had always been busy working at the shelter or tending the roses that he loved or helping a neighbor in need.

Never like this, spread out beneath white sheets, motionless and pale.

Another nurse gave her an encouraging smile and then moved outside, pulling the curtain closed behind her to give them some privacy.

"Grandpa, it's Grace. I'm here. Caro called me in D.C. and told me you were hurt."

There was no answering sound. No flutter of his eyelids.

No sign of life.

Grace sat down slowly beside the bed and took his cool hand in hers. She stroked the callused fingers, fighting tears. "I'm not going away. I'll keep an eye on the clinic, so don't worry about anything. Just rest. All you have to do is get well again. You *have* to get well." Her voice broke, despite all efforts to stay calm. "We—we all need you, Grandpa."

## CHAPTER FIFTEEN

OVER THE NEXT TWO DAYS, Grace haunted and paced, roamed and stalked. She got to know the unit nurses, the orderlies and the night cafeteria workers. Old friends from Summer Island came to offer their heartfelt wishes for her grandfather, assuring her that the shelter would stay running, the animals cared for by staff, as well as volunteers, until her grandfather returned.

Peter Lindstrom still had not regained clarity. He slept on, connected to beeping meters and IV lines that were constantly monitored. New tests confirmed that two of his ribs had been broken, but there were no signs of a stroke or cardiac arrest.

His attending physician assured Grace that this was excellent news. Ribs could and would heal. She tried to be happy with the news, but all she could think of was that he hadn't awakened. All she could see was his pale, gaunt face against the sheets of his hospital bed.

Restless, she roamed the halls, dozing for several hours on the nearby couch when she had to. Around midnight on the second night, Caro came to keep her company, ignoring Grace's protests. Later that night Jilly returned, sending Caro off to be with Gage.

After Caro left, Jilly pulled a sample-size bottle of her newest chipotle-mango salsa creation out of her big leather tote bag.

Grace had to admit, the combination was a knockout, sweet and spicy, with layers of roasted pepper and big chunks of ripe fruit. "I think that you're going to make a mint with this," Grace muttered, scooping more sweet crushed fruit onto the blue corn chips that Jilly had produced. "What does Sally think?"

"She's backing the rollout. We're going fifty-fifty."

"You always knew what you wanted in life. Even back in high school all you thought about was food and recipes and cooking tools." Grace took another mouthful of salsa and whistled softly. "You're definitely on your way."

"So are you," Jilly said firmly. "Three highly praised food books in five years and a profitable restaurant consulting business." Jilly's eyes narrowed. "It is profitable, isn't it?"

"Good enough."

"And you still have the apartment in Paris, right?"

Grace shook her head. "I let it go last year, right after James…" She stared down the shadowed corridor. "It felt like the right time."

"You had your own bank account and your own

cash, right? When James died, it didn't leave you tangled up or in debt?"

Leave it to Jilly to stab right to the bottom line, Grace thought. "My accounts are fine. We were going to make all those decisions after we were married." Grace rubbed her shoulders. "I only wish I had spent more time here in Oregon. I might have prevented this from happening to my grandfather," she said quietly.

Jilly rounded on her with a stormy frown. "Would have, could have, my ass. Don't turn into a martyr here, Grace. Your grandfather is the most stubborn person I know, and that includes me. You couldn't have changed one thing by being here."

"But maybe—"

"No buts, Lindstrom. He's a tough customer. The man will keep working eighty-hour weeks until his walker breaks," Jilly said. "And he'll be happy as a lark doing it. So suck it in and stop trying to blame yourself."

"Don't soft-pedal this. I should have been here more often. I should have paid more attention, no matter *how* stubborn he was."

Jilly made an exasperated sound. "Maybe you should have. But you did everything you could without stepping on his toes. In hindsight everyone sees 20/20, remember?" Now it was Jilly's turn to pace. "You're here right now. That's what matters. You'll stand by him until he's well. We all will. Even if he hates the help."

Tears burned at Grace's eyes as she looked at her friend's flushed, determined face. "Thank you," she whispered. "I forgot how much I counted on all of you."

"Well, start remembering," Jilly snapped. "And if I hear any more talk about you being at fault in all this, I'm going to work you over with the heavy-duty spatula I keep in my tote."

Grace forced a smile.

"Do you really have a spatula in there?"

"Damned right I do."

"Anyone ever tell you you're a bully?"

"Not to my face," Jilly shot back. "Turn around."

"Why?"

"Because that nurse down the hall is waving at you, and it looks important."

Grace immediately headed toward the nurse. "Is my grandfather awake?"

"No, I'm afraid not, Ms. Lindstrom. But there's a delivery for you at the main reception desk downstairs. A cell phone, I think. You need to sign for it."

Grace fought a wave a disappointment. "Mine was broken, and the replacement was delayed. Thanks for letting me know."

"No more long faces." Jilly ran her arm around Grace's shoulders and guided her toward the elevator. "I'll go with you."

"Your puppy isn't out in your car, is he? It can't be comfortable out there."

"Nope, he's with Sally tonight. She pretends not

to care, but deep down she loves him." Jilly soon had Grace laughing at some of the more outrageous objects that the puppy had chewed on or consumed in the last month. They were laughing as Grace picked up her package, signed the papers and opened the box.

The unit was partially charged, and as soon as Grace hit the power button, a string of unread text messages flashed onto the screen. Three were from her publisher. The rest were from Noah.

A wave of heat filled Grace's cheeks as she scanned the messages.

Hope your flight was good and your grandfather is doing better. Call me once your cell is working. At least give me a number where I can reach you.

Two hours later:

Snowing again. Lucky you, there at the ocean. Call me.

Five hours later:

Hope you are there. How is he?

At the bottom of the screen was another message.

Hello?

Grace had to smile, feeling a little giddy as she scanned the final lines.

Don't make me come out there and find you, Lindstrom... Because I will. You know I will. We have some unfinished business, you and I.

"Whoa." Jilly leaned over Grace's shoulder, trying to read the messages. "Who sent all of those text messages?"

"Just a friend."

"Sure. And that's why your face is the color of an heirloom tomato right now." Jilly's eyes narrowed. "You're seeing someone, aren't you?"

"What if I am?"

"I'll dance a jig, that's what." Jilly made a little snort. "Maybe it's bad to speak ill of the dead, but I never liked James. He was a stuffy little arse, holding forth about the *only* right way to drink Bordeaux and the *only* right way to cook an oyster. Blah, blah, blah. You let him walk all over you. The time I visited you in Paris, you wouldn't even go to the yarn store there because James considered it a waste of time."

"That's not true," Grace said hotly. "I went twice."

"After James left for Malaysia," Jilly pointed out. "You love to knit, Grace. You should have told him where to go jump."

Grace had a sudden, uncomfortable memory of Jilly's visit and James's lukewarm reception of her friend. It had angered her at the time, but somehow over the succeeding months she had forgotten. "He was edgy then. He seemed anxious to get away. But maybe you're right...." She ran a hand through her hair, wondering if James had had an inkling that his deceptions were about to become public. The last day before he left, he had been more short-tempered than Grace had ever seen him. Strange. Why had she buried that memory?

Not that it mattered now.

But it was important that she not repeat her mistake. Would that ever happen with Noah?

Impossible, a voice whispered. Because Noah was different. And because she and Noah had no chance of a future anyway.

"Aren't you going to answer that?"

"What?"

Jilly gestured to the phone, where a new text message had just appeared. "From Mr. Can't-Get-Enough-of-You," she muttered. "Why didn't you tell me you had a big, torrid love affair going on?"

"Because I don't." Grace cradled the phone, shielding the screen from Jilly, who tried to push in closer. "Back off."

"Whatever. Unless it's phone sex, I'm not interested." Jilly's eyebrow rose. "It isn't phone sex, is it?"

"Idiot. Just go away."

"You're blushing, Lindstrom. Direct hit."

"Go away." Grace felt her cheeks flush even more.

"It is a torrid love affair," Jilly whispered. "Why didn't you tell me right away? Dish, Lindstrom."

"It isn't serious and there will not be any phone sex happening today." She swallowed as two orderlies walked past, giving her quick, appraising looks. They looked back at her and then gestured in her direction to another orderly, who crossed toward Grace.

"Ms. Lindstrom?"

"Yes?"

"There's a package for you down at the first-floor information desk." His lips curved. "Flowers. A whole box of them. I'd say that someone is thinking about you a lot right now."

"FLOWERS? A WHOLE boxful?" Jilly snorted. "Not serious? Yeah, right."

"Shut up," Grace hissed, trying to ignore Jilly's laughter. "It isn't serious. I only met him a few days ago. We barely know each other."

"Yeah, just keep saying that." Jilly caught a breath as she saw the big florist's box perched on the information desk. "A whole box." Four colors of roses spilled in mounds against green florist paper, filling the air with perfume. Jilly whistled. "Probably six dozen roses in there. That's even better than phone sex."

Grace shot her an irritated look. "How would you know?"

Jilly gave a smug smile. "Life holds more than

cooking, my friend. I keep busy in Arizona. In fact, there's one firefighter who—"

"I don't want to know the details. TMI."

Jilly laughed and pushed Grace toward the desk. "She's the one for the flower delivery," Jilly announced. "I'd say it's serious, wouldn't you?"

The petite, gray-haired attendant at the desk nodded. "Only one piece of advice. Scoop him up and marry him fast." She grinned. "But if you are going to throw him back, then please give me his phone number first."

GRACE SENT JILLY off for whatever passed for hot food in the cafeteria between meals, and once her friend was safely gone, she settled down to answer Noah's messages.

Just received my new phone a few minutes ago. Things are pretty hectic, but I'm glad to be here.

Grace stood up, stretched and walked the shadowed hallway. Moments later her new cell phone chimed an incoming message.

Glad you got the phone. How's your grandfather doing?

Pale. On a lot of machines. Didn't have a

stroke. Not a heart attack, it appears. Dr. says that is all good news.

It is. Give it some time. How are you holding up?

Grace considered for long moments, then typed an answer.

Okay. My friends are here. Sad to be at hospital, but great to see them. Should have come home sooner.

No point in regrets. Take care of him. Take care of yourself too.

Grace smiled, gnawed at her lip and then typed an answer.

BTW I just got a package. A very big package. I must have a secret admirer somewhere. Whoever he is, the man has excellent taste. All the nurses are swooning. My friend wants to know when the phone sex is starting.

Flushing a little, Grace reread the message. Then she hit the send button. She paced restlessly, watching the phone.

But no answer appeared.

Deeply embarrassed, she closed her eyes, rubbing

her face. Why had she written that? Maybe it was exhaustion—and the heady perfume spilling from the roses on the table beside her.

Abruptly, her cell phone chimed.

All the phone sex you want, honey. Day or night. Glad you liked the roses. But I still wish you were here. Remember, you have one week....

Grace's heart took a giddy little whirl as she read the words. Despite the giddiness, she forced herself to stay calm and focused.

He's going to require a lot of care and recuperating time.

What about the book project?

I don't know. The animal shelter will need someone to manage it while he's gone. So many responsibilities that he handled without help or even thanks. And I'm all he's got. It's going to be on me now. So...

Grace paced some more, watching the phone. Seconds passed. Then the return message came back.

So...I'll be here. Remember that.

Grace looked up as Jilly turned the corner, holding a tray loaded with plates and cartons. "Any phone sex yet? What did I miss?"

"Yeah, we've been burning up the wires here. Too bad you missed all of it."

"Let me see—" Jilly made a lunge for the phone, and the two swung around, giddy with laughter. Jilly barely managed to get the tray down safely. "Go on. Do all the hot texting you want. I'll check out which of this stuff is edible." With a last, knowing glance at her friend, she moved off to the little table next to the vending machines.

Grace's phone chimed again.

R u still there?

Yes, at the hospital. Are you at work?

Yeah.

Grace glanced at her watch and frowned.

It's late. Why aren't you home with your feet up, nursing a cup of Irish coffee? Rolling Stones on the stereo. Or maybe Gipsy Kings...

One or two ends to tie up. Just boring stuff. But I'll go soon. And I'll be thinking of you when the music starts.

Grace closed her eyes, put a hand to her heart. She felt strange, both solid and weightless at the same time. *Alive* was the word. Amazingly alive, connected to Noah by odd, humming threads of awareness.

Her blood seemed to zing with little electric sparks as she read his message again. She smiled, then typed.

Please do. 'Night.

## CHAPTER SIXTEEN

BACK IN D.C., Noah read Grace's message again. He took a hard breath and then closed his phone. He hadn't expected to miss her this way, like a slow, dull ache in his chest. He hadn't expected anything like this low, raw edge of need that didn't let up.

But she missed him, too. That meant something. The thought put a stupid grin on his face, which he quickly wiped away. No point in stirring up nosy questions from his coworkers.

Besides, there was no point in making plans. Grace had a full plate in Oregon, and…

Noah rubbed his gritty eyes. He was just finishing his first break in six hours, swilling down a cup of bad coffee with a soggy pastry, and he wouldn't be going home anytime soon.

He looked up as his best tech analyst trotted over with the disemboweled digital circuits and wires of a new improvised explosive device, fresh from the lab. With another shipment uncovered at the Baltimore docks, law enforcement manpower was going into deep overtime.

This assignment would probably take most of a

month, Noah estimated. Right now everyone was praying that only two ships were involved.

He studied the carefully labeled wires. "So what have we got, Anna?"

The tech expert ran her fingers over the tangle of bright colors. Something about her movement made Noah think about the order and beauty of the yarns in the shop that he and Grace had visited. But this device belonged to a different world, he thought grimly. Whoever had made this IED had left a similar one in a crowded Kabul street outside a hospital with dozens of sick children inside. That cold mind had left any concept of order and beauty behind long ago.

His twentysomething tech assistant pulled out two green wires and brandished them with a look of glee. "Nothing too technical, boss. Strictly lowbrow wiring. We've seen this kind of layout before. But they've done something different with this one. See the blue wire near my thumb?"

Noah looked. In a handful of years, explosives had graduated from basic mechanics to a constantly evolving science requiring highly trained technicians in a number of fields. Every report could save a life out in the field. "Tell it to me straight up, Anna. Make it in words of two syllables," he added drily.

"Redundancy."

"Four syllables."

"Just checking that you were paying attention, boss. You look a little tired. Yesterday might—"

"I'm fine, Anna." Noah rubbed his shoulder. He'd been called out again the night before.

The tech flipped out the two green wires and then turned the device, showing a similar set of couplings in three different colors. "Four sets. Multiple redundancies. If one doesn't work, the circuit triggers the next through gravity pulls. And they didn't stop with wiring redundancy. Look under the cheap plastic they used for the housing. That's one very nasty gyroscope."

Noah leaned closer. "So if anyone lifts this baby once it's armed—or even sneezes while they're touching it—*kaboom*."

"You got it." But his tech's smile didn't reach her eyes. "Bad juju here. Oh, it's not beyond our technical abilities. The problem is that the container ship was full. There could be a thousand of these little nasties stuck in hundreds of corners. And there's always the possibility..."

Her voice trailed away.

"That more than one ship was sent to more than one dock." Noah ran a hand over his face. "Yeah. I've been thinking about that possibility."

"It's one thing to deal with a device like this in one city once a year, boss. If we get flooded with them..." She blew out a breath and shook her head.

Noah could do the math. It would be a very, very bad year for the home team if they didn't nail down some protocol fast. They needed training updates for all military and law enforcement who might come in contact with these devices. Not sophisticated, but still deadly.

He had already drafted an alert to port and border personnel across the country. If anything similar turned up, Noah wanted his team to hear about it first.

Meanwhile, his job was to try to figure out how to solve problems, and his people were the best.

Period.

Given the mountain of analysis and field time in front of him, sleep was going to be a luxury. So was a normal life.

"Good job, Anna. Give me twenty minutes to wrap up here, and then I'd like to talk about the plastic used in these devices, along with any chemical signatures that can help pinpoint locations. We need to alert border personnel what to look for and how to handle it once they find something."

"The last part's easy. They just call us," she said smugly.

"We can't be everywhere. We need to check fastest disposal techniques. Laser, simple heat? Water disruption? I need tests and answers." He stared at the gutted device, cursing softly. "We're not going to have a whole lot of time to get up to speed on these things. The FBI is going to need whatever we have, and I want our answers to be solid."

"You've got it, boss."

Noah winced as Anna moved away, cradling her device. He was only thirty-seven. He hated when these young bright types treated him like an old man. On the other hand, he wasn't getting any younger.

Right now he felt like he was about two hundred and nine.

He pulled out his cell phone and read Grace's last message. Some of his tension lifted.

"Doing a lot of texting today, boss." Anna studied him, one hand on her hip. "What's her name?"

"None of your business."

She nodded slowly. "So it's serious. I'm glad. I hope she knows how lucky she is."

Noah didn't have a clue how to answer that.

"Who is he?" Jilly pushed a carton of hot noodle soup toward Grace. "What did he say? Is he coming to visit?"

"I don't know."

"Did you thank him for the roses?"

"I did."

"Did you tell him how you feel about him?"

"I don't *know* how I feel about him." Grace sighed, knowing her friend could turn into a real bulldog if she thought it was important. She felt a momentary ache of loss. How had he left her so muddled? A month ago she had been totally determined to concentrate on her career and avoid any kind of entanglements.

"No, I didn't tell him how I feel. I told you that

it's too soon. No matter how I try, there's still the shadow of James blurring my future."

"Forget about James. The man was never right for you anyway." Jilly shook her head. "You still can't see that, can you?" Muttering, she grabbed her coat and stalked toward the elevator.

Grace wondered at the sudden anger in her friend's voice. Why was Jilly so upset?

There was no way to ask. The elevator doors were closing. Frowning, Grace glanced at her watch. She needed to go see if there was any change in her grandfather's condition. After that she would try to get some rest on the couch.

She heard a small chime on her phone, shoved in her pocket. When she pulled it out, a new line of text glowed on the screen.

So we change the game plan. One month from tomorrow. 7:00 p.m. My place. I'll bring the champagne. You bring the heat.

Grace took a deep breath, feeling anxious and off balance—but achingly *alive*.

You're totally on.

BUT AS SHE SETTLED on the couch down the hall half an hour later, Grace had a cold memory of her grandfather's face, still asleep, still without any sign of recognition. A month might be just the beginning of his recovery. It could be six months or a year before he was mobile or able to take care of himself.

Her life was going to change in ways she couldn't see or understand. Her old dreams had to give way to hard new realities.

She pulled up the knitted blanket that Jilly had brought and closed her eyes. Her grandfather had been strong before this accident, and Grace told herself that he would be strong again. But her dreams were restless, filled with darkness and the sad cry of the wind through lonely grass.

*Three in the morning*

SOMETHING CLATTERED LOUDLY down the hall. A voice rose, querulous and afraid. Grace shot up, disoriented by the sound of beeping machines and an alarm.

Two nurses ran past her down the hall.

The frightened voice grew louder. Grace realized it was her grandfather, but he wasn't making any sense. In a quavering voice he called a name over and over.

The name was Marta, his dead wife.

Grace's grandmother, dead for years now.

Two nurses were already inside the room when Grace got there. Together the nurses strained to push the struggling man back into bed. Grace was shocked to see his wild eyes, completely without recognition. "I want Marta. *Where is Marta?*" he demanded hoarsely. His hands dug at his hospital gown in confusion. "Where am I?"

"You will be fine, Dr. Lindstrom." One of the nurses pressed the call button while she tried to push him back onto the bed.

He shook his head, fighting to stand up. "Who are you? How do you know my name?"

Grace's heart pounded as she came closer, hoping that she could help calm her grandfather.

But his eyes ran over her face with no sign of recognition. "Where am I?" he demanded. This time his voice wavered in a broken sound of panic. "I want Marta."

"You're in the hospital, Dr. Lindstrom. You were hurt. You are here to recover. Do you remember anything?"

His eyes clouded. "Hurt? Where?" He looked down at his hospital gown and pulled at it with trembling fingers, tracing the heavy bandages around his ribs. Then he looked at the IV line in his arm. "I don't remember being hurt."

He stood, rigid, and his gaze fell on Grace. "I want to call the animal shelter," he said very carefully. He gestured to Grace. "Nurse, could you get me a phone?"

Grace realized he was looking at her. He thought she was a nurse, a stranger.

She forced a smile. "Dr. Lindstrom, please get back into bed. Then I'll get the phone, and you can call anyone you want."

He blinked at her, as if trying to figure out something about her voice. And then he sat down on the bed, slowly and very carefully. He folded his hands on his lap. "I just want Marta," he repeated, sounding sad and very lost. "I've lost her."

Grace forced herself not to cry. She lifted the quilt from the floor where it had fallen and stepped back as the nurses hurried to check on the IV that her grandfather had fought to pull out in his frenzy. When he was settled under the covers, he looked at her again. "I need a phone. Marta will be worrying about me."

Grace leaned down and patted his hand. The skin felt cold and terribly thin beneath her touch. "I'll get the phone for you, Dr. Lindstrom. You can call in a few minutes. Why don't you just rest for a moment?"

His eyes fluttered. "Marta," he repeated thickly. His gaunt fingers dug into the hospital blanket as he kept repeating the name, a lifeline to his past. To security and the only person that he remembered, though she had been dead for years.

Grace felt a hand on her shoulder. One of the nurses was guiding her toward the door. "You should wait outside. We'll take care of him now."

Blinded by tears, Grace found her way back into the corridor while the nurses talked to her grandfather, who kept repeating his dead wife's name. Grace sank back against the wall, her knees weak. She couldn't stop trembling. What if he never came back from this? What if the trauma had damaged part of his brain permanently?

Footsteps echoed up the hall. "What happened?" Jilly ran toward her.

"He woke up. He didn't recognize me. He doesn't remember anything," Grace said hoarsely. "He keeps calling for my grandmother, and she's been dead for years."

Grace felt Jilly tug a shawl around her, pulling her back down the hall to the nearest chair. Without a word Jilly pressed a cup of hot chocolate into her hands. "Drink that. You're freezing."

"I don't want anything, Jilly."

Her friend made a sharp sound and lifted the paper cup to Grace's mouth. "Just do it, Lindstrom. Don't even try to argue with me."

Closing her eyes, she choked down some of the hot chocolate. But nothing would make this cold, clammy fear go away. "Jilly, what if he—what if he's always like this?"

"Stop it." Grace heard the fierce determination in her friend's voice. "He's going to recover. You wake up in a hospital alone, in pain and disoriented. You're on medications and you haven't eaten. Of course you're confused. He'll be better as soon as he gets stronger. You need to believe that." Jilly's voice was rough. "He *needs* you to believe that, Grace."

"I'm trying." Grace's fingers twisted in the shawl that Jilly had draped over her shoulders. "I'm trying so hard. But if you had seen him, how thin he is now,

Jilly. How sad and frightened he was, trying to find my grandmother."

"It's awful. I wish you hadn't seen him that way." Jilly's voice hardened. She slid out of her coat and pulled it around Grace's shoulders over the thin shawl she wore. "He'll be asleep now for a while. They probably gave him medicine. You don't need to be here, Grace. You should go and rest."

"I can't—"

"You can. You're getting out of this hospital now." Grim and determined, Jilly stood up, tugging her toward the elevator.

Grace couldn't seem to concentrate. Her friend pulled her along to the front door. The cold sea wind hit her face and made Grace blink, looking around her. "I can't leave him, Jilly."

"If you stay there any longer, you'll turn into a basket case. Now be quiet. My car is right over here."

Jilly pushed her into a dusty red Wrangler. They shot out through the parking lot and onto the coast road that wound south to Summer Island.

Grace was too dazed to talk, too filled with sadness and worry for her grandfather. To her right she saw the dark outline of the ocean. She seemed caught in a nightmare, just like the dream she had had earlier. Where was she supposed to go? Where was home?

She was glad that Jilly didn't try to cheer her up with empty optimism. They both knew it was bad, and they both knew it could get worse.

Grace studied Jilly's face in the dim light. "Why were you so angry about James? Why now?"

"Because he—" Jilly hesitated. "Because the last time I visited you he tried to talk me into bed. You were at an all-day cooking workshop. He kept saying he liked my energy and my laugh. Shmuck," she hissed.

Grace just stared. "Your energy? What a lame pickup line." She swallowed, digging her nails into the seat.

"Do you believe me?" Jilly's face was pale.

"Of course I do. You wouldn't make that up." Grace stared out at the water. "At least now I know why you disliked him so much." Strangely, this punch hurt less than the others. Grace was only sorry that Jilly had been involved in the ugly mess. "But why didn't you tell me?"

"I took the easy way out because I was afraid." Jilly sighed. "I hated myself, but I couldn't take the chance that you would cut me off over it. I didn't want to lose you as a friend."

What could Grace say?

All she did was reach over and squeeze Jilly's arm. "I wish you'd told me. I'm sorry you had to wait and worry about it all this time. But we're friends forever. Remember that," Grace said fiercely.

They drove in silence. Grace finally dozed a little, lulled to sleep by the sound of the ocean and the rhythm of the motor. She sat up with a start at the sound of a car door opening.

She recognized a tall building with an ornate Victorian front porch. The library. Around the darkened street was the town office building.

They walked around a corner, climbed a little rise overlooking the harbor, past a garden that would be full of roses in the summer. Jilly hooked her arm around Grace's. "Come on. There's something you need to see."

The sea wind was sharp and familiar, a breath of home. Grace drank in the cold air, caught up in memories. She was anchored by the harbor, surrounded by the powerful force of family. She blinked as Jilly pulled her up a set of steps and then south along the pier, past a stone wall and a pair of intricately carved Chinese lions.

Jilly seemed tense and excited as she turned up a little cobblestone drive. Then she stopped, pointing straight ahead.

It was a tall building, three floors and an attic, with a steep gabled roof. A single lamp was lit in the big picture window on the first floor. "Harbor House?" Grace remembered this building. There had been a high-end gift shop here for several years and after that a wine store. Now there was nothing, and the building looked sadly derelict.

She frowned as Jilly fumbled in her pocket and pulled out keys. Hinges screeched as Jilly pushed open the door and motioned Grace inside.

"Why are we here? I don't understand."

"You'll see." Jilly pulled her inside. Caro appeared with dust on her cheeks and her hair wild on her shoulders. Gage was right behind her, carrying a broom and mop.

"What are you two doing here?"

They stopped, stunned to see Grace. Jilly rushed right past them, tugging Grace toward the room's only chair.

Grace's eyebrows rose at the peeling wallpaper and the scuffed wood floors. "What's going on?"

"Let's get a fire going," Jilly said quickly. "I have some hot chocolate in the back. There's a Crock-Pot with chili."

"We had some of it." Caro looked worriedly at Grace. "I'll go get some. I think there's bread left, too."

"I'll get it, honey. You stay here with Grace." Gage disappeared through the back room.

Nothing made any sense to Grace. She looked from Jilly to Caro and then around her at the empty room. "Why are you all here? It's just an empty shop. There's not even any heat."

"We're working on that," Jilly said, pacing nervously. "At least the fireplace is functional." She reached out, straightening a chintz curtain, the only decoration in the room. Then Jilly shrugged. "You tell her, Caro."

Caro blew out a breath. "No, you."

"Tell me what?" Grace demanded.

Jilly gave a low, reckless laugh. "We bought it." Her voice was hoarse. "It's been for sale for a year.

They finally came down to rock bottom and we bought it."

Jilly crossed her arms, staring around the room. She was silent for long moments. Her head turned as she imagined chairs and tables, rugs and curtains and paintings of the harbor. She cleared her throat.

"It's going to be a yarn store, Grace. Caro has it all planned. I'm going to make a café on the other side. We're calling it the Harbor House Yarn Café." She moved to stand next to Caro. Both of them were looking at Grace, half guilty, half defiant.

"Here?" Grace looked around her, forcing her thoughts away from her worries about her grandfather. "There's never been a yarn shop on Summer Island. Never a good pastry or coffee shop, either. Everyone drives over to the mainland. It's a ridiculous risk. But..."

"But what?" Jilly said hoarsely.

"On the other hand your espresso chocolate muffins could make a stone weep." She nodded slowly. "It might actually work."

Jilly turned to give Caro a high-five, then put her hands on her hips. "So here it is. If you're staying, we want you to be part of it with us. Sure it's a risk, and I know the timing is rotten, but what do you say, Grace? Are you in?"

# CHAPTER SEVENTEEN

"YOU'RE...CRAZY."

There was dust everywhere. A broken wooden chair leaned against the far wall, one leg in fragments. A painting hung next to the front window, tattered and water stained.

Grace sneezed. "This place is a nightmare."

Jilly raced past her, waving her hands in excitement. "That's why we got it so cheap. Because it *was* a nightmare. But the space is good and the structure is sound, and you can't beat its access to the water. Think about all that lovely tourist traffic in the summer."

"The summer is five months away," Grace said drily.

"And it will take all of five months to get this place cleaned up and decked out. I have a friend coming in tomorrow to give me an estimate on a new wooden floor. Then we're going to scrape the walls and put up new wallpaper. Something wonderful and atmospheric, a vintage print with flowers and birds. I see sage-green with nice little pops of rose-red."

"I see mildew and serious repair costs," Grace murmured.

"There's no mold and the foundation is excellent." Jilly moved on, her fingers trailing lovingly over the faded walls. She wasn't seeing the dirt and the mess. She was five months in the future, seeing new lights, fresh wallpaper and tourists who couldn't wait to spend their money on expensive pastries and luscious yarn.

Grace looked over her shoulder, back into the shadows where Gage had vanished. "What about the kitchen? This building is at least eighty years old. What about wiring?" She stood up slowly, shoved her hair out of her face and started toward the back.

Jilly blocked her way, looking uncomfortable. "You're right, it's old. I don't think you should go back there right now."

Grace snorted. "That bad, is it? Well, you wanted to pick my brain. This is what I do, so you'd better step aside and let me deliver the bad news."

After a moment Jilly sighed and turned, letting Grace walk into the dim kitchen. The walls were chipped, but not as bad as the public rooms. The counters sagged, but the wood was heavy and the bad spots could be replaced. There was only one small window at the back of the kitchen, so there would be little natural light. Grace looked up to the ceiling. An ugly fluorescent fixture hung from an old, rusted industrial bracket.

She rolled her eyes. "Are you nuts? This place

wouldn't pass a building code in Botswana. Not without about a year's work." Frowning, she made rough calculations, assessing the customer volume, food preparation speed, and what kind of equipment would be required. Since cooking school she had supplemented her income with restaurant start-up work, but she had never expected to crunch numbers for her own business.

It was more exciting than she had expected. More frightening, too.

"You have a contractor?"

Jilly nodded.

Grace did a few more calculations.

"You're going to need a commercial dishwasher. Something with good Energy Star compliance. You can save over a thousand dollars a year on electricity and water usage. You won't have that much volume, so you don't need anything huge. A nice walk-in refrigerator, too. I can get you a deal on that in Portland," Grace mused. "Over in this corner a high-efficiency pre-rinse spray valve to speed up your dishwashing process. That makes a huge bump in your water energy savings." She turned around, saw Caro, Jilly and now Gage staring at her.

"Well, what did you want me to say? It's not all organic produce and dreamy spices. What goes on back here sets the pace for everything else. You can't throw away money on energy, and you sure as heck don't want a customer getting sick because your dishwasher isn't heating at the right temperature."

Jilly burst out laughing. She slid one arm around Caro's shoulders and the other around Gage. "I told you," she said hoarsely, trying to stifle another laugh. "I told you she'd be grumpy and she'd complain. She'd find a thousand things that were wrong. But then she'd be hooked. You couldn't keep her out of this if you wanted to."

Grace looked at the three of them, saw them grinning back at her. "Oh, you said that, did you, Jilly? You knew exactly what I'd say, certain that I'd be enthusiastic." She blew a curve of hair out of her face and stared critically at the room, taking in the grimy window, the pitted wooden counters and the peeling walls. Yet even through the grime and old paint she sensed the bones of a lost beauty.

She shook her head. "It's a wreck. It will take weeks just to bring your kitchen wiring up to code, and that big front porch looks like it could collapse any minute."

But what a lovely place for knitters to sit and relax, comparing the yarns they had purchased inside...or for tables where tourists could enjoy lunch and savor the curve of the harbor and whales passing off the coast.

She crossed her arms. "The harbor view is amazing. There will be roses everywhere, spilling from the garden next door. We could put in a flagstone patio for more tables—"

*We?*

Why was she thinking in terms of *we?* The risk

was terrible. The amount of work required was daunting. And yet...

Grace realized this could be the answer she needed.

She rolled her eyes and sighed. "So when do we get started?"

THEY PUSHED THEIR CHAIRS together in the front room near the fireplace, drinking hot chocolate and arguing over appliance costs and opening menus. Jilly had a flare for creative organic produce and mixing unusual tastes, Grace couldn't deny it. Some of her recipes were drop-dead brilliant.

But there were a thousand details that would have to be taken care of before that first plate of pastry was set down in front of the café's first customer. And that was where Grace shone. She outlined a plan, making notes of suppliers and architects. She sketched out what would be required for building code approval and food safety inspections.

When she was done she leaned back, smiling. "I have to hand it to you, you can't beat the location. Jilly, you're right. In summer this strip of waterfront is always thronged, and the only other place to eat is the diner on the far side of the harbor. If you do this right, you could rake in money. The yarn shop idea is brilliant though it may have to be small at first. How about including a few other crafts, too, just to gauge the traffic and see what kind of things people want? And classes, too. It wouldn't hurt to have samples knitted up on display, available for sale. Not every-one can knit, as you know."

Caro nodded in excitement. "I thought about open craft nights and inviting some celebrity pattern de-signers. They did that when I was in Chicago and it was a huge draw. We're not that far from Portland, and I could call some yarn stores there to schedule visiting teachers to come out here."

"Good idea." Grace tapped the end of her pencil on the wobbly table that she was using to write on. "How much did they want for the building?" she asked abruptly.

Jilly named a figure that left Grace breathless. "Don't look that way. Sally and I are going in to-gether. Caro and Gage have a partial share now. They'll come in fully later, once Caro's had the baby and can go back to work here."

"How much do you need from me?"

Jilly gave another number, smaller but still enough to make Grace blink. It would take up all her savings, almost every penny. But what was life for if it wasn't to put your body and soul into real-izing a dream?

She sat back and crossed her arms, determined to be blunt. "You need to understand that my future is a big muddle now. My grandfather could get better—or he could get worse. Whatever happens, he's going to come first. I have to take care of the animal shel-ter, too. I can't give up on his dream, not when he's kept it alive for so many years."

"We know all that," Jilly said. "We'd never expect you to."

"There's something else. I think he's been pulling from his private savings," Grace said quietly. She managed a weak smile as Caro gave a little gasp. "I don't know how much is left. There may be nothing at all. I know that every cost, from food to heating and medical supplies has gone up. Whenever I asked him about it, he brushed off the question and laughed, telling me that he had made plans and everything would be fine. Now I wonder."

She felt a sudden, sick pang of fear. Her life was changing too fast, throwing new responsibilities and commitments into her path. She prayed that she was smart enough and determined enough to do the right thing.

She looked down at the wobbly table, at the hasty sketches with numbers and drawings of building layout and equipment placement. She took a deep breath and put one hand over Caro's and her other hand over Jilly's. She squeezed hard.

And knew she was doing the right thing.

"Whatever happens, I'm in. I may not have much time. My earnings may have to go to the animal shelter at first. But...I'm in."

Jilly laughed, leaning over to give her a quick hug. Caro smiled and then turned to give Gage a kiss. Grace shook her head. "We all may need our heads examined before this is over, I warn you. There's a reason that sixty to as many as ninety percent of all new restaurants fail." She knew the numbers by heart. She had seen other friends fail despite good planning and solid financial backing.

Grace couldn't bear to see her closest friends on that casualty list.

She glanced at her watch and thought about going back to the hospital to be with her grandfather. But Jilly was right. He would be medicated now. He needed rest as much as she needed downtime.

She yawned and glanced around the room. Jilly had a hot plate on the kitchen counter, and she was heating water for more hot chocolate. Gage had bought a box of doughnuts and Caro had made sandwiches to go with the chili that was left. The odd thing was, despite the dust and the dilapidated conditions, the room already felt like home. Being here felt just like growing up, when Grace had been surrounded by her strong and stubborn friends. They had stood together, laughed together, watched each other's backs and cheered on their quiet dreams and secret hopes.

Somehow they had fallen back into the same pattern.

Grace sighed. There was one place she would always be safe, and that was here on Summer Island, surrounded by her friends.

*Yes,* she thought, *this could actually work.*

She could restore her dreams here, just as this grand house, once a place of legendary beauty, could be restored to its full glory, magnificent at dawn in fog and radiant at sunset.

OVER THE NEXT DAYS the three women argued and planned with much appreciated suggestions from Gage. The planning helped to take Grace's mind off the constant worries about her grandfather.

As they stood in the kitchen, surrounded by newly scrubbed and shining floors, Grace had a sharp image of laughter and voices and sunshine streaming through the open back door. She took a quick breath, wanting to believe it was their future.

She felt Jilly drape an arm across her shoulders. "I don't know about you, but I'm whipped. Let's get a cup of tea and call it a night. You two have done way too much again." Jilly pointed at Gage and Caro. "Go home. Relax. Sleep late. I don't want to see you until dinnertime tomorrow. I'm trying a new recipe for grilled chipotle mango salmon. Chocolate éclairs for dessert."

Caro groaned. "Éclairs? That's evil. You know I can't have them. I've gained seven pounds in two weeks and my doctor wants me to be careful."

"One bite won't hurt." Jilly grinned at Gage. "Your husband can finish off the rest. Now go *home*," she ordered with a smile that took away the sting.

Caro wrinkled her nose. "Big bully. Just like in fourth grade." Caro turned with a laugh and she and Jilly bumped hips. "This place is starting to look good. Tomorrow a yarn rep is coming to set up a credit line and show us samples for new stock." She giggled. "Can you *believe* it? A private yarn showing?"

As she looked across the room Grace saw their faces blur, and somehow, whether through exhaustion or the rich pull of memories, she saw her friends the way they used to be, with braided hair or bobs. Wearing baggy jeans or khaki shorts. Keds or flip-flops.

Bound together. Sharing wild, grand dreams and wrenching fear, close enough to be sisters.

Maybe even closer than sisters.

Grace sighed, shaking off the shadows of the past. She was exhausted, drained by three more days of seeing her grandfather in the same disoriented state. She looked down and tried vainly to stifle a yawn.

"Grace, you're exhausted. I'll run you home to your grandfather's house. In the morning I'll come back and drive you to the hospital."

Grace nodded, yawning again. She pulled on her coat and then turned. The thought of going back to her grandfather's big empty house again left her cold. The silence was unbearable, a constant reminder of his illness. "No, I want to stay here, Jilly. You have a room upstairs, right? All I need is a sleeping bag." She gnawed at her lip. "The house— without my grandfather, it's just too quiet. Too sad."

"Great. You can be my first houseguest. I've got a sofa bed so you won't need to sleep on the floor." Jilly walked toward the hallway upstairs, then stopped, turning to look at her friends. "It's going to work. Together we're going to make something special here. I...I can feel it." She cleared her throat, looking a little shy. "I just wanted to say—thank you for all those years I didn't say it. You guys are the best," she muttered huskily. "You're pretty great too, Lt. Grayson." Because she was embarrassed by her sudden emotions, Jilly looked at Gage and pointed to the door. "Now get Caro home. Just because I don't sleep doesn't mean that everybody else has to keep my crazy hours." She shot a wry glance at Grace. "As for *you,* Einstein—we'll have plenty of time to discuss the romantic details of Energy Star ratings and commercial dishwashers tomorrow."

LATER, ENSCONCED BENEATH a down comforter on Jilly's sofa bed in an attic room overlooking the harbor, Grace listened to wind rattle the old windows.

The house creaked and settled. She could almost feel the sadness in the old rooms and the shadows that lingered at its grimy windows. The Harbor House had been a local landmark as long as she remembered, but a string of uncaring owners and speculators had left its beauty just a faded memory.

But no matter. They would change all that.

And in the summer, with the harbor full of yachts and pleasure boats, the view would be heart stopping. Grace held on to that golden image as she slipped down into sleep.

THE DREAM CAME SLOWLY.

Grace tossed, dimly aware of the shifting images. In that odd way of dreams, she stood on the steps in front of the Harbor House, wearing the same nightgown she had loved as a girl. In the dream, she watched a magnolia tree grow up, rich white petals opening to a brilliant sky. She watched a blanket appear, hanging from the tallest branch of the tree, intricately knitted, with cables and a dozen stitches in the style of intricate Guernsey sweaters Grace had always loved.

The cables shifted and seemed to move, almost as if alive. The deeply textured bands looked like walls or fences. Lace panels and eyelets soared like golden wings, crossing a stormy sea.

The sense of weight and meaning grew stronger. Grace felt the wind grow icy, grabbing at her hair. The blanket shook in the wind and all of its intricate stitches moved too, shadowed and restless. She reached out, trying to hold the borders and cables just as they were, but the thick stitches crumbled in her fingers, scattered like ashes.

The wind rose to a howl. She tossed back and forth, trying to block her ears.

"Wake up."

The blanket melted in her hands, dropping at her feet. There it rose and fell, still alive, lifting and twisting wildly.

A hand gripped her shoulders and shook her hard.

"Grace, *wake up.* Something's wrong." It was Jilly, her voice hoarse. "I think—I think the building might be on fire."

## CHAPTER EIGHTEEN

GRACE SAT UP with a start. Jilly's Samoyed puppy was barking furiously, his paws on the bedroom door. He scratched, wildly trying to get out.

"He's been that way for the last five minutes, totally frenzied. I hated to wake you since you were dead asleep." Jilly zipped up her thick sweatshirt and held up a heavy, long-handled flashlight. "The electricity's off again. And I smell something funny. Acrid and a little oily, like something's burning." She tossed a down jacket to Grace and then pulled on her boots. "Come on. If this place really is on fire, we need to get out."

Still groggy, caught up in the fading images of her disturbing dream, Grace shrugged on the jacket and followed Jilly to the door.

Jilly put her hand on Duffy's back, calming him. "Sit," she said sharply. "Sit, Duffy." The dog strained against her leg, alert and restless, but finally sat down as she ordered.

Jilly took a deep breath and gripped the heavy flashlight. "Okay, let's do this." She opened the door, bending to keep one hand on the puppy's back as they moved down the narrow stairway, lit only by the beam from her flashlight. The air smelled musty, and now Grace caught the odd smell that Jilly had described.

There was no sign of fire or any smoke as they reached the second floor and checked all the rooms. Duffy was growing more restless, pulling and straining forward against Jilly's grip. "Duffy, heel," Jilly ordered. At the first floor they turned, moving back through the front room, a nearby storeroom, and into the kitchen. No smoke, but the burning smell was intense.

Suddenly Duffy tore off across the kitchen, throwing his body against the back door. Jilly looked back at Grace, her face pale. "I guess we'd better go see what's making him crazy."

Grace didn't particularly like the idea of exploring in the darkness. She didn't like thinking about what could put a puppy into such a frenzy. But it had to be done, so she nodded.

She moved closer, right behind Jilly as she unlocked the back door and pushed it open. The access street behind the Harbor House was shadowed and Jilly flashed the light quickly, trying to hold Duffy's straining body as she checked her Wrangler, parked behind the rear entrance. Nothing moved in the garden across the road, barren now in winter. There were no other cars and the lights were off in the shop next door.

Something continued to bother Duffy. He growled, staring down the alley.

The sound of a banging door froze them in their tracks.

Jilly flashed her light to the small building between the two houses. As wind gusted up the alley, a door opened and then banged shut again. "The fuse boxes are in there," Jilly said softly. "The wiring is really old. Our electric and gas meters are in there, too. I think we'd better take a look."

Grace wasn't thrilled about the idea, considering how agitated the puppy was becoming. But if there was some kind of a wiring problem or an electrical short, they needed to handle it fast. As the two women walked down the back wooden steps, the oily, acid smell grew much stronger. Oddly, the puppy seemed calmer now, restless but no longer straining to pull free from Jilly's grip. He barked, nudging Jilly's leg, as if he had done his job as a guardian and expected to be praised.

Wind tossed Grace's hair, blinding her for a moment as she stared up into the branches of the big tree that grew over the driveway from the shop next door. Something about the twisting horizontal branches made her think of her odd dream. Was it supposed to mean something?

"Come on." Impatiently, Jilly shone the flashlight back into the darkness at Grace. Then she vanished into the storage shed that housed the electricity. Shivering from cold, Grace leaned over her shoulder, watching Jilly open the old-fashioned fuse box. As she did, smoke swirled out and the odor of burning oil and scorched metal became intense. One of the fuses was black, and two others were covered with oil. When Jilly raised her light, they saw two rusted cans of machinery oil overturned above the box. Dark liquid had oozed down the fuse grid. There were ridges where the oil had caught fire, probably sparked by contact with the fuses. Fortunately, the lower rows of fuses appeared intact.

"Good dog. Good boy, Duffy. You're in for a serious steak dinner today. Such a smart and brave boy," Jilly crooned.

As the dog pranced happily, Jilly closed the fuse box and glanced around the small storage area. It had been cleaned recently. There were no signs of dust or any damage to the worn wooden floor. But two more rusty oil cans had been pushed into a corner.

Jilly looked at Grace and shrugged. "It could have been worse. I think an electrician goes to the top of our to-do list. I also think I'm going to have a chat with whoever has been in charge of maintenance for these two buildings," she said grimly. "They won't be working for us, that's for sure."

AFTER TWO RESTLESS hours Grace gave up trying to sleep. It was freezing in the house without heat and she couldn't even read without electricity. But the residents of Summer Island were early risers, so

Grace walked down to the convenience store. She sent two text messages to Noah, bought coffee to go and grabbed a box of doughnuts for Jilly, who had a sweet tooth the size of Montana.

By the time she got back, Jilly was up, talking on her cell phone. Jilly took the coffee from Grace with a smile and a sigh of thanks, still talking. "Yes, I have the directions." Duffy pranced at her feet and it was clear that the two had just returned from a walk.

"Okay, great. I'll see you in an hour." Jilly closed her phone and pulled a hand-knitted scarf from the pocket of her jacket. "Not mine. Caro knitted this one for me last year. I keep trying, but I just can't figure out where the blasted needles go. So sue me." She closed her eyes in bliss, taking a last drink of her coffee. "Even cold coffee is good first thing in the morning. Thanks for going, Grace. Sorry, but I have an appointment scouting a new organic farm for local produce. I'll be gone a couple of hours. I called and whined, so the electrician said he could be here about eight. Would you mind letting him in?"

"No problem. I'll visit Granddad when you get back."

Jilly moved as she spoke, packing a notebook and a file folder in her big leather bag. "Caro and Gage are coming over later, but I didn't want to ask them. I think Caro had a hard night last night. She doesn't talk about it, but I'm pretty sure this pregnancy may be more difficult than she's telling any of us. Why don't you see if you can get her to talk about it with you? I'm having no luck at all." Jilly leaned down and scratched Duffy behind the ears. "Ready to go, big guy? Ready for a drive? Ready to smell some organic bok choy?" The puppy trotted in excited circles, clearly thrilled to go anywhere with Jilly.

"By the way, Gage wants to talk to the electrician about that fuse box. He said that he would drive you to the hospital after that."

"I've bothered them enough. I'm going to find the keys to my grandfather's truck today and drive myself. You go on. Organic bok choy should never be kept waiting," she said.

THE ELECTRICIAN ARRIVED on time, wonder of wonders. Grace remembered him from high school. He'd been good in science and chemistry and had gone off to college in Seattle. Now he was back on Summer Island, taking over the family business from his father.

As they caught up on old times and mutual friends, Grace watched him expertly examine the scorched fuse box. He gave a low whistle when he saw the black oil marks. "Good thing this baby shut down. That could have been one nasty fire. The fuses and box look up to code, but I wouldn't trust living with this in my own house. You need commercial breakers here. And whoever left those old cans of lubricant oil on the top of that ledge should be kicked in the head a few dozen times." He stared at the box and shook his head. "Now about that estimate you want. After I check the house over, I can give it to you in two ways. One is the bare basics, just to get your power running again. The other is the safe way, but it's going to cost a lot more. Only a complete overhaul will guarantee this kind of thing doesn't happen again."

*Ka-ching.*

Grace could hear the cash register racking up repair costs. "I'll take both estimates and discuss them with my friends." It was false economy to patch up the problem and then wait until it happened again, probably in the busiest time of the summer, but there was a limit to their repair budget.

A car door slammed out in the alley. She heard Caro calling something to Gage.

Grace leaned around the door and waved her hand. "Over here. The electrician is looking over our little problem." Grace prayed that it would indeed be a little problem and not the first of many surprises that would turn their dream house into a nightmare.

WITHOUT ELECTRICITY, it was very cold inside, even when the sun finally broke through the fog. Grace insisted on bringing down blankets for Caro. But Caro refused to sit down. Instead, she moved from room to room, poking in every closet, looking behind cabinets and under shelves.

Then she stood at the big picture window, watching whitecaps race across the curve of the harbor. "Jilly was up early."

"Wholesale produce was calling her name."

Caro shook her head. "I'm worried about her. She's running on fumes. You should have seen her earlier this month. She refuses to rest and even though she works with food all day, I don't think she's eating enough."

"When was Jilly ever calm?"

"This is worse. There's something she's not saying. When she thinks I'm not watching, a wistful look crosses her face." Caro leaned forward suddenly, rubbing her back and wincing. "Back pains. I read about this in the pregnancy books, but I kept thinking it wouldn't happen to me," she said drily. "Anyway, about Jilly. Her line of gourmet foods is growing faster than she expected, and there are a thousand details for her to manage. I told her she needs to hire a manager back in Arizona, but she wants to control everything herself. For Jilly, *delegating* is a four-letter word." Caro's eyes narrowed. "Maybe you can talk to her, Grace. She won't tell me anything."

Grace coughed to hide a sudden laugh. They were back to their old roles, with her as the intermediary. A decade had gone by, but some things never changed. "I'll do what I can."

"She'll talk to you," Caro said firmly. "And I think we could really make a go of this place, but I don't want Jilly biting off more than she can chew. I know she's always had the energy of two people, but she can't go on this way forever. If we aren't careful, this lovely dilapidated old house could turn into an albatross." Caro gestured out at the electrician's truck and smiled grimly. "As we've just seen." She turned, one hand on her round stomach. "Of course, I don't want you to say anything obvious to her. Jilly's way too smart for that. Just promise me you'll probe a little. You two were always close."

"Deal." Grace saw lines of strain around her friend's eyes. "Something else is wrong, isn't it, Caro? Let's have it."

"Oh, don't mind me. I'm just feeling silly and weepy today. Gage is going back to Afghanistan in nine days, and I can't seem to think of anything else." She bent her head, moving her hand gently over her stomach, as if to reassure the baby and herself that everything would be fine after Gage left. "Meanwhile, my grandmother's had a case of nerves ever since your grandfather went into the hospital. The two of them keep up this ridiculous act as if they aren't involved in a serious relationship. If you ask me, it's high time the two of them got married."

This was no secret to Grace. She was perfectly aware that Morgan McNeal and her grandfather had been seeing each other for some time. But they were always discreet, both holding on to their separate lives. She had tried to discuss it with him once, but he denied it was serious.

"I agree. But my grandfather could have a long way to go to a full recovery."

"One day at a time." Caro took a sharp breath and sank down in the nearby chair.

"Caro, what is it?"

Grace's friend took another quick breath. "Just an occasional twinge. It's my back. The doctor says the baby is riding very low now."

"That's all? There's nothing wrong, is there? Because if there is, you need to discuss it with Gage and your doctor."

"I was just in for a whole day's worth of tests. So far, everything looks fine, but we're waiting for the last results. Stop looking so upset. I'm in good health with no major vices. Everything will be fine. Women give birth to babies every day, right? There's no reason for me or you to get bent out of shape. It's going to be fine," she said firmly.

Grace was certain that her friend was trying hard to believe that, trying not to worry about her husband returning to a war zone. "If there's anything I can do to help, Caro, just name it."

"If there is, I'll ask. Now enough of this gloomy talk." Caro sat down on the sill at the front window. The paint was still chipped but now the glass gleamed from their labors.

Her gaze seemed to move over Grace's shoulder. "This room is going to be beautiful in summer, with splashes of color from yarn on the wall and the smell of Jilly's baguettes and chocolate croissants coming from the kitchen. I'd been thinking about a yarn store for Summer Island for months. At the same time, Jilly had been thinking about putting a café in here. Suddenly, there we were, talking to a Realtor and looking at wallpaper books."

She rubbed her neck. From inside a big quilted bag she pulled out bamboo needles and a half-finished purple glove. "When all else fails, grab your needles."

And Caro knitted fast, the way she had before her hand had been hurt in an accident the year before. She had always been the fastest knitter Grace knew, and effortless cables and ribs flowed beneath her needles. With each stitch, the tension in her shoulders relaxed. Her breathing became calmer, steadier.

Grace knew the feeling. Anyone who had knitted for any length of time knew the feeling. Knitting soaked up anxiety like a magic sponge. Even watching Caro knit made Grace more relaxed.

"So what's happened with that big project you were working on in D.C.? Wasn't it a digital reference, something very high profile? You never did give me the details."

Grace forced a smile. "It went to someone else. Probably just as well. Between my grandfather and the café, I'm going to have every minute taken." She ignored a quick stab of regret. This was the right thing to do, she thought.

Caro pulled out a new ball of yarn, looking

thoughtful. "And what about your mystery man with the roses? He sounds nice."

"Jilly told you?"

Caro nodded serenely. "I wormed every detail out of her, right down to the phone sex."

"There *wasn't* any phone sex. We're just—oh, I don't know *what* we are. We're both busy and then I had to leave before we could work things out."

"But you're going to see him again, aren't you? Why don't you invite him to visit?"

"One day at a time, remember? I don't have much free time at the moment. And don't you and Jilly go into matchmaker mode on me."

"I wouldn't dream of it. You're quite capable of making your own decisions. In fact, you're the most calm and sensible person that I know."

The conversation moved on to generalities. Through it all, Caro knitted on. She finished her glove and then pulled out a new workbag.

"What are you making?"

Caro held up her next project, intricate panels of ribbing and seed stitch and cables. "It's going to be a blanket for the sofa, and I'm making it big enough for the three of us. Me, Gage and the baby." She smoothed the soft teal wool between her fingers. "It matches the wallpaper Gage and I picked out." Caro looked up, smiling as footsteps crossed the back kitchen.

Caro put down her knitting as her husband and

the electrician walked in. Both of them were dusty, and Gage had an oil streak down one cheek.

They looked exceedingly pleased with themselves, Grace thought.

"There was an exposed line near the sidewalk. Lots of faulty wiring, too. We took care of it." Gage held up a knotted piece of wire, frowning. "Drew wants to show me a new breaker box in his workshop. It could help get you by here until all the wiring can be updated. But if you want me to stay—"

Caro laughed. "Go check out your breakers. And when you're done, maybe you and I can drive Grace to the hospital to see her grandfather."

"Absolutely." Gage nodded, but it was clear he was already thinking about wiring and fuse boxes.

*Men,* Grace thought. She looked down as her cell phone rang. It was a local area code, but not a number she recognized. "Hello?"

"Ms. Lindstrom? This is Woodvale Hospital calling."

Her fingers tightened. "Yes, this is Grace Lindstrom." Grace tried to prepare for what would follow next.

"Ms. Lindstrom, I have someone here who wants to talk to you."

There was a rustling on the line. And then Grace heard the deep, familiar voice.

Not so strong now. Not nearly as decisive as she had always remembered.

Now he was slow, hoarse, every word rough with pain. "Grace." Peter Lindstrom took a long breath. "Honey, I—I'm sorry about the problems I'm causing. I don't want to bother anyone." He gave a shaky cough. "I...I remember you were there at the hospital. I didn't recognize you. But now my head hurts and everything is strange here. I need to g-go home. Will you come and get me?"

## CHAPTER NINETEEN

PETER LINDSTROM WAS awake but agitated when Grace reached his room.

"Grace?" The old man's voice broke. "I'm all confused. You were gone. I remember it was in a big city. Not New York." Panic tightened his face. "Where were you? You're always going somewhere."

"Washington, D.C., Granddad. I came straight here as soon as I heard." She set down her purse and placed a covered cup on his rolling table. "Janie at the ice-cream shop was open early to make some repairs. She remembered how much you like their—"

"Pineapple sherbet!" The vet's eyes lit up as he inhaled the tropical scent. Then his delight faded. "But I'm in the hospital, Grace. This morning they wouldn't let me have coffee or real tea. The herbal thing wasn't bad but I always have coffee or real tea. I probably can't have sweets."

"It's all right. Your doctor approved this." Grace struggled to speak calmly. She didn't want her grandfather to see how much his appearance worried her. He looked as if he had shrunk, thin and weak against the pillows. His skin was sallow and his hair in disarray.

She forced a smile. "Go on. I dare you. Besides, this will melt if you don't eat it."

"I never could resist a dare. It has long been a source of trouble in my life. Marta told me that." He seemed to struggle to focus. "Why don't you have it, Grace?"

"I've already eaten, Granddad. You go ahead."

"Well, if you insist…" He managed a faint smile, then straightened up in his bed. "Now this feels like old times." He took a bite and rolled his eyes. "Just the way I remembered."

At least he could remember some things. She had to believe that all the rest would return eventually.

Her grandfather continued to eat his dessert, saying nothing until the cup was empty. He always approached his favorite treat like a little boy, stretching out the careful, measured pleasure in a way that reminded Grace how hard his childhood had been. This had been one of his few indulgences in a disciplined and controlled life. He had waited patiently for Saturdays and the fruit sherbet. Trips for ice cream had been a long-standing tradition for them.

Grace shook off her nostalgia. "Sorry, Granddad, I didn't hear you."

He stared up at the ceiling. "I said I apologize for this, honey." A frown worked over his face. "I didn't want you to come. Then that nice young woman said you had to know. Sorry." He closed his eyes. "My head hurts. I can't remember why. What…what happened to me? Why can't I remember?" He was growing agitated.

"It will all come back to you, Granddad. For now, you need to rest."

"No. I need to know what happened."

Grace sat next to him and placed her hand over his, explaining that he had had an accident at the clinic. He wouldn't forgive vague explanations about his prognosis, so she gave the truth but kept the details brief. "Your ribs will take the longest to mend, but like everything else, they will heal." She rushed on as he opened his mouth to blurt out more questions. "Yes, the animal shelter is in good hands. Your staff took over, along with Caro's grandmother. That's why Morgan hasn't been over to see you yet. She's been busy organizing your friends onto a volunteer schedule so the place will keep running as well as it always has."

His eyelids closed. He sighed deeply, as if all his burdens had finally been lifted. "I'm…very relieved. I knew Morgie would help. But I wish I could see her."

Grace kept talking in a soft voice. "I'll be doing my share, too, but Morgan would have a fit if I tried to take over, and she'd be right. She knows exactly what you would want done for the animals…."

A tear fought to escape and Grace blinked hard. *She* should know what he'd want done, but she'd never been home long enough to find out. She should know all the details of her grandfather's daily routine so she could take care of him properly, but she'd been too wrapped up in her own life to notice how much he was aging.

Guilt made her sick as she stared at his pale features. "I'm so sorry I wasn't here to help you more, Granddad. I should have been."

"You should not." His voice was precise and determined, sounding just the way she remembered it.

Startled, Grace studied his face. "What do you mean?"

"I mean you should have been doing exactly what you were—building your life, filling it with wonderful people who matter to you." He seemed to rouse, his focus clear suddenly. "The thought of my granddaughter hovering over me day and night, as if I was helpless and needed constant care like an invalid." He poked a finger at the air. "Appalling."

"You mean you don't want me here?"

"Of course that's not what I meant. I love to see you. But you have your own life now. I only want you here if it doesn't create a problem for you." The vet closed his eyes again, sounding very tired. His eye cracked open. "I want your promise on that. You can leave now. I'll be fine."

"It's not a problem. I have plenty to do here." Grace had considered her friends' proposition for Harbor House thoroughly during her sleepless nights. This new venture would solve all kinds problems and give her something to do while she cared for her grandfather, since his recovery could take months. She would be home, where she wanted to be, doing what she loved.

Except Noah was on the other side of the country.

Grace looked down and saw that Peter was sound asleep, looking weak but at peace. And she realized his cool fingers were wrapped tightly around hers, almost childlike.

She didn't expect the storm of love and protectiveness that hit her as she listened to his quiet breathing.

When his grip finally relaxed, Grace walked out into the hallway. Closing her eyes, she sank back against the wall, trembling. Most of what she felt was relief that her grandfather was lucid again, even briefly.

She had so much to be thankful for. But it would be a long road back. And his weakened condition meant a whole new set of responsibilities for her.

"Honey, are you all right?" One of the intensive-care nurses crossed the hall, studying her face. She glanced at the name on the door. "That's your grandfather, Dr. Lindstrom, right? The vet from down the coast?"

Grace managed a nod, wiping her eyes furiously.

"First of all, crying is nothing to be ashamed of. Having a relative in the hospital hits us all hard. But your grandfather is doing extremely well. Don't get upset because he's forgetful. It often happens after head trauma. He's going to look weak and pale until he gets out of the hospital and starts exercising again. All things considered, he's in amazing shape."

Grace forced a smile. "I know you're right. I know that he's being well cared for, too. And I'm so glad that he finally recognized me today. But he's so changed. So thin." She took a deep breath. "I hate seeing him this way. Now I can't seem to stop all these emotions."

The nurse nodded. "It's traumatic, but don't bury your feelings. If you need to cry, cry. If you need to get angry and kick something, get angry and kick something. The very best thing you can do right now is to find people you love and tell them how you feel. Tell them that you love them. That kind of honesty is the best medicine in the world," the nurse said firmly. "And I won't even charge you for it."

"Thanks. I'll keep it in mind." But Grace didn't want to talk to anyone about how she felt. She couldn't stop worrying about her grandfather or the big changes ahead of both of them. The responsibility of keeping the animal shelter on firm ground made her doubly worried. And Grace's friends had their own problems. She wasn't about to burden them with hers.

*Find someone that you love.*

Somehow, without knowing it, her hand slid to her pocket. She reacted with raw instinct, no longer fighting the emotions flowing through her. She had to talk to someone. Denial wouldn't help her or her grandfather. She had lost a fiancé—and then lost him again when she learned the extent of his betrayals. Her career had been her solace during that dark time of pain, but with her grandfather so ill, there would be no more research that would take her away from home for weeks. She still had her restaurant consulting work, and eventually she might find a few jobs in Portland or the upscale restaurants of the Willamette Valley to supplement income from the Harbor House when it opened. Over time she could build up local contacts, but it would be slow.

More changes. More shifting ground beneath her feet.

Overwhelmed by looming uncertainties, Grace closed her eyes. She had always dreamed bigger than one town and one state. Her heart had always led the way, calling her down little paved streets on Paris's Left Bank or the back roads of Asia. She loved the obscure and the exotic. She savored the excitement of waking up every day in a new town, sometimes a new continent, wandering through markets with spices she had no names for.

But she loved her grandfather deeply. There was no question that she would stay and help him, even though he would frown and try to talk her out of it. As long as he needed her, she would stay. It would be hard for both of them to accept the changes to come. He would hate his loss of independence, hate his new weakness. Physical therapy would be a trial. How was she going to manage him and the animal shelter and still do her share at the café?

She gave a little jump at a chime from her cell phone. A text message flickered on the screen.

Hey. Haven't heard from you in a while. Everything OK?

Threads of warmth worked through her. It was hard to face these new emotions and harder still to share them, but Grace knew the nurse was right. She needed to reach out to someone she could trust.

Even if he was on the opposite side of the continent. She took a deep breath and began to type. Not sure.

Your grandfather?

Lucid, thank heaven. We just talked. But he's so pale, nothing like the man I remember. And right now...all I seem to want to do is cry. I feel so stupid. Helpless. I think I'm a mess.

She pressed the send button, then leaned back against the wall and closed her eyes.

She missed his voice, missed his laugh. Suddenly she ached to feel his arms around her. She needed to feel safe, but her world was changing too fast.

Not stupid. NOT helpless.

There was a pause.

At hospital?

Yes.

Grace's phone rang. She recognized the Washington, D.C., area code of the caller. "Hello?"

"You're not helpless and you're not a mess. You could *never* be a mess. You're the most sane, stable and well-balanced person I know. Let's get that straight right now."

His voice calmed her on almost a physical level. Grace felt his strength and absolute confidence in her. They flowed out to her, real and true despite the distance. That knowledge made some of the tension leave her shoulders. "You wouldn't say that if you could see me now. My hair is a wreck. I'm wearing a black sweatshirt that's two sizes too big because that's all that my friend Jilly had to loan me. Yeah, I'm a mess." Her voice fell. "It's really good to talk to you. I miss you, Noah."

"Me, too, honey." He cleared his throat and Grace heard a chair creak nearby.

"If you're busy, I can call back later."

"Now is fine. Tell me what's happened and what I can do to help."

Grace felt her heart lurch at the tenderness in his voice. She wanted to see him, to touch his face and hear his laugh. She hated being so far away from him. "Noah—I can't leave, not for several weeks.

Maybe longer. It all depends on my grandfather. But do you think…would you consider coming here? One day, two days or even a week. Whatever you want." She took a ragged breath. "I miss you. Did I already say that?"

"You did. I'll come. Just as soon as I can, I promise. But I've got things to tie up here. I'm not sure how long that will take."

"Whenever you can get here is fine, no pressure. I'll be ready. I'll even cook for you." She smiled into the phone, restored to balance. Then she took a deep breath and told him all about her grandfather and the new café and the Harbor House project. If her voice wavered a little during the telling, Noah made no comment. When she was done, she heard the sound of the creaking chair as he leaned back.

"That's some island you've got. Friends like that will stick by you. And from what I know about your grandfather, he's a stubborn old moose. He'll recover. In fact, he'll probably outlive all of us. Now tell me more about this house you plan to restore."

GRACE WAS CHUCKLING ten minutes later when she hung up. She didn't put her phone away immediately. Holding its weight made her feel as if she was still connected to Noah.

She gripped the cool metal, trying to hold tight to this precious new thing they had found. Even if their relationship went no further, Grace wanted him in her life, whether as a friend, a confidante or as a lover.

But the truth was that she wanted him to be all three.

FOG WAS BURNING away above the ocean when Grace turned into the parking area at the Summer Island Animal Shelter. She sat without moving, remembering all the other times she had come here. Usually there were three or four cars parked in the rough gravel area, but now she saw at least three dozen. As she turned off the motor, a young couple and their teenage son walked by. The father was lecturing the boy about the responsibilities that came with being a volunteer and how much the animals inside needed their help, now that Dr. Peter was sick.

Two more cars pulled up. A young girl got out of one, and Grace recognized the daughter of an old friend. The girl saw her and waved, then climbed the steps to the front door, followed by a teenage boy carrying a big bag of dog food.

Grace took a deep breath. She had such deep and fixed memories of this place and all the time she had spent working here with her grandfather. She knew that he had hoped she would follow in his footsteps one day and go to veterinary school, but Grace's dreams had carried her on a different path. Her grandfather had never argued with her about that choice, but she had always felt guilty that she couldn't be what he had hoped. At the least she would see that his beloved animals were well tended until his return, whenever that might be.

For a moment she felt a lump at her throat. It had been a struggle for him to finish a sentence and impossible for him to stand up unassisted. He had so far to go.

But she pushed the dark thoughts out of her mind. He had improved steadily the past few days, and there was no reason that he wouldn't keep right on improving with good care.

Meanwhile, the animal shelter looked to be in excellent hands. Two more cars had pulled up. She saw a pair of high school students dumping trash in the back. A trio of teenage girls and their parents were cleaning out animal cages nearby, scrubbing them down with the long gloves and heavy brushes that Grace remembered from her own childhood chores. There were always chores here, always another cage to clean. It was time for her to get started.

INSIDE, EVERY ROOM was full of volunteers tackling the hard jobs that came with caring for almost seventy animals. She recognized some of the faces, longtime residents of Summer Island. Others were not so familiar, probably children and relatives. Working together, they flew through the jobs that had usually taken her grandfather and his small staff many hours.

Grace watched in amazement, aware that everyone here had come because of her grandfather. It was a gift of thanks to a man who had never asked for any.

As she walked down the hall to her grandfather's office, Grace waved to the tall college student who helped supervise the shelter. Andy Wilson was in his senior year of college, and after that he was bound for vet school. But right now, all his spare time went into helping Dr. Peter. When he saw Grace, he jumped up from behind his desk.

"Grace, it's great to see you! I just heard from a friend who works at the hospital that your grandfather is doing a whole lot better today. I can't tell you how worried I was." He waved her to a seat and then crossed to pour her a cup of coffee, adding a healthy dose of cream, just the way she liked it. "Man, have you seen anything like this? When I got here around seven the parking lot already had ten cars and it's been growing every hour. Do you believe it? The word is out about your grandfather and people just began showing up to help." He ran a hand through his long hair, then pointed to the local men unloading heavy feed bags from a storage area in the back of the shelter. "I didn't have to ask anyone, Grace. It's—well, amazing. Everyone here on Summer Island owes him. He's helped more people than I can count, but he never mentions it. That's just his way."

Grace nodded, fighting tears. "I know. He never asks for help."

"Sometimes he got mad if I offered to take over

for him." The boy turned, blinking a little as he looked out the window. "He helped me so much." He cleared his throat. "At the beginning of my sophomore year, my scholarship was cut. I was working two jobs, but it wasn't enough. Your grandfather insisted on loaning me enough to get me through the year. I argued, but he wouldn't have it any other way. Yeah, I owe him. Everyone here owes him. And by the time he's out of the hospital, this whole facility is going to shine from the baseboards to the ceiling," he said fiercely. "I hate that he had to be hurt for this to happen, but he refused anything except the most necessary help before."

"I understand only too well. And this will make him so happy. Anything for the animals. I'll be sure and tell him when I go back to the hospital." Grace finished her coffee and stood up. "Isn't there anything I can do to help? The last time we talked on the phone, he told me there were all kinds of small repair jobs that needed to be done."

"We're finally taking care of them now." Andy followed Grace to the door. "But that water heater took us by surprise. I mean, we both knew it was ancient. It's been here as long as this building has been here, but it never looked unstable."

He looked at Grace, frowning. "I should have kept a better eye on things. All I can figure is that the power went out in the storm. We had a small quake here the same night, pretty rare for Oregon. He must have gone down in the basement, looking for the backup generator. Maybe he tripped or maybe one of the metal legs of the water heater collapsed and knocked the shelf unit over on him." Andy made a flat sound of anger. "I still feel sick when I think of him down there in the cold all night, alone and bleeding." His face looked strained. "He insisted on doing too much. If I had fought harder, none of this would have happened."

He was clearly upset, Grace realized. She moved quickly, blocking his way. "It's not your fault, Andy. I know just how stubborn my grandfather can be. Thank heavens you found him the next morning and had Caro and Gage help get him to the hospital. Maybe we should all be thankful for this wake-up call. Now things are going to change and he'll have to accept more help, like it or not. Since I'm going to be here, I'll make sure that he doesn't overwork."

Andy stared at her in surprise. "You? You're going to stay here on Summer Island? But I thought your writing—well, I know you travel a lot."

"Not anymore. It's time I came home." Grace waved at an old friend from high school and then squeezed the hand of a mother and daughter who lived down the street from her grandfather. Her eyes burned as the little girl held up one of the puppies, her hands gentle with love, saying she hoped that Dr. Peter would be back soon because she missed him.

Her grandfather would have been very proud.

Reluctantly, Grace looked down the hall at her

grandfather's office. "I want to go through his papers and records, Andy. Did he keep them in his desk?"

"I think so. He never let me help with that."

"I think he was getting behind in some of his bills. I'll need to check on that. His truck may need maintenance, too." Grace shot him a quick smile. "But before that, I expect you to give me a list of everything I can do to help you around here. It's been a long time since I've scrubbed out a cage, but I haven't forgotten how, believe me."

## CHAPTER TWENTY

GRACE TURNED OFF her car and yawned, eyeing her face in the car mirror.

Right now she looked as tired as she felt. There were dark circles under her eyes and her hair was shoved back in a rubber band, wisps escaping around her face. She could feel the welts on her hands, along with bruises from the leg of a table she had tried to pick up the night before. She hadn't done this kind of manual labor in years.

Meanwhile, her grandfather was making progress. Grace spent long hours at his side, encouraging and explaining, building his morale. Every day he recovered a little more strength. His memory was better, and he understood what had happened to him. Yet he hated being dependent on others, and his mood could change in an instant. He grumbled at having to use a wheelchair and he grumbled at having physical therapy. Then Andy, his young assistant at the clinic, had gotten permission to bring one of their favorite dogs for a brief visit in the hospital lobby. Grace's grandfather had been in high spirits for a week afterward.

But he still worried about her. She put on a touch of lipstick and added a few quick strokes of color to her face to hide her exhaustion, wondering what kind of mood he would be in today. She hadn't been in the room for thirty seconds when he zeroed in on the circles under her eyes.

"You look tired. Those people are working you too hard. Tell them your new book can wait. It's just not worth ruining your health." His eyes narrowed. "But...where are you working now, honey? Is it in New York? No, not there. Someplace else. I can't seem to remember."

Grace didn't tell him the truth, that it was her work here in Oregon that had put dark circles under her eyes. Instead, she managed a smile. "It was Washington, D.C., Granddad. You remember that I told you about visiting the Smithsonian. But I'm not working there now. I've moved back home."

His frown deepened. "So you're staying in our house? You didn't tell me that."

"No, I'm not staying there." Grace had been very careful about what she told her grandfather. Since he still had bouts of confusion and panic, she had tried to avoid any subjects that might worry him. "But I've been by every day to check on things. I'm staying at the Harbor House with Jilly now."

The old man's frown deepened. "That place is a wreck. There probably isn't any heat."

"We're fine, Granddad. Caro's husband and the electrician are taking care of everything. I've even got my own room on the third floor. You wouldn't believe the view of the harbor from my window."

Peter sank back slowly. "Well, if that's really the way you want it. It is true, no place has a view like the old Harbor House." His eyes rose to the window, looking west. Grace had the sense that he had drifted off.

"Granddad, do you need anything? I'll bring you your favorite ice cream tonight. But what about magazines? Books to read?"

He cracked one eye open. "Oh, no, I don't need anything, honey. I have my new veterinary journal here. I've been reading it when I can. At least, I've been trying to...but it's slow work." He shook his head. "I don't know when things got so complicated in my profession."

His profession hadn't changed since the accident. It was his own mental abilities that were different.

He yawned and closed his eyes. "Get some rest, honey."

Grace leaned over and squeezed his hand. "You, too. You'll have plenty of time to catch up on your journals once you're home."

"I'd like that. It's so noisy here. I know they try hard, but the food...I won't bother them. It's just food." He yawned again.

Then he struggled back from sleep, staring at her. "Don't work so hard, Grace. You always were working on something exciting. We both need to slow down. You be sure and tell them that back in New

York—or in Boston. Wherever it was. They need to stop working you so hard."

And then he drifted back into sleep.

Grace reached over and took his hand, feeling the cool skin that was still too frail. No, she wouldn't tell him the truth, that she was running herself ragged here in Oregon. She wouldn't mention that the plumbing had broken again at the animal clinic and she'd worked four hours with Andy, cleaning up a flooded storage area. There had been bills to pay, paperwork to file, and pet food to order. Then one of the younger dogs had escaped. She and Andy had stumbled around in the darkness, clutching flashlights, for almost twenty minutes before they'd cornered the frightened animal.

Maybe she *should* go back to Washington, Grace thought. That would be a piece of cake compared to what she was doing now.

Except she was enjoying the sheer variety and spontaneity of work to be done every day. She had always enjoyed working with her hands, and now she savored her daily interaction with needy animals at the shelter. Often abused or cruelly abandoned, they flowered in response to a little human love. They knew Grace now. When she appeared, they responded with instant excitement, their keen eyes bright with love. Every day her heart melted all over again.

She understood exactly why her grandfather couldn't give up his long hours at the shelter.

"How is he doing?"

Grace turned to see Caro's grandmother peeking inside. Morgan McNeal's silver hair fell in stunning waves around her shoulders. Her makeup was flawless, as always, and she wore a set of handmade glass beads around her neck. "I couldn't stay away any longer."

Grace stood up and moved quietly to the door, giving Morgan a hug. "Better. He has his ups and downs. He still forgets a lot of things, but the doctors assure me he's getting stronger every day."

Morgan ran a hand across her eyes, and the look of tenderness she had for Grace's grandfather was so intense that Grace felt like an intruder. But there were things that had to be said.

She put a hand on Morgan's arm. "When are you two getting married, Morgan? This relationship of yours has been going on forever. Don't think you're fooling anyone because everyone on Summer Island knows that you two are involved."

Morgan sighed. "I know they do. But it's your grandfather. Peter wants things done properly. He's always been afraid it would upset you if our relationship changed. He keeps saying we need to wait."

"*Me?* My grandfather is insisting on this charade because he doesn't want to bother *me?*" Grace ran a hand through her hair. "That's ridiculous. I'd be delighted to see you two together officially. Everyone on Summer Island would. You've both been alone too long."

Morgan rolled her eyes. "That's what I keep telling him. But your grandfather is as stubborn as a rhino. Something always comes up, or he's worried about the clinic, apologizing because some new project is taking up all his time. I keep telling him that we don't have forever. We're not young things any longer." She smiled, but there was sadness in her eyes. "And it seems as if I was right. If I'd insisted on him marrying me, we would move in together, and I could keep a better watch on him. No more late-night trips to the clinic to check on a sick animal. And no more carrying bags of feed or heavy cages by himself. He's going to have to hire someone younger and let them do the running. He should be using that good brain of his to teach, too. I keep telling him all that, but he never listens."

So it hadn't been Morgan's idea to wait, but her grandfather's.

"I think he is silly to wait, too. But as for feeling guilty, don't. If anyone is to blame here, it's *me*. I should have been keeping a better eye on him. I know exactly what he's like and how he refuses to ask for help. I've been too focused on my own career, caught up in my research and my traveling—"

Caro's grandmother cut her off. "You were doing exactly what your grandfather wanted you to do. Don't you sink into a guilt-fest. One of us is quite enough."

"More than enough," Grace said firmly. "I'm glad that we can agree on that. And for the record I think you're the best medicine that my grandfather could have. He's been restless today, trying to catch up on his veterinary journals. The stubborn idiot."

Morgan chuckled. "That he is. And it's part of the reason I love him so much. What would we do without him?" She sighed and squeezed Grace's hand. "You really don't mind? I mean, the two of us are as old as Methuselah. It seems ridiculous for us to upset both households to get married now, at our age."

"Why? You deserve your happiness. You should be together, enjoying yourselves. You're both so busy. This way you'll be able to spend your free time together whenever you can. I intend to tell my grandfather that as soon as he is stronger."

"I don't want him having another problem like this." Morgan tilted her head, studying Grace's face. "Why are you working so hard? They should give you more time off between your projects." Morgan's eyes narrowed. "By the way, your grandfather told me that you were just getting started on a big project. How is that coming?"

Grace ignored a pang at the lie she was about to tell. "Oh, my research has been going very well, right on schedule. But I may not be involved much longer."

"Really? Well, don't let them push you around. You should get more rest. You can't burn the candle at both ends. It doesn't work."

"I'll keep that in mind, Morgan."

Caro's grandmother laughed a little sadly. "No

you won't. Young people never do. You think you have all the energy and all the time in the world. You think no one knows half as much as you do. Believe me, when I was your age I was just the same way. But things change." She sighed. "Remember that."

There was a noise inside the room. "Morgie, is that you? Why don't you come inside? Grace just left. She's going to bring me some of that ice cream I like. Or maybe she already brought me some. I'm getting confused. Morgie, are you out there?"

"Go on," Grace said. "Otherwise he'll be fuming over his vet magazine again. I'm sure he'd much rather look at your face."

"Thank you for your blessing." Morgan gave a self-conscious laugh and then turned around, vanishing into the room.

Grace smiled when she heard her grandfather sitting up, followed by Morgan's giggle and what might have been an emphatic kiss.

WONDERFUL SMELLS CAME from the kitchen.

As she sniffed the air, Grace put down her bag of groceries and went in search of Jilly. Her friend was on one knee, scraping a cabinet. She took one look at Grace and shook her head. "You look terrible. You're working too hard."

Was everyone going to tell her she looked awful? "Not as hard as you."

"Seriously, Grace. It's not your grandfather, is it? There's nothing wrong at the hospital?"

"No, Morgan was there when I left, and the two of them were like young kids. She will make certain that he's in good spirits. And I would seriously appreciate it if you and everyone else would stop telling me I look awful," Grace muttered.

"Touchy, aren't we?" Jilly smiled wickedly. "Somebody isn't getting enough phone sex. Maybe I should go get your cell phone and call up that hunk. Noah, isn't that his name? Maybe I should tell him that—"

"If you touch my phone, I'll murder you." Grace was already tugging off her jacket, searching for the old sweatshirt she wore to work in the kitchen. "And now if the jokes are over, maybe you'll tell me what's on the list for this afternoon. I finished cleaning the shelves last night. I scrubbed the floor, too."

"I saw how much you did. That's why you're taking a break. Come into the kitchen and admire my new table. I have chocolate espresso brownies in the oven and your knitting bag is in the corner."

Grace felt her exhaustion lift. "Chocolate brownies? The ones you make with the nuts and that amazing gooey center?" She trailed after Jilly toward the far door. "And whipped cream?"

"Bingo."

Grace was afraid she might have drooled. "This could be good."

"Better than good. There's a box of yarn over there with samples. Caro opened it and went into some kind of trance. She fondled every one," Jilly said. "Talked to the yarn for probably ten minutes."

She put a hot plate of brownies on the table along with a canister of freshly whipped cream. "Your turn, Lindstrom. Go fondle the yarn." Jilly raised an eyebrow. "I'll be over here fixing a shelf. Try not to drool, will you?"

IT WAS HEAVEN to sit and do nothing, heaven to savor Jilly's newest decadent dessert and feast on the glorious spring colors of the new yarn samples. Sated with brownies, Grace picked up her needles to finish a scarf for Jilly, who had no idea the gift was for her.

"So what's the update on the hunk?" Jilly stuck her head out of a cabinet. "When is he coming to visit?"

"No date yet. He's very busy."

"What kind of job?"

Grace rubbed her neck. "Government work. He's on call and goes out on emergencies."

Jilly sat back slowly. "What kind of emergencies?"

"Oh, this and that."

Jilly studied her grimy hands, frowning. "You don't know what he does, do you? It's secret. Is he some kind of spy? Secret Service maybe?"

"I don't *know*. He told me what he could, but it wasn't much."

"And that doesn't...bother you?"

Grace stood up, piling yarn neatly back into the

sample box. "Or course it bothers me. I *hate* wondering, not knowing where he is or if he's...hurt." Grace rubbed her forehead, feeling a headache begin.

"Oh, honey, I'm sorry. I didn't mean to be a pain. I just want him to be good for you. You don't smile enough, do you know that?" Jilly rubbed Grace's shoulders. "Only when you talk to him on the phone." She drummed her fingers on the table. "So get him out here. Call him again. Go make passionate love out at Lover's Point." Jilly smiled a little wistfully. "Find out if he's the one."

NOAH STOOD UP and stretched, shaking his head at the chaos of wires, fuses and timing devices ranged over his work space. Another day, another bomb, he thought grimly.

"You closing up soon, boss?" Anna, his tech expert, studied him carefully, one hand on her hip. "Don't you have to text your lady friend?"

"I'll handle my private life, Anna. Just get your new forensics report on my desk first thing."

"Will do. But here's a tip, boss. We women can be tricky. We don't like it if a man forgets about us."

Noah ground his teeth. "I sent her roses, Anna."

"Good call. But that's just an opener. You need a follow-up plan."

Noah rubbed his neck and smiled thoughtfully. "I have six of them. She's a knitter. She's got a surprise coming."

Anna's eyebrow rose. "A knitter, huh? She must

be good with her hands. Sensual, too. All that merino and angora and cashmere. Why don't you blow this place and go find her? Those wires aren't going anywhere."

She left before Noah could shoot back a smart answer. But she had only voiced the thoughts circling through Noah's head for the past week.

He missed her laugh, her cool, focused intelligence. He wanted to feed her more s'mores with his fingers, Noah thought wryly.

"You still here, McLeod?" Noah's boss looked in, his coat draped over his shoulder. "Nice work at that forensics task force today. Your presentation got noticed. It might mean more funding for us."

"Thank you, sir." Noah sat back, frowning. "You know I have some private time coming, sir. I thought after this new case report is completed, I'd take a week off."

Noah's boss didn't move. "A week? Half of our people are still at that EEC briefing."

"How about two or three days then?"

"I could probably manage that. Not easy, but possible. So where are you going? Too cold for fly-fishing in Montana." Ed Merrill pulled on his coat. "Tell me it's a hot beach in the Caribbean. Clothing optional."

*Oregon,* Noah thought. And he hoped that clothing would be very optional. "Not sure yet, sir. I'll put in a formal request tomorrow."

"I'll shoehorn it through. I wish I could get away, too. This weather is killing me."

Noah glanced outside. "Don't tell me it's snowing again?"

"And another storm predicted." Noah's boss shook his head. "Didn't they get the memo about global warming?"

GRACE'S PHONE CHIMED. She put down her knitting and grabbed the phone.

How's life at the beach?

Not bad. Jilly made brownies that would wake the dead. I'm actually doing some knitting. I almost forgot how.

No way. You're too good for that. My mom loved the pattern and the yarn. She's got two squares done already. Says thanks for recommending.

Excellent. Tell her hello. My grandfather walked across the room today. We helped him, but still… Progress.

Great news. You should celebrate.

Grace looked at her greasy top and torn jeans. Her nails were beyond any hope of repair. Meanwhile, there were two boxes of old fixtures to clear out of the storage area.

I'll keep that in mind. Still busy?

A little this, a little that.

Grace didn't want to push. He'd come if he could. She stopped, one finger poised over the phone. Before she could answer him, another message appeared.

Put in for leave today. You change your mind?

She rubbed the center of her chest, feeling her heart take a sharp dive. Heat swirled through her cheeks.

No way. I've got a menu all planned. Three kinds of chocolate and an organic single-origin espresso from Bolivia. Killer stuff. We'll go park at Lover's Point and watch the sun come up.

She closed her eyes, wishing she could see his face.

Keep the coffee warm. Here comes the sun. We'll see it together.

# CHAPTER TWENTY-ONE

"WHAT ARE *YOU* GRINNING FOR?"

"Me?"

"Yeah, Lindstrom. *You.* A major Cheshire-cat version." Jilly poured herself a fresh cup of coffee. "You just spoke to the Flower Guy, right? When's he showing up?"

Grace gave up trying to hide a grin. She leaned back in her chair—and almost collapsed backward.

"Whoa. Careful. Get those raging hormones under control."

"I am not—that is, my hormones are *not* raging." Grace closed her eyes. "Frothing a little, maybe." It felt wonderful to froth, Grace thought.

To dream and imagine and hope.

She could start making plans for Noah's arrival right away. "Jilly, I need that recipe for dark chocolate ganache with organic espresso bits."

"Coming right up. Anything else? Truffles? A magnum of champagne, maybe?" Jilly asked.

"A great *guy* meal would be good. I was making Noah chipotle coffee chili when we got interrupted. That's my favorite, but I need something new."

"Mac and cheese. Best comfort food around. And don't screw up your nose on me. I can cook highbrow, but guys don't want all that shredded herbs with truffles and three-color oil stuff. Mac and cheese made from scratch. One bite and he'll be eating out of your palm," Jilly said smugly.

"And you know this *how?*"

"Cooking isn't the only thing you can do in a kitchen." Jilly gave a silken smile. "Remember that."

Grace made a mental note to pursue this avenue of discussion later. Something was going on with Jilly and Grace was going to get every detail.

She glanced at her watch and sat up quickly. "It's not that late, is it? I have to be back at the hospital tonight and——"

The doorbell rang.

Jilly flipped a towel over her shoulder. "You expecting anyone?"

"Not me."

"I told Caro to stay home and rest tonight. She's doing too much," Jilly grumbled. "If she thinks she's going to clean more cabinets, she's wrong." Scowling, she flung open the front door. *"What?"*

A woman in a brown uniform raised an eyebrow. "Delivery for Grace Lindstrom. Smells like roses to me. Of course, if you want me to take it back to the truck——"

*"No."* Grace reached around Jilly for the box.

"Sign here. Enjoy the flowers."

Jilly sniffed as Grace carried the box back to the kitchen. "I don't smell flowers. Who's it from? The hunk again?"

Grace slit the tape and pulled away layers of pink tissue paper and then sighed.

A single ball of perfect pink cashmere lay in the box. A single pink rose in a protective cellophane sleeve lay beside the delicate yarn.

Jilly peered over Grace's shoulder and sniffed. "Well. Yarn and one perfect rose. This guy could be worth keeping."

Grace couldn't answer. She lifted the yarn to brush her cheek, feeling a silly smile starting to form. "Yarn." He had remembered the kind she liked. The exact color, too.

"You're starting to drool," Jilly muttered. "I'll go find a vase. One of us needs to be practical."

The doorbell rang gain. Grace reached it before Jilly this time. A different delivery person held a small box. "Grace Lindstrom?"

"Right here."

"Need a signature."

Grace took the box, feeling the silly grin spread all the way to her toes.

"Careful. I think you're starting to levitate," Jilly murmured.

It was another ball of yarn, slightly darker. The same cashmere. A matching rose lay beside it.

Jilly's breath caught. "Does this guy have any brothers?"

FOUR MORE BOXES came in the next hour. Each with a rose and yarn in a slightly different shade of pink. They were all lined up on the kitchen counter, matched with a rose in its vase.

"Smooth," Jilly said after a long time. "Not many guys would be smart enough to send yarn." She shot a glance at Grace. "You're smiling again. I'm glad for that. As for me, fresh produce is calling. I can't take Duffy this time because they have sheep. He'd run them ragged and all my produce dreams would be ruined."

"Not a problem. I'll keep him here with me."

"Be careful with those old boxes. No one has been back there in the storage area for months. They may have spiders and all kinds of crawling things."

"I'll survive." Grace was definitely light-headed. "I'm going to text Noah, then get right to work. I want to start something special tonight with his cashmere."

They came. All six boxes. They're beautiful, Noah. You shouldn't have...

NOAH HAD TWO KITTENS on his lap and a puppy under his arm. He juggled them carefully as he read

Grace's message. He scratched Ivan's head and smiled.

Glad to hear it. The bad boys say hi. Ivan just chewed through another shoestring. That makes three this week. I'll call tomorrow. Watch for another box.

## CHAPTER TWENTY-TWO

BY THE NEXT afternoon Grace's back was aching and she had bruises down one leg where a pile of old boxes had fallen on her. The cleanup work continued, dirty and tedious. The storage room was full of boxes and old papers, with dust everywhere.

Duffy stayed right beside her while she worked, exploring every dusty corner and sniffing the old boxes as soon as Grace pulled them down off a shelf. She brushed a strand of hair out of her face and smeared dust all over her cheek. She didn't want to think about how she looked. Frankly, she was too tired to care. There was no one except Duffy to see her anyway.

"You don't care about how I look, do you, sweetie?"

The dog wagged his tail and jumped up, licking her face and smearing more dust across her cheeks. Laughing, Grace gave him a good scratching and then turned to survey the boxes neatly stacked by one wall. Another hour and she should be done.

Her stomach growled, but Grace was determined

to keep going. Then maybe she would make a peanut butter and jelly sandwich.

Gourmet cooking had faded to a wistful memory. Between hospital visits, work at the animal shelter and cleaning jobs here at the house, she was lucky to have enough energy to toss a salad.

Duffy bumped her leg and looked up at her, tail wagging. "I know. I'm here with the people I love doing work that has meaning. What's a few lost gourmet meals against that?"

As Grace swept, she wondered where Noah was and what he was doing. She wondered if it was dangerous. There were a hundred little things she wanted to tell him—stories about growing up on Summer Island, funny things that Duffy had done.

Most of all she wanted to see him. She imagined him walking up the front stairs, looking good enough to eat. He would smell like wind off the sea and his eyes would range over her in the intense way that always made her heart skip.

Enough fantasies. With a sigh she stretched her cramped muscles, counting the boxes stacked on the far wall. Then she froze.

One of the boxes moved.

*Just a mouse, Lindstrom. Nothing to get hysterical about.*

She moved closer, Duffy right behind her. "Stay," Grace whispered.

The mouse shot out from behind a box and Duffy leaped. Grace tried to jump out of the way, tripped on Duffy and fell sideways, hitting the floor with her right knee.

The old floorboards gave way and her leg plunged down through a hole in the splintered wood.

Grace threw her arm out, trying to balance as the floor made another ominous sound. What if the floor gave way? What if—

She concentrated on crawling forward over the splintered wood. Wriggling, she reached for an old plank balanced against a box. Keeping her movements slow, she gripped the wood and drew it slowly closer.

Something broke free beneath her. Both legs dropped through the cracked floor and dangled crazily.

Duffy barked madly, aware that something was wrong, and Grace tossed her cleaning rag through the kitchen door to the kitchen. The dog shot away to continue the game they had begun earlier.

She had five feet to go to reach the edge of the doorway. Meanwhile, she could feel a new crack forming.

A splinter dug into her palm. She bit back a sound of pain, wriggling out of the hole and forward inch by inch. Sweat streaked her face as she thought about falling into the widening hole. Down and down. Her fear made her think about her grandfather, tired and weak, trapped and frightened in his own way in his lonely hospital bed.

Duffy bounded back, barking at her from the

doorway, the cleaning rag in his teeth. "Stay, Duffy." Grace's voice shook. She inched onto one elbow and crawled carefully through the kitchen doorway, away from the splintered wood and then collapsed.

Duffy raced forward, barking wildly, licking her face. Grace didn't have the strength to push him away as his wet tongue slicked her face. Tears gave way to ragged laughter. She had never been more happy to be alive.

Abruptly, Duffy bounded away, dancing in excitement as Jilly elbowed open the back door. She was laden down with produce boxes, frowning at Duffy. "What's up with him?" She didn't wait for an answer, stacking fruit boxes and fresh bread on the counter. "I had to go to four different farms before I found what I needed." The dog raced around Jilly's feet, while she rubbed his head. "He's really wound up." She glanced over her shoulder at Grace. "Why are you lying on the floor?"

"You don't want to know." Grace sat up slowly.

Jilly's eyes narrowed. "Your jeans are ripped." She stalked across the kitchen. "What happened?"

"There's a hole in the floor back there in the storage area. I fell." Grace took a shaky breath. "I closed the door so Duffy wouldn't get in."

"A hole?" Jilly's voice rose shrilly. "Are you hurt? Is it bad? Why didn't you tell me?"

"There's no need to yell."

"I'll yell if I want. Sit right there and don't move. Not an inch." Jilly strode toward the stairs, calling back over her shoulder. "I have a first-aid kit. Duffy, bite her if she moves."

From long experience, Grace knew that Jilly talked tough, but she was fiercely loyal to her friends. Grace also knew that friendship didn't come easy. After growing up in foster care, Jilly had been adopted by a family from Summer Island. She never talked about the years before she was adopted—not to anyone. Eventually her friends had stopped asking.

"Aren't you going to check on the hole?" Grace tried to move her bruised ankle and winced. "It's a real mess back there."

"The mess can wait. I hate to think of you here alone, hurt. From now on no more working alone. I'll call my contractor to make a thorough inspection in that back room tomorrow." Drawers slammed down the hall. "Where did I put that stupid thing?"

Grace closed her eyes, trying to relax. She heard her cell phone chime. With shaky hands she pulled the phone off the nearby table.

I can be there in a week.

Grace's heart skipped wildly. A week? Feeling a little faint, she reread Noah's message.

"Eureka." Jilly came back, brandishing a white plastic box. "Let me see your leg."

"He's coming, Jilly. *Here*. To see me." Her bruises were all forgotten. Grace rubbed a hand over her chest, feeling the slam of her heart. "Noah," she whispered. "Finally." She flopped back onto the floor, gripping the phone. "I think I may faint."

## CHAPTER TWENTY-THREE

JILLY PEERED AROUND the doorway to the kitchen, shaking her head. She gestured to Caro and frowned. "Look at her. She's been in there for an hour. Last night she put up new wallpaper in the bedroom."

Caro peeked over Jilly's shoulder and saw Grace bending over the sink, a bandanna tied around her hair. "What's she doing?"

"Cleaning the sink. *Again.* If it wasn't so pathetic, I could almost laugh. Manic behavior is supposed to be my specialty," Jilly said quietly.

Caro frowned at Jilly. "And you think it's funny? What are we going to do? We can't let her go on like this. Now she's scrubbing the sink with a manicure brush."

"I was going to give her five more minutes. I just needed a good clear memory so that I can toss it back in her face next month, when she calls *me* obsessive." Jilly smiled guiltily. "I was going to stop her, okay? She's a little crazy because the Flower Guy is coming. I've got a hunch that this is the one." Jilly squared her shoulders. "Come on. Let's go stage a cleaning intervention."

They walked into the kitchen together. "You with the manicure brush. Step away from the sink," Jilly ordered.

"What?" Grace stood up, rubbing her back. "Why are you staring at me like that? I'm just doing a little cleaning."

"A little?" Jilly grabbed a coat from the table and tossed it to Grace. "You're cleaning the sink with a manicure brush. Get a grip, Lindstrom. This isn't a home makeover show. If the guy is half the man you think he is, he won't notice anything, not the peeling wallpaper, not the chipped floors. All he's going to be looking at is you."

"But—"

"But we're going for a walk on the beach. Get your coat on." Shaking her head, Jilly wrestled the manicure brush from Grace's dirty fingers. "And this thing is going right into the garbage."

"You have the coffee, right? And those chocolate croissants?"

Grace stared around her at the pristine kitchen. It had been a crazy week, but the house was finally beginning to take shape. A bouquet of roses gleamed in a crystal vase on the counter, a recent gift from Noah. Toile curtains hung at the little window. Her fingernails were chipped and her hands were a mess of cuts, but the house radiated with life.

Good thing for it, too. Noah was due in five hours.

"Yeah, yeah. Coffee's in here. Croissants are proofing." Jilly hitched one hip against the table, her eyes narrowed. "When are you going to get cleaned up? I suggest a nice long bath in those perfumed salts that Caro is always waving around."

"I have a few more little things to finish here."

Jilly stared grimly at her friend. "It was funny at first. I enjoyed having ammunition against you in the future. But this is unnatural. You're not like this. You don't obsess. You don't brood and over-react. That's strictly *my* department. And no more coffee." Jilly intercepted her cup. "You're starting to twitch."

"I am completely under control," Grace said loftily. "Now if you would kindly leave, I would like to finish. That grout behind the faucet needs another scrubbing."

The front doorbell rang. "If that's a door-to-door salesman, I'm going to make him regret his choice of profession." Jilly stalked to the front room and peeked through the side window. She cleared her throat and looked again.

"What's wrong? Who is it?"

"No one that I ever saw before." Jilly gave a low whistle. "Trust me, you don't forget a face like that. Or a body like that one."

The doorbell rang again, but Jilly still didn't answer it. She turned around slowly. "Change of schedule. Unless I'm very mistaken, that's your Flower Guy out there on the porch."

Grace's heart stumbled. She felt as if she was glued to the floor. Then she remembered Jilly's delight in practical jokes. "Very funny. You're a real scream today."

Jilly gave a little shrug and then shot another look outside. "Definitely one great-looking man out there."

"Honestly, Jilly."

The doorbell rang again. Grace blew out a little breath and ran a hand through her hair. "This isn't funny."

Jilly went for the door, and then everything happened at once. Grace tried to straighten her old sweatshirt—and Duffy galloped straight between her feet, barking at the tall stranger who threatened his household. In the rush, Grace lost her footing and stumbled forward.

Her hands met soft black wool, stretched taut over Noah's hard shoulders. His arms closed around her, tightening, pulling her against him.

Safety.

Home.

"Noah," she rasped. "You're—early." The scent of leather and some kind of citrus with a hint of the sea wind clung to his hair. She gave in to blind instinct, leaning closer, hoarding each impression, afraid to miss anything.

Afraid to believe that he was finally, truly here.

She gave a reckless laugh as he lifted her higher, swinging her up against his chest and carrying her across the room to deposit her in the big wing chair by the window.

She couldn't take her eyes off him. Laughter lit his face, along with satisfaction and something that might have been downright mischief. A woman could get hooked on that combination, Grace thought. A woman could learn to depend on those strong arms and on the husky, infectious way he laughed.

But she was a mess. She hadn't changed and her hands were streaked with dirt. All her careful plans were going up in smoke, and it wasn't fair.

"I was cleaning." She tried to pull free, her face flushed. "My hair is a nightmare—" Grace touched his face wonderingly. "You're here. You weren't supposed to be here until seven."

"I got an earlier flight." He picked a piece of string out of her hair, smiling slightly. "I should have called."

"No—I'm glad." Grace was staring at his mouth, struck by a wave of heat. "It's just—I have a new dress. Shoes. I was going to soak in bubbles. Do my nails." She swallowed as his hand opened over her waist.

She closed her eyes, wanting more.

Wanting to touch him now. Without even thinking, she leaned in, her fingers tightening on his chest.

"Well then." Behind them Jilly cleared her throat. The front door opened. "I'm going out for a few hours. There are fresh sheets on the bed on the third floor. The rug is thin, but the view will stop your heart. There's coffee in a thermos and quiche in the refrigerator. If anyone's interested."

Cold wind rushed in, playing through the room, rich with the sound and smell of pine trees, wind and the sea. Duffy barked wildly.

And then Jilly was gone.

Grace looked up into Noah's eyes, her heart pounding. She touched his mouth and his chin and the curve of his eyebrow. "It's not fair. I wanted everything to be ready. All those plans." She felt his hand tighten around hers. "I've got dirt up to my elbows, and I'm wearing this stupid, awful sweatshirt, and I wanted to be elegant and sleek and so beautiful you couldn't take your eyes off me," she whispered. "I had it all p-planned."

"I can't," Noah said roughly. "And you are."

"No." She pulled free, digging at her hair. "It will only take me a few minutes." She started for the stairs. It was all supposed to be so different. So smooth and effortless. Just like in her dreams.

And then she stopped. What was she doing?

She turned around slowly. "I'm an idiot. It doesn't have to be perfect, does it?" She took a long breath and looked at him, really seeing him for the first time.

Seeing the cut just above his eyebrow, not quite healed. Seeing the humor in his eyes and the need he wasn't afraid to show. "Jilly was right." She took a deep breath and walked down the stairs, straight into his arms, resting her head against his chest. "Those things don't matter." She gave a shaky laugh. "Oh, Noah. I missed you. I missed this."

"Me, too." His arms tightened. Callused fingers opened against her waist. He pulled the bandanna away and let it fall so that her hair tumbled around her shoulders. "And just for the record, I love your hair."

Grace looked up and kissed the edge of his mouth. "Welcome to Harbor House." She traced his cheek, seeing the lines on his forehead. "You're tired. When did you last sleep?"

"Last night."

"The truth."

He shrugged. "Can't remember. An hour on the plane, I think. It's been a crazy week."

How hard had he worked to clear his schedule and make this time for them? she thought guiltily, knowing he would never admit it. Grace kissed his mouth again, lingering. "You're going to sleep."

"I'll be fine."

She shook her head, sliding her arm through his. "Upstairs. Big bed with cool white sheets. Down comforter. We have all the time in the world."

Noah tried to stifle a yawn. "I don't need—"

"Stop arguing." They walked slowly up the stairs, arm in arm.

No haste. Tender and somehow familiar. As if they had done this before. He kissed the nape of her neck and she sighed with a sharp swirl of desire. She thought about him and that soft bed.

"Just for an hour. Wake me up."

"Absolutely." Grace had no intention of waking him. At the top of the stairs she opened the door and folded back the down comforter. "I'll be here."

"I was supposed to sweep you off your feet with roses." Noah sank down on the bed and Grace saw the way he rubbed his right shoulder. "You were supposed to be enchanted."

She pushed him down, one hand to his chest. Pulled off his shoes, watching the tension begin to leave his eyes. "You did. And I am. Now close your eyes and rest."

SHE HAD A QUICK SHOWER to remove the day's grime, smoothed her skin with the lotion she had kept just for him. Then she tugged on a soft knit gown and a matching robe and sat down in the chair beside the bed. And she watched him sleep.

Just watched.

Seeing the single light from the hall glint on his hair. Seeing the way his chest rose and fell, his restless fingers opening to move on the quilt.

All the little details stored away. Whatever happened, she would have this. As shadows changed, growing into twilight and then night, she drowsed. Finally, she slipped off her robe and climbed in beside him, smiling to feel his fingers slide around her, pulling her into the curve of his body, his mouth gently nuzzling her hair.

As if they had always slept this way.

## CHAPTER TWENTY-FOUR

FIRE REACHED OUT in an explosive inferno.

Smoking oil and burning metal surrounded him.

Noah came awake in a rush, dragged in a shuddering breath—and knew in the same moment that it was only a dream.

There was no IED in his hands, clicking down to lethal zero.

A different kind of danger lay in his hands. Smooth skin. A perfect curve of hip and thigh. He whispered her name, let his breath out slowly.

It wasn't supposed to happen this way. Exhaustion had caught up with both of them at the worst possible moment, he thought.

And yet it was just as it should be. Expectations changed, but not the dreams or feelings beneath. He touched Grace's chipped nails and the welts on her hands, signs of how much work she had done. He already knew desire, knew the hot stab of need, but now he was overwhelmed by a sharp wave of tenderness.

He eased off the bed, pulled on a shirt and his

jeans. He straightened the quilt over Grace and then headed downstairs.

First coffee.

Then he planned to have a look around.

HE WAS UP ON A CHAIR, examining the back of the coffee machine when feet padded across the floor. A tall woman in gray sweats stared up at him, a hand on her hip. "Something wrong?"

"Just checking some wires. I heard a noisy humming behind the back somewhere."

"Nothing was burning, I hope." Jilly stared at the counter outlet, frowning. "This house is pretty old."

A big white puppy raced through the door and barked loudly at Noah. "It's okay, Duffy. He's a good guy." The woman studied Noah. "I hope."

"Nice dog. Duffy, is it?" Noah reached out a hand slowly and let the dog smell him thoroughly. "And everything looked fine. A spoon was wedged under the back feet. It vibrated whenever the heating element came on."

"No kidding. A spoon? I never could figure out what was making the noise."

Noah stepped off the chair and held out his hand. "Noah McLeod. You must be Jilly. We didn't really get introduced earlier."

"You were busy with more important things." Jilly's eyes crinkled. "Nice to meet you, Noah McLeod." The big puppy danced around her bare feet. "Sit, Duffy." She smiled in satisfaction when the dog dropped into position as ordered. "Good baby," she crooned. "So where's Grace?"

"Exhausted. Let her rest." Noah ran a hand along the freshly polished counter, studying the room. "Great house. Nice crown molding along the doorways. Grace told me you're going to renovate it for a yarn store and café. How old is it exactly?"

"Eighty-two years, the papers say. I've been doing some research in the old newspaper archives. If I can find a president or a movie star who stayed here, I figure we'll be in clover." She leaned against the doorway. "You know anything about renovations?"

"Some. My brother and I did an overhaul on his house last year. I have some experience in wiring and electricity," he added casually. "I thought I would look around while Grace slept. Unless you'd rather I didn't."

"Be my guest. Poke all you like." Looking thoughtful, Jilly pulled some dog food down for Duffy and filled his bowl. "Wiring and electricity," she murmured, scratching Duffy's head. She started to say something else, then shook her head. "Just don't go in that back room. The door is locked because there's a hole in the floor. Grace fell in there."

Noah's eyes narrowed. "How bad?"

"Some bruises and a cut. It could have been worse. Now the rule is no working here alone."

Noah didn't like the sound of any of this. "Is the house structurally sound? What does your building contractor say?"

"No problems in that area. There was a particular section of floor that was never properly joined. That was the problem."

"I see." Not exactly reassured, Noah stared up at the ceiling, wondering what other surprises the house had in store. "Sorry if that sounded rude. When I helped my brother, we kept turning up all kinds of building problems. Old houses can be dangerous."

"Not this one. The contractor checked everything out. We have all the reports, a time frame for work and money budgeted for his repairs."

"That's a good plan." The coffee machine light came on. "I filled the machine. Caffeine withdrawal." Noah gave a sheepish laugh. "Like a cup?"

"Sure." Pleased, Jilly sat back and watched him prowl the kitchen, enjoying the sight of a man who knew what he was doing.

A man in worn, thigh-hugging jeans with probably the best pair of biceps she had ever seen.

She coughed and forced away the thought.

Definitely time to go.

"Well, if you'll excuse me, I'll take mine to go, thanks. Duffy and I have big plans for the night. You can tell Grace I'm dropping by the hospital to see her grandfather, so she shouldn't worry about him. I'll call her if anything's new. After that we're going to visit a friend in Portland. Make her eat. She's been working too hard, eating too little." She took the cup from Noah, poured it into a travel mug and gave a little wave. "Have fun. The house is all yours. Tell Grace the chocolate croissants are in the fridge."

She gave a wicked little grin. "Don't do anything I wouldn't do."

AN INTERESTING WOMAN, Noah thought. Scrappy and stubborn, she would be an unshakable ally and friend. He was glad that Grace had a friend like Jilly.

He was thinking about the old house, considering possible problems, when he heard the scuff of bare feet on the stairs. He had a faint warning in the brush of a light perfume, gardenia and citrus. Then he turned and saw Grace blinking at him from the doorway, her eyes dazed with sleep, her body wrapped in a long blue knit robe with a blue satin belt.

One look and the desire roared into angry overdrive, slamming him in the chest until it was hard not to wince. Somehow he managed to stay calm, pulling down another cup for coffee and searching out sugar, milk and a spoon for her.

Anything so he didn't have to look at her sleepy, vulnerable eyes and the soft mouth he was aching to kiss.

"I fell asleep." She stifled a yawn, half irritated and half embarrassed. "You should have wakened me."

"You were out for the count. I got my second wind and came down to look around. It's a great house."

She ran a hand through the sexy disorder of her hair and smiled, looking just a little dreamy. "It is, isn't it? Wonderful old molding and views that go on for miles. It will be amazing when all the work is done."

He nodded. "Your friend Jilly made chocolate croissants. I put them on the counter while the oven is heating."

Grace blinked at him. Color swirled through her cheeks. "This is strange, having you here talking about the oven and croissants. Very good," she said quickly, "but strange. I could get used to it."

He could get used to it, too, Noah thought. He wanted to see her like this, smiling and sleepy, for the rest of his life. "Sit down and have something to drink. I'll put the croissants in the oven."

She wandered to the table, added milk to her coffee and then frowned. "Where is Jilly?"

"She's visiting a friend in Portland. She said to tell you she is stopping to see your grandfather and will call you later." Noah slid the croissants into the oven, then turned back. "So we've got the house all to ourselves, it seems."

"So it seems." Grace toyed with her coffee, added more milk, then toyed with the cup again.

"Sit down and relax."

When she started to pull out a chair, Noah caught her hand. "Here," he said, drawing her down onto his lap with a quick tug. "Tell me what happened when you fell," he said quietly.

"Did Jilly tell you about that?" Grace fidgeted, avoiding his eyes. "It worked out okay. We closed off the room."

"It could have been worse. Promise me you'll be careful."

Her eyes darkened at the sound in his voice. More of that enchanting color swirled through her cheeks. Noah was shocked at a sudden urge to rip away that blue belt and see how she looked underneath. He had dreamed about it for a few centuries already.

Because he was losing the battle, he focused on feeding her one of the strawberries from the refrigerator.

"I—thank you."

"Have another. She also said you aren't eating enough."

"I'm eating fine." She stopped to take another strawberry he held to her mouth. In the process, sweet juice spilled between her teeth, darkening her lips.

Noah couldn't take his eyes away, brushing the spot slowly with his thumb. He drew the sweet juice into his own mouth.

A fresh wave of color flamed through her face. Noah realized she had to feel the effect she was having on him. Every time her hips moved, the brush of her body made him harder.

"Can I get you something else? I saw bottled water in the fridge. Some kind of juice—"

"Nothing." Her voice was husky. She seemed to

be staring at his mouth. "I was going to feed you an amazing meal, then sit with you by the fire and find out everything that's been happening. About the kittens, about Ivan. About your parents and your job. But the whole time I was sleeping, I felt your arms around me. And I realized how much I wanted them around me again, Noah. Upstairs. Under that big down quilt." She gave a soft laugh. "I can't believe I'm trying to seduce you up to bed."

She was doing a very successful job of it, he thought. His body was responding completely.

"You're working too hard. You're worrying too much." He ran his hand along her ankle and up her leg. "Tomorrow you can tell me how I can help. But tonight...I'm happy to be seduced."

GRACE WAS TOO BUSY looking into those dark, intense eyes to hear him at first. Too busy thinking how good it felt to have his arms around her.

She had learned something in the weeks since she had last seen him. She had come to understand that life had its own currents and timetables. Sometimes life could know what you wanted and needed even though it was still a mystery to you.

When his hand brushed a drop of strawberry pulp from her lip, she felt something pull loose inside her, freeing her from her old rules and old cautions.

He lifted her hand to his lips and kissed each knuckle, then the sensitive palm. Time seemed to slow. The moment trembled between them, alive with possibilities. But how did you know you were making the right choice, seeing the real person and not the one you wanted to be there?

You didn't.

The answer was just that simple. You took a deep breath and opened your arms to all that made you feel alive. That's what her grandmother would have told her.

You had to start somewhere. Otherwise you lived half a life, always watching from the sidelines, never jumping in yourself.

"So a woman could seduce you?" she said huskily.

"The right woman." He traced her cheek. "A woman who would climb into a Dumpster in a snowstorm to rescue a lost cat. A woman who isn't afraid to take a risk when she follows a dream."

She looked up slowly. Savoring the hard lines of his face. The keen, brooding eyes.

The strong, expressive mouth.

She closed her eyes as his lips brushed the curve of her wrist. "I was lost when I saw you in that alley." Noah gave her a slow, heart-stopping smile, and Grace felt her breath catch. How could one smile do that to a person?

"I think—"

"Don't." Noah kissed the curve of her forehead. "Don't think, Grace. Tonight, just close your eyes and let me touch you. Feel all the things that my hands will whisper. Listen to the dreams and the promises." Slowly he traced the arch of her lip.

"Thinking won't get us where we need to go, but this will."

He seduced her with a slow, hot kiss. He wooed her deepest fantasies, showing her his own. Never hurrying. Never pushing. Only offering.

He was a brave man. A complex man, Grace thought. A man who would never be easily read or quickly understood. With a man like this you could throw your heart out the window without a thought. A man like this would catch it and keep it safe.

One night, she thought.

She realized that her choice had already been made, had truly been made for days. Trusting Noah was the easiest thing she had ever done. And she was brave enough—or stubborn enough—to take all that he offered.

She whispered his name and brought her mouth to his. Silence hung heavy between them. Then she took a slow breath. "Who's seducing whom here?"

"So far it's neck and neck," he said hoarsely.

Wind hissed and growled up from the sea, rattling the windows and the eaves. Noah didn't seem to notice. His breath was thick as his hands moved to the belt of her robe.

"I was going to be civilized and give us both more time." His hand slid under her hair, massaging her neck. He bit the curve of her earlobe gently. "But when I touch you, I forget about being civilized."

"Civilization can be highly overrated."

Her eyelids fluttered as his lips brushed the warm hollow behind her ear.

"This is going to get hot fast." He kissed her eyelids, one after the other, then took slow possession of her mouth again. Slow and rough, he whispered how many ways he loved her and how he meant to show her all of them tonight, while the storm whipped the harbor.

Grace swam through the current of his words. Like a dreamer, she dove into the depths of his voice, following sweet-rough waves of whispered emotion.

They started at the bottom of the stairs, mouths searching, both a little drunk as skin met skin in swift shocks of discovery. At the top of the landing, Grace yanked his shirt free, not caring that she tore off two buttons in the process. She sighed when she ran her hands over his flat waist.

It was more than she had imagined, feeling him this way. She seemed to be melting right out of her body, nerve to his nerve, every inch alive and on fire with wanting. And they hadn't even reached the second floor yet.

Rain drummed on the windows as they staggered up another flight. This time Noah tugged one shoulder of Grace's robe down and drew a raw breath when he saw there was nothing underneath. One hand to the wall, he leaned down to take her with his hungry mouth, moving over her with restless skill. The robe fell lower, snapped at her waist and Noah drew her breast into his mouth, tasting and goading until Grace realized she had never known desire, not even close, until Noah's mouth burned over her skin like this.

He made her feel achingly young—and darkly experienced. The combination was another assault on her senses.

They managed six more steps. Their clothes fell forgotten while they claimed and took blindly, then gave back in double measure. Outside the storm hurled wind and rain at the old walls, but for all its problems, Harbor House had been built in earlier times by men and women stout of heart and clear of vision. There would be problems and repairs to come with the old house, but it had stood against decades of storms. This wind would find no opening.

They lost track of anything but each other. With a low sound of pleasure, she shoved him back against the wall, savoring the hard angles of his chest with her hands. Her mouth followed. She nuzzled her way slowly down where the buckle of his belt intrigued her. Her hands trembled when she pulled the belt away and opened the top snap of his jeans.

His muscles clenched. His breath tore into a low groan. "Grace."

Her fingers worked under the soft denim, seduced by warmth and hot muscle. He was hard as her fingers closed around him. Need left her blind and giddy.

Noah gave a strangled laugh and caught her wrists with hands that trembled. "It's my turn, honey."

"No, I want to feel you."

"Later. All you want."

Grace sighed in regret as he lifted her. Her back against the wall, she shivered in waves of pleasure, trapped beneath his clever, callused hands. He gave and took, stirring her unspoken need until her body melted against him.

"We're not going to make the bedroom, are we?"

"Doesn't look that way."

She felt his heart hammer. He knelt on the old carpeted stairs. His fingers slid beneath the last bit of cotton at her hips, and her robe fell away, baring creamy skin already sheened with sweat.

His eyes brooded, savored. He whispered her name, the word smoky with the weight of his desire. He kissed her stomach and then his tongue trailed lower until his mouth found her. His hands dug into her thighs, holding her when she trembled, when she gasped in shock as need slammed her up into explosive pleasure.

Noah's hands opened on her hips. He whispered hoarse praise across her skin and then tongued her sleek heat, slipping inside her. Grace's body rocked in another race of pleasure as Noah taught her a dozen kinds of hunger with his mouth and hands. She had never felt more beautiful or more loved. She had never trusted anyone more.

Her body sang, drawn tight in chords that only he could create. She gasped as he skimmed and searched, and she locked her trembling arms around his neck, breathing his name.

The old house seemed to float in restless silence against the roar of the storm as she shuddered, speared her hands into his hair with a raspy cry and fell.

## CHAPTER TWENTY-FIVE

NOAH TOOK A RAW, shuddering breath.

She had amazed him. She had awed him, open and generous with her body and her trust.

She, who had every reason to shy away from trust.

He felt her knees tremble in the wake of passion and he stood, bracing her when she would have fallen. With her body anchored safely, he listened to the howl of the wind from the sea, feeling more than a little savage. Her breathless climax had hit him with a surge of emotions. Possession, desire, unimaginable joy.

He was determined to weave their lives together, no matter what it took. He knew the process wouldn't be easy. His job was a cruel master and for now personal attachments would always have to yield to emergency calls. For her part, Grace had serious commitments to her grandfather, to her friends and to her own dreams. She would always stand by to support the animal shelter that belonged to her beloved grandfather. After Peter Lindstrom recovered....

Noah's grip tightened as she nuzzled his neck. Would he lose her to the dusty roads and far-flung cities, when they drew her away in search of some new exotic type of plant or rare spice?

Neither of them could change what they were.

But both of them had to try.

It would be easier if their lives were less complex, but in the end life had its own gifts. He and Grace would find a path to their future.

Her eyes flickered open. A glorious haze of color swept her cheeks. "Noah. I haven't felt so…hungry. Dizzy. Amazingly alive." She took a shaky breath. "Not ever."

"I like the sound of dizzy and amazing. How about we go for unforgettable next?"

"You didn't…" She glanced down at his thighs. "I thought you would."

He brushed a wave of hair from her cheek. "We've got all the time in the world, honey."

She wet her lips, looking tousled and hungry and restless in a way that had a fresh ache building, threatening his control. But Noah wasn't about to be hurried. He had waited forever to find her and they were going to have all night to follow this restless dream into being.

Suddenly he saw Grace shiver as a cold wind gusted up the stairs. Only a fool would have gotten so carried away, nearly taking her on the stairs.

Cursing, Noah swept her into his arms and strode up the last flight, leaving their scattered clothes behind. "You're freezing. I want you in a bed. I want soft covers and lots of room."

She flushed again. Her smile grew. "I was hoping you'd say that."

Sheer seduction, he thought.

He laughed as he crossed the top landing. Behind a freshly painted blue door he found the bedroom where Grace had led him to sleep earlier that night. He hadn't noticed much before. Now he saw a single lamp shedding half-light from a chipped side table, and a rug that was probably twenty years old. But the bed made up for everything, tall and graceful with twisting wood posts and crisp sheets topped by a thick quilt.

Grace wrapped her arms around Noah's neck and kissed him hard. When he tried to let her go, she gripped the waist of his jeans and pulled him down so they hit the down quilt together in a tangle of legs and a burst of laughter.

But the laughter stilled when Grace rose to her knees and moved across him, cupping his face. "I love your mouth. I love your chin, too. It says don't mess with me, but then your mouth says, mess with me all you want. And I want to mess with you a whole lot. Here. Here."

Noah closed his eyes, following the road where she was taking them, his body hard with need.

"Definitely...here." She inched down the worn denim and studied his stomach, her eyes shimmering. Noah twisted, pressing her beneath him.

He started to pull off his jeans, but Grace caught his hand.

"I want to do that. I want us both to know that I'm here completely. No regrets or reservations," she said gravely. "I've never felt half the things you make me feel. And that's why I need to do this." She pulled his jeans free and then the white cotton beneath.

Grace leaned down, her fingers trembling. Every move she made felt perfect to him. When her mouth opened, Noah bit back a groan, wrapping his leg across her naked thighs and lifting her up to ease his fingers against her.

Her back arched and she opened to him, gasping his name, pressing down to find his body waiting.

She closed around him sleekly and Noah lifted her, moving in a rhythm that left them both crazy and panting. The blind call of release throbbed through Noah's blood. He fought for control, to savor every second of her wild, joyous giving, so aching in its beauty. Then her legs tightened around him and her nails dug into his shoulders. She raised her head. He saw her eyes darken, dazed with her climax.

Noah's fingers snaked through hers. He let the pleasure rock her and then he took her up again, driving deep until she shuddered and closed around him, their joining complete.

Only then did Noah let himself follow her down, deep into the brooding need and chaos, her name on his lips, their fingers entwined.

A FEW LIFETIMES LATER, Grace let out a shaky breath. Her hand moved slowly to Noah's shoulder. "I may be breathing again. In case you're interested."

"Breathing is good." Noah heard the rasp in his own voice. With the last of his energy he pulled her closer and guided her head to his shoulder. "I try to do it all I can."

Rain drummed at the old windows. In the quiet room neither spoke.

There was no sense of withdrawing. No awkward searching for words. Instead, they seemed to breathe together, testing this new space, growing even closer in their linked silence.

Noah snaked one arm across her waist. "I love your waist. I love your hips. I love how you fill my hands." His fingers opened, enjoying her curves. Funny, he had always liked petite women. It had become a kind of habit.

Yet now all he wanted was long legs and real curves. Full breasts and strong arms. All he wanted was Grace, with her broken fingernails and her cool strength.

He smiled when her palm spread possessively on his stomach. She traced the ridged muscles. "I can talk again. But none of the words seem good enough."

Noah simply nodded. "I know what you mean."

Grace slid to her side. She traced his mouth, then kissed his ear. She feathered the hollows with her tongue, smiling when Noah's breath caught. "What happens next?"

"Your choice, honey."

"Hmm." She brought their bodies together. He was already hard, already filling her as she breathed his name in husky surprise.

Her gasp turned to a sigh as he lifted her higher, thigh to thigh. Her head fell back and her nails drove into his shoulders. She bit the curve of his ear, moving to meet him, lost in passion.

Then she took him home inside her, past the shadows and the memories of old loss, past betrayal and regret, giving herself completely, trusting all that they could become together.

The rain grew less intense. The wind stilled to a sigh. Fog crept over the harbor and across the snug houses that hugged the coast. A first gray shimmer of dawn touched the sky.

Beneath the thick quilt Grace and Noah slept, their bodies curled together, and in the wake of the storm the journey to weave their lives together began.

# CHAPTER TWENTY-SIX

"YOU SHOULD BE RESTING." Gage Grayson frowned at his radiant wife. "It's nearly eleven."

"I won't melt. Besides, I'm almost done here." Caro Grayson gave the wooden mantel another swipe with her grandmother's favorite lemon oil, finally satisfied when the smooth grain glowed. "That's done. Now I'm going to knit for a bit."

"You should go to bed and try to sleep, honey. I know these last few days haven't been easy for you. I can feel you toss and turn."

Caro started to deny her growing restlessness, then took a deep breath and touched her husband's cheek. "Okay, I admit it. My back hurts more than ever, and if I get any bigger I may not be able to stand up without help. I hate feeling so big and clumsy. But I hate complaining about it, too. So now that I've admitted the truth why don't we put it to rest? It won't change anything, Gage. Knitting calms me down and right now I need that badly."

Neither one mentioned the other source of Caro's worry. Her husband was going back to a war zone in less than forty-eight hours. The certainty of the danger waiting for him there weighed on them both, especially with Caro's delivery date only two weeks away.

"How about I make you some of that herbal tea your grandmother dropped off? The one with the chamomile."

"I'd like that." With a little grimace, Caro slid into her favorite recliner near the fire. Bogart circled the room and then came to lie near her feet.

Gage tucked a big, hand-knitted afghan around her. "What do you think about this guy Grace is seeing? Noah something or other."

"Noah McLeod. Jilly said he seems reliable. Grace lights up when she's with him, according to Jilly. After what she's been through, I'm glad for anyone or anything that can make her laugh again. But who's to say?"

Gage stirred the fire. "I've got friends I can call to check him out."

"Grace won't like it." Caro looked uncertain. "I don't want to interfere in her private business."

"You're looking out for a friend. Nothing wrong with that. She'd do the same for you," Gage said calmly. He leaned down to scratch Bogart's head. "You want me to rub your back?"

Caro shot him a radiant smile. "That would be lovely. But I want to knit a little first."

"Okay." Gage rummaged in the kitchen and then returned with his wife's tea. "By the way, watch this. I've been teaching Bogart a few things." Gage tossed a treat in the air, and the dog shot to his feet, eyes alert. But instead of going for the food, the big dog ran into the bedroom and returned with a pair of Grace's slippers in his mouth. He ran to her chair and dropped the slippers in her lap, looking very pleased with himself.

"That's wonderful, honey. What a good dog you are, Bogart." Grace scratched the dog's favorite spot, smiling as the dog slumped, nuzzling her hand and whining. She glanced at Gage. "What does that mean?"

"He doesn't get the treat until you have your slippers on and you're sitting down with the afghan. He's going to be acting in my stead, making sure you don't overdo it. Every time you give him a treat, he checks on you. It will be a good system for you both while I'm gone."

While I'm gone.

The moment he said the words, Gage regretted them. Neither of them needed to be reminded that his leave was running out. Within hours he would be driving along the curving coast road, headed back to Portland.

Grace turned away, leaning down to look at her knitting. But Gage wasn't fooled by her sudden attention to her wool. "Honey, you know that I..."

"Don't. I can't talk about it, Gage." Her voice broke. "We have to do this and talking won't change anything."

"Caro." Gage knelt beside her and cupped her

cheeks. A single tear glistened. "Cry if you need to. It hurts me like hell, too."

"I don't want you to remember me crying. I want you to have the very best to take with you. Over there," she said. "Oh, Gage. I'm going to miss you so much. I don't know how I can bear it."

His arms closed around her and he held her as her body shook with the sobs she could no longer hold back. Their fingers linked and she squeezed hard, as if she was trying to hold back the hour of departure that was coming too soon. Bogart barked, squeezing up against her, tail banging in Gage's face, and Bacall bounded across the room to see what the fuss was about. In one leap the white cat jumped onto Gage's shoulders and began to purr.

"Hail, hail, the gang's all here," Gage said after a long time. "It's all going to be fine, honey. I can feel it. I've had these dreams lately—images of you near a white fence with a big tree. It's some kind of field, and there's a big farm table out in the middle, full of great food. It feels like summer and all your friends are there."

"There's a big tree up in the meadow above the sea. It was my favorite place growing up. Maybe that's in the dream."

"See? It's a good omen." Gage squeezed her shoulder. "It's all going to be fine." He brushed the tears from har face. "Believe it."

He rested his head on her hair. They didn't move for a long time. Even in their pain, they gave strength to each other, anchored in the unbreakable threads of their love.

When Gage finally went to make a call to check on Grace's grandfather, Caro snuggled against Bacall. She shed a few last tears, hidden in the cat's soft fur. She didn't believe in premonitions or dreams, but she was going to work hard to believe in those that Gage had seen.

And that he would be home soon.

GAGE WAITED UNTIL Caro was asleep before slipping out his cell phone and moving quietly to the living room. He dialed and waited impatiently.

The man answered on the first ring. He launched into a report with no preamble. Just the facts and only what was required. He was exactly as Gage remembered him from Afghanistan.

"No problems noted. I'm parked down the back street. So far, three perimeter checks. Everything's quiet."

Gage relaxed. It wasn't a war zone here. No snipers on the cliffs.

But nothing got past his friend Tyler. A fellow Marine from Afghanistan, Tyler was a man of few words. He had saved their squad more than once in mountain ambushes.

Gage owed Tyler, and Gage always repaid his debts. Tyler was at loose ends, back in the States after a medical discharge courtesy of an artillery round that had blown out his right eardrum and torn up his shoulder. Though his friend would never mention it, Gage knew that Tyler needed a mission and purpose. The Marines had been his life for eighteen years. Shifting gears to find his way as a civilian was not going to be easy for a hard case like Tyler. The answer had come to Gage during a long, restless night.

He wasn't about to leave Caro here alone, about to deliver and involved in a complicated and expensive renovation of the old Harbor House. She had good friends and close family nearby, but Gage needed to know that she was safe at all times and that someone he could trust was close in case of a problem. Tyler fit the bill.

He would watch over Caro like a bulldog and she'd never know he was there.

Gage felt slightly guilty about the arrangement. He didn't like being deceptive with his friend and his wife. To Tyler, he had implied that Caro's health was a little bit worse than it was, aware that a personal request like this would be just the morale builder Tyler needed. Gage didn't want Caro to feel as if he didn't trust her or have confidence in this new undertaking at Harbor House. It was just the opposite. He knew his wife well enough to guess that she would tackle any challenge head-on and ask for help only as a last resort. The same held true for her two friends. All three of them were tough, stubborn and capable women. But with the baby due in weeks, Caro needed extra protection, even if Gage had to provide it by deception. All he had told his wife was that Tyler was a fellow Marine from Afghanistan, describing the hostile action in which Tyler had saved his life. That one conversation had been enough to ensure that Caro welcomed the ex-Marine with open arms, no reservations and no questions asked.

Tyler would have a home on Summer Island as long as he needed it, and that was exactly what Gage wanted.

He hated leaving Caro, hated knowing he would miss seeing their baby being born and witnessing the miracle of the new life their love and commitment had created. But nothing would change his duty and commitment to his country. He would board his plane and not look back, keeping his focus on his men during the difficult weeks to come. He had heard hints of a new campaign to cut terrorist supply routes through the mountains. Word was that it was going to be a long, protracted struggle.

He was ready. Whenever, wherever. He would see the mission through.

To know that Tyler was here close by, keeping a close eye on things, was going to make leaving a whole lot easier.

"When do you head out, Lieutenant?"

Gage frowned at the term of address. Tyler was out of the military now. He would have to start getting accustomed to civilian behavior and informality. "No need to call me Lieutenant, Tyler."

"Yes, sir."

Gage looked out the window, smiling slightly. "You're a civilian now, Tyler."

"So they tell me, sir." He didn't sound happy about it.

Something soft bumped Gage's knee. He looked down and scooped up his white cat. Bacall purred louder, rubbing her head against his chest.

"Everything okay, Lieutenant? What's that noise?"

"Relax, Tyler. It's just my cat. Bacall doesn't sleep any better than I do these days. And I fly out in thirty-six hours."

Silence fell, both men caught up in dark memories. At the other end of the line Gage could hear the sound of wind and the muffled slap of waves. He knew that Tyler was bunkered down somewhere near the water, but he didn't ask for details. No one was more thorough than Tyler. He could vanish in plain sight, and he always got the job done.

His wife would be in good hands here.

"In that case, I'll sign off, sir. You've got better things to do than shoot the breeze with me."

The line went dead.

The man had no social skills whatsoever, Gage thought wryly. He was a definite hard case. But even hard cases needed friends and a place to belong. They needed a family most of all. Finding Tyler a family was another thing on Gage's very long to-do list.

But right now he had to get upstairs to bed. Caro never slept well these days. He didn't want his wife waking up alone any sooner than she had to.

## CHAPTER TWENTY-SEVEN

JILLY WAS IN THE KITCHEN cooking when Noah and Grace finally wandered downstairs, looking very satisfied—and very hungry.

She made a point of not mentioning the beard burn on Grace's neck. She also made a point of not mentioning the nail marks across the Noah's neck, just above the edge of his T-shirt.

They had definitely had an interesting night. She was pleased that she was only a little bit jealous. "So, what will it be, blueberry and sour cream pancakes or huevos rancheros? Everything's ready to go. I stocked up yesterday."

Noah glanced at Grace, one eyebrow raised.

"The eggs sound wonderful. I know how great you make them. Then again your pancakes are amazing too, Jilly. How about…both?" Grace ran a hand through her hair and smiled crookedly. "I have the most outrageous appetite this morning."

Jilly managed to bite off the smart-ass reply that shot to her lips. No point in embarrassing Grace. Or Noah. "You've got it. Have a seat. I brought a folding table down from the attic and set it up in the front room, overlooking the harbor. It's still a little cloudy, but the worst of the storm is past. And I've got some great news."

She whirled an apron deftly around her waist and flipped a hand towel over her shoulder. "My contractor friend has already been here. He says the hole is contained, and the whole storage room needs to be gutted, but structurally things are sound. He doesn't think it's going to be a big problem. The sooner we get it done, the better, so he's working up a complete bid today. I should have a figure soon. You may want to pray, however. We're going to need it."

"That sounds reassuring." Noah slid his arm around Grace's waist. "Isn't there something I can do to help?"

"Yeah. Go sit down. No one interferes when I'm cooking." Jilly made shooing motions with her towel.

They walked out hand in hand and Jilly saw Grace tilt her head up for Noah's kiss.

Oh, Jilly remembered how it felt.

Heaven one minute and hell the next. As far as she was concerned, being in love was highly overrated. Fortunately, she wouldn't be in love again anytime soon.

When she finished cooking, she served plates of food nonstop, dishing up a stream of cooking anecdotes that were largely humorous at her own expense. Next came her ongoing problems with subcontractors and repairmen. Lawyers came in a close

second. "And don't get me started on the food critics."

Soon she had Noah and Grace laughing until they
were red-faced, unable to believe the bizarre dis-
guises that food critics used to hide themselves in
a restaurant where they were known, as well as the
crazy lengths that chefs went to in order to court
those same food critics. Her entrance into the food
world had been an eye-opener, and Jilly certainly
had battle wounds from encounters with food critics.

Out of the corner of her eye, she saw that Noah
and Grace were holding hands under the table. What
mattered most to her was that Grace looked radiant,
calm and rested.

Duffy barked suddenly. Feet stamped across the
back wooden stairs. The big puppy launched into a
mad charge straight through the kitchen in a flurry
of excitement when Gage opened the door and held
it for his wife. With the skill born from experience,
Gage moved in front of Caro, cutting off Duffy's
crazy charge before the dog could leap against her
chest.

Gage sank down on one knee, rubbing the puppy's head. "Hey there, Duffy. Are they giving you
enough steak? You look a little run-down today. I've
got Bogie and Bacall out in the car. How about you
and Bogie and I take a run on the beach while Mom
here puts her feet up?"

Jilly could have sworn that Duffy knew the names

of Gage's two pets, because the puppy threw back his head and howled happily.

Gage laughed. "I'll take that for a yes, bud."

While he snapped on Duffy's leash, Gage shot a look through the door at Noah. "Everything okay in there?"

"Excellent," Jilly said. "You want me to introduce you?"

"After our walk. Bogart has been all wound up this morning. I'll wear them out and then you can make the introductions." He frowned, studying Noah's head.

The air seemed heavy. Testosterone popped. Men sizing up other men, Jilly thought, rolling her eyes.

Gage opened the door and let Duffy outside for their walk. "Catch you in a few minutes," he called back. "Don't let Caro start cleaning cabinets or going up and down stairs, Jilly. Her feet and back are bothering her again. Make her sit down and rest."

He closed the door fast, before he could hear his wife's sharp protest.

Smart man, Jilly thought. But then it would have taken a smart man and a very good man to capture her friend's heart.

Concerned for Caro, Jilly launched into action. She cleared a place at the table, set out a steaming pot of herbal tea and glared until Caro sat down. After making introductions, she stacked food in front of Caro and tapped her foot until her friend took a bite of everything.

"You're just as good a cook as you always were," Caro said. "These pancakes are killer, don't you think, Noah?"

"No doubt about it. Probably that explains why I just ate seven of them."

Caro took a sip of tea, looking thoughtful. "Maybe we should have a special breakfast at the café here. An early-bird menu, with knitting on the side for people who have a busy day ahead. You know, a workout for your fingers before the day begins. Those pancakes would be amazing, Jilly."

"Good idea. I'll put it down in my BlackBerry. I've got some ideas for publicity, too. I thought every Friday between noon and one we could have some dessert item heavily discounted at three for the price of one. But the clincher is, they have to bring two extra people. That's an easy way to bring in bodies. One person pays and two of them eat for free. Who would say no to that?"

"Not bad," Caro said. "You really do have a promotion brain up there, hidden behind the chef's toque, don't you?"

"You make it sound like a social disease," Jilly snapped, huffing back to the kitchen.

Caro shot to her feet and followed her. "I didn't mean it like that, Jilly. We know you're doing twice the work of any normal person. We couldn't do this without you."

After a moment Jilly sighed. "Sorry. I'm a little prickly worrying about that floor repair. But you need to go back and sit down, remember? Go keep Grace and Noah company while I finish in here."

Caro rubbed her back. "As if they'd notice. Love is in the air," she said with a quiet laugh. But she pulled out her knitting bag and went back to the table.

By the time Gage returned, the three were deep in a discussion of vintage stair rails and crown molding.

Thick as thieves, Jilly thought.

Gage was carrying his other pet, Bacall, a beautiful white cat with striking blue eyes. Bogart, his golden retriever, charged off after Duffy to explore the house.

"They're definitely wound up today." Gage sauntered into the front room and leveled a searching look at Noah. "I'm Gage. Nice to meet you."

More of that undefined testosterone, Jilly noted.

"Do you want to have a look at the power box? It's going to need a major overhaul, and I've been kicking around some ideas with the electrician."

Noah nodded and pulled on the sweatshirt hanging behind his chair. "Sounds good to me." He leaned over to kiss Grace and then followed Gage through the kitchen. The two were deep in a discussion of transformers and wiring specs when the door closed.

Jilly sniffed. "First they'll go look at the wiring. Then I give you odds they'll stop at Gage's truck. They'll discuss the carburetor or the fuel injection system or the antilock brakes and they'll probably be out there for an hour. Men," she muttered.

Grace stood up and stretched lazily. "But they do have their uses."

"That's obvious."

Grace flushed. "Stop looking at me that way, you two. Noah is nice—no, he's fabulous. When I'm with him I feel wonderful. But it's too early. Don't start ordering place cards for a wedding reception."

"Wouldn't dream of it." Jilly smiled broadly at Caro. "Wait—what's that sound I keep hearing?"

"I don't hear anything." Grace leaned close to the window. "Just the wind."

"The wind...and the sound of wedding bells," Jilly said firmly. As usual, she had the last word.

"NICE JOB ON THE CARBURETOR." Noah leaned an elbow on the hood and studied Gage. "And you can stop checking me out. I'm going to do what's best for Grace. I won't hurt her."

"Glad to hear it. She's had a tough time. She doesn't need another upheaval." Gage reached down, muttering as he wiped a drop of oil off his sock. "I knew I shouldn't have worn these. Caro knitted them for me. They're my favorite pair."

"No kidding. Grace hasn't offered." Noah rubbed his neck. "Those look comfortable."

"Like walking on air," Gage said proudly. "By the way, it's too bad that she hasn't heard about that big digital project yet. It would be a great fit with her research skills."

Noah's eyes narrowed. "She heard. And she got it. But she opted out because she was worried about her grandfather."

"But she told Caro—" Gage stopped, tossing the cleaning rag from hand to hand. "I see. She wanted to protect her grandfather. She didn't want him to know and feel bad about the choice she made. Women are something." Gage glanced at Noah. "They can be very complicated sometimes."

Noah decided he liked this Marine. "Tell me about it."

"ARE THEY STILL OUT THERE?" Jilly emerged from the kitchen, up to her elbows in flour. "I thought I heard the sound of wrenches banging."

"Still out there. They've got the hood up on the truck now. Gage took something out, wiped it with a rag, and Noah put it back in."

"Men," Jilly muttered. "Show them a *Playboy* magazine or a carburetor cap and their brains turn to mush and ooze out their ears." She raised a hand abruptly when Caro started to stand up. *"You. Sit.* Anything that needs to be gotten, Grace or I will get it. No arguing."

Caro sat down in the big rocking chair near the window. She closed her eyes and rubbed her back.

"How much does it hurt?" Grace asked quietly

after Jilly vanished back into the kitchen, banging pots and baking trays. "The truth."

Grace had seen her friend's frown. It was clear that Caro was feeling all the discomfort of the last weeks of pregnancy.

"It only hurts when I breathe," Caro said. "Some days are better than others, but I take it as a good sign. It won't be long until I have this baby."

There was a firmness and certainty in her voice that made Grace feel a quick, sharp pang of envy. Caro was glowing, looking every inch the way a healthy and confident mother-to-be should. What would it feel like to be carrying the child of the man you loved? Grace wondered.

And what would it feel like to know he was leaving within hours, going back to war?

The thought left her sick with worry, but she hid her feelings. After pouring Caro another cup of herbal tea, Grace pulled out the scarf she had been working on for Jilly. "I mangle one more stitch, I'm tossing this thing out the window. It's rated as an easy pattern, nice mindless knitting, but I seem to make a mistake every other stitch."

"You're just distracted, and it's easy to see the source of your distraction standing outside. He is one gorgeous man. So enjoy it. Relax and go with the flow."

Grace gave a dry laugh. "It's not easy. In my family, going with the flow was not a prized state of mind. I love my grandfather and respect all his years of work and dedication, but an easygoing man he is not."

"Then it's time that you helped him start. Give him a few lessons. He's going to have to learn to relax when he comes home from the hospital," Caro pointed out quietly.

"I know. I've already talked with your grandmother about how we're going to keep him busy. Andy, from the clinic, has already set up a little woodworking shop in our garage. I know that's the one thing my grandfather always wanted to do. Now he won't have any excuses."

"That's a great idea. I'm sure you could convince Andy to spend some time with him, too. I'm not sure that either one of them has much of a social life outside the animal clinic," Caro added.

More pans rattled in the kitchen. Jilly emerged, wearing a smile of triumph. "My new French *macarons* are done. After they've cooled, I'll add the ganache filling. Trust me, you haven't known temptation until you've tasted an espresso-filled *macaron*." She leaned toward the window. "Are those idiots still out there under the hood?"

Grace followed her glance. "Now they've got parts from the motor lined up along one fender. They'll probably be out there quite a while."

Duffy raced into the room, came to a halt beside Jilly and whined sharply. "What is with you, Duffy?" Bogie trotted up beside him. "Not food time yet, fellows. I'll take you for a walk later. But for now, get this." She tossed a rope toy and the two raced off.

"Seriously, I'd like your opinion on the *macarons*," Jilly said. "I want to see if I used too much dark chocolate."

After a short pause, all three women laughed. "Too much chocolate?" Grace grabbed Jilly's hand towel and flicked her with it. "Impossible. You should know that by now."

Duffy shot back through the room as the kitchen door opened. Gage scratched the puppy's head. "What's with him?"

"Don't have a clue." Jilly took the rope toy from Duffy and tossed it again, smiling as the dogs raced off again.

Gage sniffed the air. "Something smells good." He crossed the room to his wife. "Honey, the electrician is downstairs. He found some old blueprints of the house that he wants to show me. They're back at his office. It could make a difference in the renovation plans." Gage leaned down, touching his wife's cheek. "Will you be okay here for an hour?"

"Of course. You two go on. I'll just sit here and knit. That smell happens to be the decadent cookies Jilly has just made. I may not move for the rest of the afternoon."

"You're sure?" Gage hesitated, studying his wife's face. "I'd feel better knowing more about the structure of this old place. You're all going to be spending a lot of time here."

"I'll be fine, Gage. Go on with Noah. Take several of Jilly's *macarons* before you leave. They may be gone by the time you get back."

"I think we can manage to save a few," Jilly muttered. "I've made six dozen." She shook flour off her hands, glancing out the window toward the harbor. "That's strange."

"What?" Gage looked over her shoulder. Out in the harbor the water was smooth and leaden, with no waves. Beyond the lighthouse the horizon was a hard, flat line.

Jilly shrugged. "I don't know. The harbor—it's so calm. I'm not used to seeing it that way."

"It looks good to me. Better than a storm. We've already had three big ones in the last two weeks." Gage gave his wife a kiss. "I'll be back soon. You take it easy, honey. No lifting, understand?"

"I promise," Caro said, sticking out her tongue at him. "Nothing heavier than a few *macarons*."

CARO HEARD THE SLAM of the door and her husband's feet on the stairs. She forced herself not to look out the window, not to search for his retreating back. It was a small test and a small victory. She knew the real test would come soon, when Gage left for Afghanistan.

She closed her eyes and rubbed the aching spot in her lower back. For a moment her hand opened and her knitting was forgotten as she felt the sudden surge of movement just below her heart, where a tiny foot kicked restlessly.

*Be safe, little one. He'll come back to us. You'll see.*

She heard the sound of a motor and then Gage's truck moving off down the street.

He *had* to come back to them.

She picked up her knitting and eyed the plate that Jilly held high, filling the air filled with luscious scents.

Grace snagged a *macaron* and took a quick bite. "Jilly, these are pure decadence, and your meringues have perfect little edges. I have a French recipe in one of my books, but yours are different. You have to tell me how many egg whites—"

She didn't finish.

Dishes rattled on the kitchen counter. Wood creaked in the walls and over the front porch and the glass panes shook at the front windows. The floor of the old house seemed to sway sharply.

Jilly spun around, looking confused. "It can't be the floor. They said it was stable." Duffy shot toward her, barking furiously, his whole body rigid.

And then the earthquake struck in earnest.

## CHAPTER TWENTY-EIGHT

THE WALLS CREAKED as the house was plunged into darkness. Caro caught a shaky breath, leaning against the wall. "Power's out. Must be an earthquake—I can't remember the last time we had one." She pressed one hand to her chest, over her hammering heart. "We have to get outside. Right now." Behind her a window shattered in the kitchen.

"You go first," Jilly said hoarsely. "Duffy!" Jilly grabbed the frightened puppy's collar and swung around toward the front of the house. "Caro, go. We'll be right behind you. Call Bogart."

At Caro's call, the big dog shot past, circled Caro's feet, and then stopped short. He stared into the darkness and whined.

"Bogie, honey, come on. We have to go." Caro grabbed for his collar, but the retriever pulled free, scrambling toward the door off the kitchen. "No!" Caro called. "Bogie, stay. Don't—"

She blanched as she heard Bacall's high-pitched meow from down the hall. "Sweet heaven, the cat must be back there somewhere. Bogart knew. We have to—"

"You have to get out *now*," Jilly snapped. She pushed Caro toward the door, one hand firm at her back. "Take Duffy's collar and go outside. We'll get the other two out. Go, Caro."

The walls creaked ominously. Caro touched her stomach protectively and turned toward the front door. Voices seemed to echo from a distance, along with the sound of powerful motors. The front door hinges rattled.

"Hurry up," Caro called.

"We'll be right there." Grace walked blindly through the darkness, wincing when she hit the table. By touch alone she found her knitting bag slung over her chair and dug out her lighted knitting needles from an interior pocket. With one quick flick of the switch, the room glowed in pale blue light.

Jilly moved behind her, pointing at Bogart. The dog was right outside the partially open door to the storage room, growling low in his throat.

"Here, you take one of these needles. Let's get him out of here." Grace shot ahead of Jilly. When she held up her lighted knitting needle, she saw Bacall's white shape inside the storage room. The cat was pressed rigidly against the wall.

A new crack stretched ominously in her direction. As the floor creaked, the little cat tried to leap away. She hit the wall, stunned, and toppled in a wild struggle toward the splintering hole, down into the darkness.

GAGE SLAMMED ON HIS BRAKES as the first wave hit.

An oak tree toppled in front of him and leaves rained down over the windshield. "Earthquake," he said hoarsely.

Noah jumped from the truck, racing down the center of the street. A branch hit the cement beside him, toppling a fence. Windows broke somewhere nearby. Grimly, Noah leaped over the tangle of branches and fallen wood and kept going, with Gage close behind.

Another tree fell. Noah pulled up the hood of his sweatshirt and kept running, his face grim. He saw a figure charging up the back steps of the Harbor House. "Who's that at the back stairs?"

"A friend," Gage snapped. "If there's a way inside, he'll find it. Head for the front."

"I don't understand," Noah said curtly.

"Trust me and go for the front."

Something hissed overhead. Gage bit back a curse as a power line swayed crazily, then plummeted straight toward them, raining white sparks over the ground and blocking their way to the front steps.

The figure at the back steps leaned out. Gage gestured sharply to the back door. "Tyler, get inside. Get them out. We'll work our way past this power line up through the next yard and then back around through the front."

At least he prayed they could get in.

Gage felt sweat dotting his forehead.

"Copy that, Lieutenant." Tyler gave a two-finger wave and then disappeared.

THEY HAD TO GET THE CAT.

The floor was still shifting and Grace wouldn't leave her.

She heard Caro's awkward steps as she pulled Duffy toward the front door. Meanwhile, Jilly was trying to hold Bogart, who was barking wildly. She vanished, then called out from the kitchen, "Salmon. Bacall loves it. Let's pray that it works."

Jilly reappeared with a wedge of fish and a big produce basket. Holding her lighted knitting needle up, Grace led the way to the storeroom.

She leaned toward the frantic cat. "Come on, Bacall. Everything will be fine, honey. Come and get your treat."

She dropped the fish into the basket and lowered it into the crack, afraid that her weight would make the hole bigger. But the cat was frozen, crouching on a beam just below the floor edge.

"Hurry," Jilly snapped. "Try again."

Grace took a breath and inched toward the hole, feeling sweat drop into her eyes as she lowered the basket slowly. "Come on, Bacall. Come here to the basket. You're going to be fine, baby." Grace stretched flat, forcing down a wave a fear as the floor creaked beneath her.

"Reach over your right shoulder," Jilly whispered. "I've got a rope. Thread it through the handle of the basket and you can lower it down to Bacall. But don't go any closer to that hole."

Grace dropped the rope twice before she managed to knot it into place. Carefully, she lowered the basket toward the beam where the cat huddled in terror, her white tail fluffed wide, her eyes huge. "Come on, honey. Right over here," Grace whispered. "You can smell the fish, can't you?"

The floor moved as another tremor hit.

"Jilly, you should go out," Grace said quietly.

"Like hell. Get that basket down and grab her. I'll be right here to hold you if..."

*If the floor collapsed.*

Jilly blew out a breath. "But she's too terrified to move."

*Just like me,* Grace thought wildly. "There has to be a way. Jilly, didn't Gage leave his knit hat on the table? Maybe if we drop his hat in the basket..."

Jilly ran for the hat while Grace talked quietly to the panicked cat. It seemed like an eternity before she felt Jilly's hand on her shoulder and then the brush of wool against her hand.

"Give it a shot." Jilly held up a real flashlight from the kitchen. She sucked in a breath as the sudden light filled the storeroom.

Bacall had backed up to the very edge of the wood. One more movement and she would go over.

NOAH JUMPED OVER the fallen fence that circled the Harbor House. With Gage right behind him, he clambered up onto the front porch, then pushed aside a broken table. The front door opened with a squeal of hinges.

Caro appeared, gripping Bogart's collar, her face white with strain. The man Noah had seen at the back stairs had his arm around Caro's shoulders, guiding her outside.

Noah heard Gage's sharp, indrawn breath as he lunged and caught his wife to his chest. "Thank God you're safe." He shot a glance at Noah. "I'm taking her to the truck, away from falling debris. Tyler, I'll come back after—"

"No. Stay there with her," Noah ordered. He shot a glance at the tall man near the door. "I could use some help."

"You got it," the man called Tyler said. "Go take care of your wife, Lieutenant. We'll handle things here."

Bogart did not want to leave, and Gage had to pull the whining dog down the slope away from the house. A fire truck rounded the corner, sirens flashing, and the dog howled in a frenzy.

"Better hurry." The man at the door glanced up and cursed as another glass pane broke free and shattered onto the porch.

Noah jumped the pile of glass. "Where are they?"

"Back there." The tall man gestured toward the back of the darkened house. "They're trying to rescue a cat." He lifted a big tactical flashlight from the pocket of his jacket. "Straight ahead. Watch for broken furniture."

Noah followed the sound of voices from the hallway, passing broken dishes and several overturned chairs. When he crossed the kitchen, he saw Duffy standing protectively next to Jilly. Jilly swung around, her eyes widening.

Then he heard Grace's low, reassuring voice, and a wave of relief hit him in the chest. She was safe. She sounded completely calm.

Noah nodded at Jilly and then moved toward Grace. His hands clenched when he saw the widening crack in the old wood floor.

"That's it, honey. Just a little bit more, and you'll be in the basket. Come on here to Momma Grace."

Tyler shone his light over Jilly's shoulder. Noah saw Grace lying prone, her body stretched at a heart-stopping angle over the widening crack in the floor. She held a big basket out toward the white cat huddled on a broken beam just under the floor.

"Go with Tyler," Noah whispered to Jilly, never taking his eyes off Grace. "He'll help you with Duffy. I'll get Grace and the cat."

Jilly gripped Duffy's collar, staring from one man to the other. Then she took a hard breath and nodded. Tyler simply lifted the dog over his shoulder and rushed Jilly out toward the door.

Without a word Noah knelt behind Grace and gripped her waist, holding her securely in case the situation went south fast. With his other hand he gripped one leg of the heavy butcher-block table just inside the door. It wasn't a great backup plan, but it was the best he could manage on short notice.

"Noah," Grace whispered. "I'm feeling a little precarious here."

Down in the hole, the white shape moved.

"That's it, honey. Get into the basket. We'll have you out in a few seconds. Good girl." Grace began to pull up the basket, slowly rising onto her elbows. The floor creaked ominously.

Noah grabbed her belt, pulling her backward in a quick, powerful movement. With the basket anchored between them, he swung Grace up into his arms and raced for the front door.

"Noah." Grace's voice broke. "I was so…afraid. The floor—"

"Shh. You did great, honey. Just great."

Upstairs another window broke. A pot clanged as it dropped onto the kitchen floor. The front door hinges creaked and the big door tilted sharply.

Gage's friend was right outside, and he caught the weight of the big door on his shoulder, holding it while Noah squeezed past. "The other woman is down at the sidewalk," he said to Noah. "The front rails are down. Take the left side of the porch. And stand clear of that fallen power line. The firemen haven't capped it yet."

"What about you?"

"I got it."

Noah gave a quick nod and crossed the porch, intensely aware of Grace's hands at his shoulders and the slam of her heart against his chest.

It seemed to take forever to climb over the shaky rails, lift Grace and the frightened cat over to safety and drop to the yard. The big oak had fallen, its branches covering the ground. Two firemen motioned him away as they worked near the fallen power line.

"I'll take the cat. You've got your hands full." Tyler ran by. With a faint grin he scooped up the basket with Gage's cat under one arm and ran off like a crazy quarterback as more firemen fanned out along the debris-filled street.

# CHAPTER TWENTY-NINE

GRACE WAS DIMLY AWARE OF CARS filling the street, parked in crazy angles.

She saw Gage standing protectively in front of Caro, who was now seated inside a fire truck, being examined by one of the firefighters. Other than being pale, she looked fine.

Relief made Grace giddy.

Noah pulled her against his chest. She heard the hammer of his heart, almost as loud as her own. "You're crazy brave, you know that?"

"Not brave. I was terrified," she whispered. "But I couldn't leave Bacall behind. I couldn't let her be hurt."

"Of course you couldn't. Maybe next time you could ask for help though. I can't take too many shocks like the one I had when I saw you out on that beam," he said hoarsely.

"Sorry."

"To hell with sorry." He kissed her, his grip suddenly tight, his breath shuddering.

And Grace fell into the kiss, drawing on his strength and the desire that flared almost in the same breath. She wanted to stay. She needed to lean. With the danger still pounding in her blood, she needed to touch him and be touched.

But there were too many questions that remained. The earthquake could have damaged her house, the shelter, even the hospital where her grandfather was. She had to check, to be certain they were safe.

"Noah, I have to—"

"I know." He smiled wryly. "You have to check on everyone else. Let's go find a car. Where to first—hospital, animal shelter or your house?"

"The shelter is on the way to the hospital. I know my grandfather will want a full report. I'll call and check on him while we drive." She looked over her shoulder at the Harbor House. A fallen tree covered the front lawn and most of the front porch. All the ornate old railing was down. Broken glass glistened over the lawn. Jilly was talking to Gage and Caro, pointing to the roof. She turned, white-faced, as if she felt Grace's gaze.

"But first I need to talk to Jilly and Caro," she said softly.

So much loss.

They had invested a part of themselves in this crazy venture. They had planned and sweated to set their dream in motion, and twenty minutes of nature's fury had swept all their work away to nothing.

At least the old house was still standing.

Noah watched her walk to her friends, staying

back just where he was. They needed their time to grieve and to support, to build their strength for the next battle. They stood together, silent, shoulders stiff as firefighters raced up toward the house.

Noah felt Grace's sadness seep out into the silence, joining the sadness of her waiting friends.

They were strong, he told himself. They had each other, with a bond that was nearly tangible. Proud and tough, all of them. But when the adrenaline faded and the knowledge of the loss hit hard, Noah wanted to be there to hold Grace. There would be questions to ask and answer, plans to make.

This was home for her now. He didn't want to be on the far side of the continent while she chased a dream here by the sea. He had been pondering the possibilities for weeks.

It wouldn't be easy.

Building something that lasted forever never was. And forever was what he wanted.

Noah heard Gage crunch over the fallen branches, sliding his fists deep into his pockets as he stared at the wreckage on the front yard.

"They're all safe," Noah said. "It could have been worse."

Gage nodded grimly. "I keep telling myself that. But it was too close. Too damned close. And now there will be repairs, structural damage. Who knows where it will stop, or if the whole place is even safe to repair. Maybe..." He shook his head. "I wouldn't say that in front of Caro. But I'll say it to you. I don't want them in danger." His voice hardened. "And I'll be leaving soon. Will you be going back?"

"I can manage a few more days. I'll do everything I can."

It wasn't the answer Gage wanted. They both knew it.

They stood in the slanting sunlight, and the broken windows looked like haunted eyes.

NOAH INSISTED ON DRIVING Grace's truck, determined that she should rest.

She took quiet, jerky breaths that told him the adrenaline was still ripping through her, leaving every nerve raw. This was the dangerous transition time when you tried to fit the memories of danger back into the neat, orderly boxes of your regular life.

Most of the time it didn't work. Bad things happened then, Noah knew. He had experienced that state all too often.

So he did the only thing he could—listen. Not offering empty hope and not telling Grace that everything would be fine. The house could be a total loss. They wouldn't know anything for sure until a structural engineer checked everything out. Noah would get a few names from a government contact back on the East Coast. He wanted the very best people to ensure the safety of the woman he loved.

Meanwhile, Grace moved restlessly in the seat. She put one arm on the windowsill, then put it down again. "Tell me again why you're driving and not me."

"So you can rest. Not that you're doing very much of it. You've been through something pretty traumatic. It might leave you with the shakes. That's what adrenaline does."

"Oh. Right. I'm talking with the adrenaline expert. Except I still don't know exactly what it *is* you do. I don't know who you do it for, either. I only know that you seem to have experience with dangerous things. No. Forget I said that." She sat stiffly, then raised a hand. "I'm *not* going to ask. You'll tell me if you want to or if you can." She didn't give him time to answer, glaring out the window. Noah saw sadness fill her face as they passed another ancient tree, now overturned, roots upended and once strong branches shattered.

"Just don't tell me that we can walk away from the Harbor House, because we can't. It wasn't my idea at first. It was Jilly and Caro who had the plan." She drummed her fingers on the dashboard, frowning. "But as soon as I saw what they had planned, as soon as I realized what this place could be, I was in completely. You have to understand, it's not just a building or a café. It's a place to belong. Jilly never had a home. She grew up in foster care and had a tough childhood," Grace said quietly. "Caro—well, she lost her parents when she was young. I lost mine, too. It's been a bond that we never talk about." She cleared her throat. "I guess we're all looking for a home. The Harbor House was going to be all that and more. Everyone on Summer Island has memories of that rambling, beautiful house. It means something to anyone who has spent a summer here. Walking away from a dream like that just isn't an option."

Noah didn't answer.

Grace shot him a look. "Anything to say?"

"Nope. You've said it all right so far. Dreams don't come often. When they do, you need to reach out for them with both hands. You need to grip them tight and see where they take you."

Noah was doing that right now. Only his dream had brown hair, a stubborn nose and a body that made his heart skitter. "So go on. What are you going to do next?" She needed to talk, not to dam all her feelings up inside. Even if it was underhanded, Noah meant to make her talk. "Are you going to take time to think things over? At the very least, it's going to be expensive to make the repairs. Maybe you should walk away."

"The *last* thing we'll do is give up." She shot him a fierce look, and her hands locked together at her waist. All the tension of the day focused, caught in the space of her fingers. "I already told you, walking away isn't an option. Weren't you listening? Don't you understand why—" She stopped and gave him a crooked little smile. "Oh, I see. You're baiting me. Testing for a commitment. Very clever."

She drummed her fingers on the dashboard again,

frowning at the coast road. "So what will we do next? We'll regroup. Analyze. Get estimates. Plan. I'm good at planning." She jammed her hand through her hair. "Probably we'll cry a lot. We worked so hard in there, Noah. All those broken dishes, ruined shelves, shattered windows. All the hours we put in, wasted. It feels like someone tore off my arm."

He reached across, rested his hand on hers. "It's going to be tough, honey. But you're tough too. And you have two strong friends to back you up. My bet's on you."

"So you're really not going to try to talk me out of this?"

"Could I succeed if I did?"

If she backed down now, Grace wasn't the woman he took her for.

"Of course I won't back down. What I meant was, aren't you going to try? You know all the clichés. Biting off more than you can chew. A house that's turning into a money pit. More dreams than common sense." She gave a tight, shaky laugh. "That's what any sane person would say, right?"

Noah didn't answer. He had to let her work through this for herself. He had to let her be strong for herself. It was the best gift he could give her.

"Of course, we're not complete idiots. If the house is ruined, then it's ruined. If there are beams miss-ing or structural disasters, well—I guess we'll walk away. We'll turn around and close our eyes and let them bulldoze the whole thing back down to dirt.

Then we'll move on." She took a deep, shuddering breath. "Oh, God, please don't let it come to that. I really, really hope it won't come to that," she whispered.

A tear trickled down her cheek. The sight of that single shining sphere drilled right into Noah's chest. He wanted to stop the car, pull her into his lap and kiss away the pain.

An ambulance raced past, siren flashing, another reminder that although the earthquake had passed, its effects were still echoing.

Grace sat stiffly. "I'm lucky to be alive. I'm lucky that no one was hurt. I know that. Whatever happens, we'll deal with it. But I can't bear living three thousand miles away from you, Noah. You're part of my dream, too." Her voice came in a rush. "I want to reach out with both hands and grip what we have, Noah. I won't walk away from that dream, either."

Noah's hands tightened on the wheel. How had she gotten out the words first? If the disaster hadn't struck, he would have already told her exactly how he felt. They would have been making plans for their future. He needed to do that now.

He was about to pull over onto the grass beside the road when Grace leaned over and gestured. "There. Turn left where the road forks. The animal shelter is right up that twisting little road." Her shoulders were tense as if she needed to prepare herself for another shock.

She pulled out her cell phone and dialed, frowning when she got an out-of-service response. "Still no cellular service. I need to call the hospital."

"Aftereffects of the earthquake. Use the landline in the animal shelter."

Noah turned up the driveway and saw half a dozen cars parked in the gravel lot, but no ambulances or fire trucks. That was a good sign. There also didn't seem to be any fallen trees or downed power lines. The building was halfway up the hill, with the ridge behind it. Maybe it had been spared.

But his personal conversation would have to wait until she had checked on the shelter.

Grace barely waited for him to come to a halt, jumping down and running over the gravel. As soon as he turned off the motor, Noah followed. He heard the frenzied sound of barking.

By the time he got to the door, Grace was talking with a lanky young man who looked harassed, gesturing toward the back of the building. Everything was clean and neat. There were no fallen shelves, no broken furniture. Noah followed Grace down the hall, listening to the noise grow louder. The man— Grace called him Andy—glanced at Noah.

"Why don't you give us a minute or two? You're a stranger, and right now every animal in the place could use a jolt of valium. We don't want to add to any stress."

"No problem. I'll be right out here."

Grace gave him a grateful smile and then pushed open the heavy door. The sound of barking and shrill meows grew deafening. She and Andy joined four other people who were moving from cage to cage, checking locks and security of the wooden structures. One Chihuahua threw itself wildly against the mesh door of the cage in a panic, and Grace knelt down. Noah could almost hear her speaking with quiet reassurance. Andy reached into his pocket and gave her a dog treat, which she maneuvered through the holes in the cage.

The little dog stopped barking, and treats were dispensed all along the row. Blessed silence returned. At the far wall Grace sat down and opened a cage, gently lifting out a collie puppy who appeared to know her well. As Grace spoke, the little tail began to wag. The dog licked her face furiously, gobbling down two treats.

Noah saw her gesture to Andy and say something that Noah couldn't hear. The young man opened two more cages and two more dogs, no longer panicked but ecstatic, raced around Grace in wild circles.

Noah decided he would vanish for a few minutes and do a quick structural check on his own. In his line of work, he had been taught to look for major warning signs of damage, cracks or sagging that dictated an immediate evacuation.

He found a flashlight and took his time circling the building, leaning down to check every inch of the foundation, pulling aside bushes so he wouldn't miss any cracks. He found no shattered windows or broken cement.

The building seemed to have been spared. Of course, they would need a real analysis by an expert. That should go to the top of their list. But for now, Noah felt more optimistic after what he had seen— and what he hadn't seen.

When he walked inside, Grace was waiting for him in the hallway. The collie puppy nestled in her arms, tail wagging. "Everything looks good in here. Some traumatized animals, but they're calming down. You want to take a quick tour?"

"Sure." Noah noticed the natural way she held the dog, the way she spoke calmly while her fingers moved with slow reassurance through the dog's fur.

Years of experience in each touch, he thought. She had watched and learned well. Yes, her grandfather would be very proud of her.

"Andy, meet Noah. He's visiting from D.C. I hope…we'll be seeing a lot of him here."

"Nice to meet you, sir." Andy raised an eyebrow but asked no personal questions. "Oh, I almost forgot to tell you, Grace. Caro's grandmother called from the hospital. She said their phones have been down, but things are fine. She was going to take your grandfather down to the cafeteria for some ice cream. While I had her on the phone, I spoke to Dr. Lindstrom and gave him a full report on the animals. He was worried that some of them might have been hurt. He was worried about you, too, Grace. I told Morgan that you'd call soon."

"My cell phone's out. Is the phone still working here?"

"We got power back right before you arrived. Be my guest. I'm going to finish checking the cages in the other room. Then chow time." He slanted Noah a thoughtful glance. "If you're in the mood, I could use a hand back there."

THE ADRENALINE WAS FINALLY wearing off.

Noah had been right about that. He had been right about a lot of things.

Grace put down the phone, glad that she was sitting down. Her knees felt weak and shaky, and she would have killed for a cup of coffee. But she had managed to reassure her grandfather about her own safety and the state of the animal shelter. Despite the earthquake tremors he had felt, he was calm, and Grace knew much of that calm was due to Morgan, who had been there to distract him during the ordeal.

He had asked her about the Harbor House and whether it had been hurt. Grace had tried to be reassuring. But now that the call was over, the anxiety returned in a flood. What would they do if the repairs were too expensive? And what if it was beyond repairing? What if—

*No.*

Grace closed her eyes. She had meant exactly what she had told Noah. They would plan and analyze, then face the realities. And if one dream ended, another dream began somewhere else. Her grandfather's accident had taught her that much.

But right now she wanted a puppy in her arms. She wanted to feel a wagging tail and the lick of a warm tongue. She wanted comfort in a restless body.

She wanted—

Her breath caught.

Noah was flat on his back in the middle of the floor, surrounded by barking dogs. Andy had opened the cages of some of the more docile dogs and half a dozen of them had raced out to explore. Noah was holding a package of dog treats up in the air, laughing as a German shepherd sat down in the middle of his chest, barking noisily.

Noah just kept laughing and the fight for the treats continued.

As she pushed open the door, Noah's eyes met hers, glinting with humor and intelligence and more than a little mischief. Grace felt the emotion build, felt the love sweep over her and overwhelm her.

But there were still things they had to discuss.

"Well—I've got more calls to make. Catch up with you later." Andy cleared his throat and left, closing the door carefully.

She sat down on the floor next to Noah, pulling the big dog from his chest. "We need to talk. I want to make plans. And I can't when I'm worrying about you." She took a short breath. "I can't stand not knowing if you're safe."

Noah sat up and cupped her face with hands

that weren't quite steady. "I'm careful. I'm trained, honey. Somebody has to do the job. But it won't be for much longer." He brushed the tear from her cheek and kissed her, whispering her name. "I was transferred. I was going to tell you this morning. I thought maybe—" Noah smiled as the collie puppy tried to burrow between them, looking for more treats. "I thought you might come visit."

"Transferred where?"

"To Paris, for three months. Then I can consider other options here in the States. Probably most will be administrative. While I'm in France, I was hoping you could come and show me the ropes. Versailles. The Louvre." His hands tightened. "I'll only be there a few months. And after that—we'll work out the rest. I love you, Grace. I don't want to live three thousand miles away from you, either. I want us to make this work."

Her hands slid into his hair. "Say it again."

"Versailles. The Louvre—"

"No. The part about loving me. I'm listening with all my heart, because it's whole again, Noah. And I'm feeling the kind of love I'd given up on, the one that lasts through six kids, twelve grandkids and a house you grow old in together. But say it again first." She looked down, laughing as the collie wriggled into her lap and licked Noah's chin wildly. "We both want to hear you say it."

"I love you. I loved you from the moment I saw you rifling through that Dumpster. I love how you didn't care that you ruined your coat and shoes to do the right thing." His mouth curved. "I even loved you when you cheated."

"Wait. I didn't cheat."

"Snow down the collar. A definite foul. Then you tripped me during our snowball fight."

Her eyes glistened. "I didn't trip you."

"Yes, you did. You knocked my feet right out from under me. I went down hard for the count and never got up again. I was a broken man."

His easy grin told a different story.

"You didn't act broken." She traced his cheek.

"Funny thing, I discovered I liked it. I wanted you to keep on kicking my feet out from under me." Noah scooped the puppy up and rested him on his shoulder. The dog barked once and then sat happily, watching the activity from his perch.

Feeling safe, just the way Grace felt safe.

Noah scratched the dog's head, his smile fading. "I was going to wait for a better time. I wanted candlelight and a few dozen roses to say this…" He took a breath, his eyes very dark as he dug in his pocket and took out a small velvet box. "Will you marry me, Grace? It may be too soon or too much to think about now, but—"

He opened the box. A ring of twisted silver with three yellow diamonds gleamed against the velvet. "It was my grandmother's. I've been carrying it around with me, trying to find the right time to ask you. But it never came." His eyes turned grave. "Of course if you don't like the setting, we could—"

"Yes." She took a shaky breath and leaned closer. "Yes, of course I'll marry you. And I love the ring," she whispered. "It's perfect just the way it is."

*We're perfect together just the way we are,* Grace thought.

Noah didn't mind the dog hair or the puppy breath that surrounded them. He looked as if he was having the time of his life.

So did the dogs racing around him.

You could always tell about a person by the way animals reacted, Grace thought. They knew who was a friend. They knew whom they could trust.

A giddy feeling filled her chest. She had been in stage three of infatuation before. Now in one smooth movement she had soared all the way to stage ten. The real thing.

He slid the ring onto her finger. "You're sure?" he asked.

She pulled him down and kissed him. "I love you. I've never been more sure of anything in my life." Hearing the break in her voice, the puppy barked and leaned over Noah's shoulder, licking her face.

Noah slid the puppy gently to the ground. "I told you I wouldn't make it easy to forget us. How we felt together." His arms slid around her waist. "How well we fit." He pulled her closer and kissed her with aching tenderness. "Like this."

Grace felt her heart dive straight to the bottom

of her chest. "Prove it," she whispered, enjoying the glorious danger of throwing her heart into his keeping.

Knowing there was no safer place on earth than right here in his arms.

\* \* \* \* \*

*Come back to Summer Island....*
*Look for THE ACCIDENTAL BRIDE*
*coming soon from*
*Christina Skye*

### Grace's Gorgeous (But Understated!) Tea Cozy

*Materials:*

*Bulky weight wool yarn*
*Size 10 needles (which will make a lovely, dense fabric. Perfect to keep your Earl Grey warm for hours.)*

Cast on 96 stitches and then connect to join in the round, keeping your stitches straight and not twisted. (Hint: check twice. Do *not* ask how I know this.)

Slide in a stitch marker before the first stitch in the joined row.
Begin knitting in the round.

Rows 1–3: Slip marker. Stockinette stitch, knitting all stitches.

Row 4: Begin *Friendship stitch* row—this pattern is a version of trinity stitch, which Grace finds much faster to work. And we all know that fast can be good!

(See Friendship stitch explanation below.)

*Knit 3 stitches together, keeping the knitted-together stitch on the left needle. Then yarn over. Then knit the first knitted-together stitch again and slide off the left needle.*
*So you decrease three stitches into one and then immediately increase back to three.*

Slip marker.
[Friendship stitch, knit 3], repeating all in brackets, to the end of the row. This is Pattern Row A.

Rows 5–7: Knit around.

Row 8: Pattern row B.

Knit 3.
[Friendship stitch, knit 3], repeating all in brackets, to the end of the row.
Note: Your Friendship pattern stitches will not line up with those in the earlier row, which makes the lovely, understated pattern.

Rows 9–11: Knit around.

Row 12: Pattern Row A.

Continue in 12-row pattern above for 5 inches.

(Note: measure your chosen teapot before you go any further. If it is smaller than 5 inches high to the top of the body, not including the lid, end your pattern rows sooner. If it is taller than 5 inches, work a few more rows in pattern before you begin decreasing for the top.) This way, you create a custom cozy for your favorite teapot!

Decrease for top:

Knit 3 together around to the end of the row.
Knit 2 rows even.

Bind off loosely in knit stitch.
This leaves a lovely ring of friendship at the top of your cozy. Grace says this represents the bonds she holds with her dearest Summer Island friends.

Happy knitting from Grace and the girls on Summer Island!

Grace will also be posting variations and updates at www.christinaskye.com/SummerIslandknitting. Be sure to drop in for a visit and lots of new knitting patterns, interviews and videos. Monthly contests, too. Just sayin'.

A note about the suggested yarn:
Grace used Imperial Yarn's Native Twist Soft Spun Singles. (www.ImperialYarn.com)

This is a chunky yarn, very minimally processed. Jeanne, the co-owner and keeper of Imperial Stock Ranch's amazing history, calls it "barely yarn"! But the rich story of the West clings to every strand and fiber, dating back to local Native American camps, where women followed the sheep paths, pulling clumps of wool off the brush where the sheep grazed. They used the unprocessed wool to line their baskets or make clothing. Native Twist is a very natural fiber in an array of wonderful colors. It feels rustic and wonderful, right from the ranch that Grace loves. She prefers canyon-shadow-blue or peach blossom for her tea cozies.